PRAISE FOR
HOW TO END THE AUTISM EPIDEMIC

"J.B. Handley is arguably the world's most thoughtful, sophisticated, knowledgeable, and indefatigable activist for children's health and safety. As a frontline leader for fifteen years, Handley has led the big fistfight against the Pharma Cartel to force the issue, broadcast the science, and expose the lies behind the vaccine policies that have created an epidemic of chronic disease among our children. Handley has helped bring the issue of toxins in medical products and regulatory corruption to a tipping point. Handley's advocacy has lifted the curtain of lies behind which the autism epidemic has sprouted. When we end this cataclysm, it will be thanks to the dogged character of people like J.B. Handley who have refused to rest in his battle to support parents, protect children, bring justice to injured families, and to punish those responsible for one of the worst scandals in American history. Please read this book and decide for yourself if you still believe that vaccines are 'safe and effective.'"

—Robert F. Kennedy Jr.

"I honestly believe J.B. Handley wrote the book that will end the autism epidemic. As I sit here now, in stillness, I want to jump up and down with excitement, but I'm holding back rivers of tears. He breaks down the scientific information in a way that doesn't intimidate the reader. And he lets us know it's okay to be angry. His soul, his fight, his love for his son radiates off the pages. Wow. Bravo, bravo."

—Jenny McCarthy, author of *Louder Than Words*; coauthor of *Healing and Preventing Autism*

"This book is inspired, powerful, the unadulterated truth, and a must read. We have sacrificed too many children at the vaccine altar while our blind belief in the CDC and AAP, government, and the media has prevented us from seeing the conflicts of interest that enable big business and Big Pharma to profit at the expense of our children's health. *How to End the Autism Epidemic* is one family's story, but it is sadly also a story shared by millions of families. A beautiful normal baby, vaccinated, and then lost to autism and all the horrible medical conditions associated with immune devastation and brain toxicity. Thank you, J.B., for sharing your story and wisdom. Parents and future parents: Read this book now, and say No to business as usual and the status quo. If your pediatrician has not yet done his or her own research and is just parroting the 'vaccines are safe and effective' marketing phrase, it is time for you to get a new pediatrician."

—**Paul Thomas**, MD, coauthor of
The Vaccine-Friendly Plan and *The Addiction Spectrum*

"I encourage everyone to read *How to End the Autism Epidemic*, which has the potential to spark a thoughtful and thorough review of how we can stop vaccine injuries among our nation's children. A dedicated and passionate advocate for medical freedom, J.B. is also a father who has lived the experience no parent would want to endure. His life's work is making sure everyone gets the information they need and vaccine-injured children and their families get the justice they deserve."

—**Tim Knopp**, Oregon State Senator

"As parents our job is to be concerned about our children's health. Yet every day in doctors' offices around the country, American parents are told we are being 'irresponsible' or 'selfish' just for asking questions about vaccines. We all want to keep our children safe and healthy, both from infectious diseases and from overexposure to toxins. It's reasonable to be concerned that there are too many vaccines on the schedule and that medications like antibiotics, acetaminophen, and ADHD drugs are being over-prescribed. What's a worried parent to do? For starters, read this book! Sharing his personal story as the father of a boy with autism and taking a close look at the most recent and rigorous science, Stanford-educated J.B. Handley shows how the CDC's aggressive childhood vaccine schedule is connected to the astonishing rise in autism in the United States. *How to End the Autism Epidemic* is a direct challenge to the American public health establishment and a gift to the millions of parents who find themselves caught in the crosshairs—uncertain of what to think or do—of the seemingly intractable debate about vaccines."

—**Jennifer Margulis**, PhD, author of *Your Baby, Your Way*;
coauthor of *The Vaccine-Friendly Plan*

"I have been thinking about the toxicity of aluminum for thirty-five years. It is my life's work. Before we completed our recent research on aluminum in brain tissue in autism, I could not see a direct link between human exposure to aluminum and autism. I certainly saw no immediate role for aluminum adjuvants in vaccines in autism. The missing link was a mechanism whereby the brain would be subjected to an acute exposure to aluminum, for example, as occurs in aluminum-induced dialysis encephalopathy. Pro-inflammatory cells, some originating from blood and lymph, heavily loaded with a cargo of aluminum in brain tissue in autism provided that missing link. We all tolerate the toxicity of aluminum adjuvants in vaccines. Unfortunately, some of us are predisposed to suffer, as opposed to tolerate, the toxicity of aluminum adjuvants, and this may cause autism.

"Autism is a disease, and it is not inevitable. J.B. Handley's elegant synthesis of what we know and what we need to know argues that autism could and should be preventable. I agree with him."

—**Professor Christopher Exley**, PhD, fellow, Royal Society of
Biology; professor of bioinorganic chemistry, Keele University

"J.B. Handley tells it like it is. His new book is a masterful synthesis of all the latest threads of autism: the controversies, the science, the legal and policy battles, and the human dimension of the 'movement' that has inspired so many of us to become parent activists. Peppered with jaw-dropping new developments—including depositions from major vaccine science luminaries—Handley weaves a compelling narrative and cuts through the noise to make a powerful and convincing case. Read it. Process what he's telling you. And then stand up and do something about it. The health of generations of children is at stake."

—**Mark Blaxill**, coauthor of
The Age of Autism, *Vaccines, 2.0*, and *Denial*

HOW TO END
the
AUTISM
EPIDEMIC

HOW TO END
the
AUTISM
EPIDEMIC

J.B. HANDLEY

Chelsea Green Publishing
White River Junction, Vermont
London, UK

Editor: Brianne Goodspeed
Copy Editor: Eileen M. Clawson
Proofreader: Deborah Heimann
Indexer: Deborah Heimann
Designer: Abrah Griggs

Printed in the United States of America.

First printing August, 2018.
10 9 8 7 6 5 4 3 2 1   18 19 20 21 22

Our Commitment to Green Publishing
Chelsea Green sees publishing as a tool for cultural change and ecological stewardship. We strive to align
our book manufacturing practices with our editorial mission and to reduce the impact of our business
enterprise in the environment. We print our books and catalogs on chlorine-free recycled paper, using
vegetable-based inks whenever possible. This book may cost slightly more because it was printed on paper
that contains recycled fiber, and we hope you'll agree that it's worth it. Chelsea Green is a member of the
Green Press Initiative (www.greenpressinitiative.org), a nonprofit coalition of publishers, manufacturers,
and authors working to protect the world's endangered forests and conserve natural resources. *How to End
the Autism Epidemic* was printed on paper supplied by Thomson-Shore that contains 100% postconsumer
recycled fiber.

Library of Congress Cataloging-in-Publication Data
Names: Handley, J. B., author.
Title: How to end the autism epidemic / J.B. Handley.
Description: White River Junction, Vermont : Chelsea Green Publishing, [2018]
   | Includes bibliographical references and index.
Identifiers: LCCN 2018023415| ISBN 9781603588249 (paperback) |
   ISBN 9781603588409 (audiobook) | ISBN 9781603588256 (ebook)
Subjects: LCSH: Autism in children. | Vaccination in children. |
   Vaccination—Complications—Risk factors. | BISAC: MEDICAL / Health
   Policy. | MEDICAL / Public Health. | MEDICAL / Immunology. | SOCIAL
   SCIENCE / Disease & Health Issues. | HEALTH & FITNESS / Health Care Issues.
Classification: LCC RJ506.A9 H263 2018 | DDC 618.92/85882—dc23
LC record available at https://lccn.loc.gov/2018023415

Chelsea Green Publishing
85 North Main Street, Suite 120
White River Junction, VT 05001
(802) 295-6300
www.chelseagreen.com

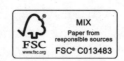

MIX
Paper from
responsible sources
FSC® C013483

Contents

Introduction   1

PART ONE
The Lies about Vaccines and Autism

1   "There Is No Autism Epidemic"   15

2   "Vaccines Are Safe and Effective"   41

3   "The Science Is Settled"   84

4   "The Reward Is Never Financial"   105

PART TWO
The Truth about Vaccines and Autism

5   Emerging Science and Vaccine-Induced Autism   141

6   The Clear Legal Basis that Vaccines Cause Autism   170

7   The Critical Mass of Parents All Saying
the Same Thing   209

PART THREE
A Reckoning to End the Epidemic

8   They Would Have Told Us   221

9   Next Steps: A Twelve-Point Proposal   233

10   Treatment and Recovery   242

Epilogue   249

Acknowledgments   251

Notes   253

Index   275

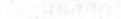

Introduction

There really are places in the heart you don't even know exist until you love a child.

—Anne Lamott

When we were newlyweds, my wife Lisa and I knew we wanted three or four kids. We planned to have kids every two years and see how we felt after each one. Our first son, Sam, was born in 1999 in Berkeley, California, and by early 2001 a family routine was settling in. We understood what it meant to be parents. Sleepless nights were routine. Our personal hobbies took a back seat. Dates and romance became rare events. Despite the chaos, it felt like the right time to expand the family.

Jamison took longer than expected. When he finally arrived in August 2002, a little more than thirty-three months younger than his big brother and almost a year behind "schedule," I was overjoyed. Two boys? My sons would always have each other. A lifetime of wrestling matches, shared sports, and being dudes together was imminent. I couldn't wait to watch and share in the fun. It was a euphoric time.

But on the night following Jamison's two-month "well baby" visit—during which he received six separate vaccines—his health deteriorated rapidly and never rebounded. He developed eczema all over his body. He didn't sleep for more than twenty minutes at a time. After a few sleepless nights, I had to move out of the master bedroom and sleep with Sam so I could make it up for work the next day. Lisa endured the crazy nights alone, waking with Jamison every time, trying to feed him back to sleep.

As time went on, Jamison developed dark circles under his eyes. His stomach became distended, and he was really skinny, almost emaciated. He sweated like crazy at night. The eczema persisted. He was constantly leaning on furniture (we later learned he was trying to ease the pain he was feeling in his gut), and he had frequent ear infections. He was always on antibiotics.

Our life, and our family, began to collapse. By late 2003, as Jamison's health continued to decline, I would call home from business trips to brutal reports from Lisa about Jamison's health. After one trip I returned home to California to a Post-it note on the kitchen counter from Lisa. "Went to Portland, sorry." She had fled home to Oregon with the kids to be with her parents.

I remember the moment when our nanny said something. She was nervous. She was only twenty-one years old, a college junior. "I'm worried about Jamison," she told me. "He's not playing with things the way he used to." I disregarded this comment—from the person who spent hours a day with my son—not yet ready to face the fact that something was terribly wrong.

A few months into 2004, our family bottomed out. Now eighteen months old, Jamison was sick, needy, never sleeping, and his behavior was changing for the worse. He'd run along walls, back and forth, turning his eyes to the side. He was spinning in circles, playing with toy trains in odd ways, stuffing himself with foods loaded with carbohydrates, alternating between diarrhea and constipation, and looking sicker than ever. He had been an early talker, but now his words had disappeared. Why was he no longer saying "juice" or "ball" or "doggie"?

"There goes our son with autism," Lisa declared. She was half-joking, trying to rationalize his odd behavior. She didn't know what "autism" meant, and neither did I. Wasn't that the guy from *Rain Man*? She knew something was wrong, though. Inside, I was starting to worry, too. It wasn't normal, the things Jamison was doing. The specter of the "A word" began to hang over our house.

Getting an appointment to have Jamison screened for autism was excruciating. The University of California, San Francisco, medical center and every other place we tried had multi-month waiting lists. When UCSF had an unexpected cancellation, we rushed in and got our answer: autism, the severe kind. The presiding doctor, famous in her field, told us to expect institutionalization. And probably no speech. Good luck; it will be a hard road. We asked about diet and some other things we had been reading about, and she said it was just a placebo for parents. My well-mannered, intelligent, socially savvy wife told the famous doctor to fuck off, in what would become the first of countless acts of rebellion against the medical establishment and its determinations of our son's life.

For a while Lisa and I told no one. We'd suppress our cries to try to show Sam, now four years old, that we were OK. As soon as he was napping or sleeping, we'd cry until the tears ran out. Every morning I woke up believing it was a nightmare. I was in a daze; the world had stopped making sense. Why was this happening to my son? So many dreams were being shattered at once about his life and his future. I felt my vision narrowing as the grief took over. Jamison was slipping away. He stopped recognizing us or acknowledging our comings and goings. It was unbearable.

I called my parents, living in Virginia, and said, "I need you right now." They arrived the next day. When I met them at their hotel, I fell into their arms and wept. They would give Sam love and care while Lisa and I figured out what the hell we were going to do for Jamison. Autism had arrived.

Dr. Lynne Mielke greeted us in the waiting room of her office. She looked with concern at Jamison; he was doubled over on a small ottoman in the waiting room, applying pressure to his gut, as he often did. "Poor baby," she exclaimed, "his belly must really be hurting him." Lisa and I looked at each other, puzzled. We'd never thought about that simple explanation. It would be the first of many things Dr. Mielke would teach us about what had actually happened to our son.

Lisa had dragged herself to the computer first, while I still wallowed in misery. She started reading. "You need to read this stuff; kids are recovering!" she yelled at me. I finally joined her. Recovery? That certainly sounded better than the prognosis from UCSF. We set up two computers, side by side, in a narrow home office so we could research together. Two Stanford geeks, putting their well-honed research skills to work. There we sat, late into the night or into the morning, rubbing elbows and comparing notes, for weeks on end.

The things we learned challenged all of our beliefs. We learned there were two camps in the autism world. In the first camp, autism was a genetic condition, sort of like Down syndrome. If you had autism, you always would. Parents would be well served to accept their child's fate and maximize the joy in life that they could. The second camp was the opposite. Autism was an environmental illness, mostly (but not only) caused by a recent massive uptick in the number of vaccines given to kids. Autism was essentially a label for a set of symptoms that included many other "comorbid" conditions, such as allergies, gut distress, poor sleep, and malnutrition. If you treated many of these physical symptoms, some or all of the things we call autism could disappear. Recovery from autism was very possible in this world, and there were doctors claiming that they were doing just that: recovering children with autism.

This information was deeply disturbing and confusing. Naively, we returned to our pediatrician and UCSF with this newfound research. They told us everything we were reading about vaccines and special diets was nonsense. We didn't understand. Both sides couldn't be right. How could there be experts telling us something that wasn't true? What the hell was going on?

As Lisa and I read, researched, talked, listened, and considered the arguments and information coming at us, what we came to was this: The "autism is genetic" story didn't make sense. There is no "autism gene," and the genetic research done up to that point provided no answers and still doesn't today. Moreover, the rate of autism has reached epidemic levels, and there's no such thing as a "genetic epidemic." Mark Blaxill, an autism parent, said it well, "You can't explain all of this as a genetic disorder since the dawn of time."[1] There had to be a cause.

The second camp—that autism is primarily environmental—made so much more sense to us. Jamie was so sick all the time! We'd watched him decline, time and again, after vaccine appointments. We went back over his pediatric appointment history and the symptoms we'd seen emerge; they corresponded completely. The parent stories we were reading online sounded exactly like Jamie's story, and many parents were also reporting their children were recovering, once they found the right type of doctor, usually a "Defeat Autism Now!" or "DAN!" doctor. We chose to see the DAN! doctor closest to our California home, Dr. Lynne Mielke down the road in Pleasanton.

The American Academy of Pediatrics (AAP) has never recognized that children can recover from autism. In 2004 DAN! doctors were viewed as medical outcasts and shunned by the mainstream community. This made us very wary. We'd see Dr. Mielke, but we'd proceed with extreme caution; the last thing we wanted to do was cause Jamison additional harm. What if the UCSF doctors and our pediatrician were right? What if it was all quackery?

Dr. Mielke didn't fit the picture our mainstream doctors had tried to paint. She had gone to Indiana University's medical school and then completed her psychiatry residency at UCLA. She'd been a practicing psychiatrist until she watched her younger son disappear into autism after his vaccine appointments, just like Jamison. Desperate to help him recover, and armed with a medical degree, her research led her to the DAN! movement growing across the country. As her son's symptoms started to improve, she decided to open a clinic to help other children. Dr. Mielke was polished, professional, and organized. Our first meeting with her left us utterly flabbergasted.

Unlike the pediatricians and UCSF diagnosticians who had dismissed our questions about the vaccine-autism rumors and special diets that we were gathering during our research, Dr. Mielke quickly confirmed them. "Yes, it's the vaccines. For most of the kids, that's what pushes them over the edge," she told us matter-of-factly. What was her evidence? Hundreds of patients with the same story as her son and Jamison and the medical tests to support the theory that vaccine injury—not genetics—was creating a generation of children with more autism than the world had ever seen.

More importantly, she was also bearing witness to many of her patients improving, and some recovering completely, by following what was known as the DAN! Protocol, a combination of diet, nutrition, and detox that had been spearheaded by the San Diego–based Autism Research Institute. She wanted to do tests on Jamison that our mainstream doctors hadn't even considered, and she was particularly focused on healing his gut. Why hadn't the other doctors even mentioned that?

We decided to give it a try. Dr. Mielke's son and our son had the same backstory. We would only do interventions that posed no risk to Jamison's health. Removing gluten and dairy posed no risks. Within two weeks of our first visit with Dr. Mielke, a combination of diet, nutritional supplements, cod liver oil, and probiotics had flattened Jamison's belly, and he'd stopped leaning on furniture. Eye contact started to return. The dark circles under his eyes were going away. His awareness of the world around him was returning.

Encouraged, we became students of biomedical treatment for autism, which means you treat the medical symptoms a child with autism is experiencing, like poor sleep, gut distress, food allergies, or recurrent ear infections. Elbow to elbow on our matching computers, Lisa and I researched everything that might work to save Jamison. He had just turned two, and we felt that recovery was a real possibility for him. He was getting better and better.

You'd think witnessing Jamison's health improve would make us ecstatic, and in a sense it did, but our feelings were also far more complex than that. Watching Dr. Mielke's prophecies bear out in Jamison's improved health was like falling down a rabbit hole and losing faith in the world we thought we knew, all at once. How could we be getting advice from autism experts that was so contradictory? How come UCSF didn't seem to care if a doctor just thirty miles away was recovering children from autism? Why weren't these doctors all talking to each other and sharing ideas and information?

More unbearable than the thought that Dr. Mielke and the hundreds of other DAN! doctors across the country were wrong was the feeling that she was right. Were vaccines the primary trigger for an epidemic of autism? Were we really doing that to kids? The scale of damage was nearly incomprehensible. This would be a recurring theme for us on this journey. We'd meet highly intelligent parents, doctors, and scientists who would tell us that, yes, that's exactly what's going on. It was two different realities.

The mainstream press paints this issue as crazy, desperate parents looking for someone or something to blame, but that's not accurate or fair, and it doesn't help kids. Over the course of fifteen years, I've been astonished by the things prominent scientists, doctors, politicians, and parents have said about the connection between vaccines and autism. The community of people who know the truth has grown massively since Jamison was diagnosed. For many the knowledge required them to pay the ultimate price: witnessing their own child decline after being vaccinated. Many of these highly educated, intelligent people would tell me, "I never would have believed it if it hadn't happened to me."

In retrospect I shirked my duty to research vaccines properly. You don't think of a vaccine as a medical procedure, but that's what it is. I hadn't done a shred of primary research about vaccines prior to vaccinating my children. I remembered being vaccinated as a kid and thought, "I've been vaccinated, and I'm fine." I trusted the authorities, who all seemed to be saying that vaccines were safe and effective.

I had no idea that in 1986 vaccine makers were given blanket indemnity from liability by the US Congress. I didn't know the vaccine schedule in the United States had tripled since the mid-1980s. Or that the US government had paid out $3.6 billion for vaccine injuries. Or that other developed countries gave many fewer vaccines, and had much less autism. I didn't know the hepatitis B vaccine, often given on day one of life, only provided protection for four years. Or that autism, ADHD, asthma, and allergies were all skyrocketing, and that their rise corresponded to changes in the vaccine schedule. I couldn't know that biological science would show how a vaccine can injure an infant's brain—because it hadn't been published yet. And I certainly had never read the many published studies showing how vaccines can result in autoimmunity and neurological damage.

Most significantly, I believed the narratives that appealed to emotion and trust in authority that we often hear about vaccines. Herd immunity, for example: Nobody wants to be the selfish parent who puts everyone else at risk. Vaccination is important, not only for our own kids but for the health of the community, especially the vulnerable, right? Well, no one really knows because we've never come close to achieving herd immunity through vaccines. Ever. Dr. Russell Blaylock, a retired neurosurgeon, explains:

> *That vaccine-induced herd immunity is mostly myth can be proven quite simply. When I was in medical school, we were taught that all of the childhood vaccines lasted a lifetime. This thinking existed for over 70 years. It was not until relatively recently that it was discovered that most of these vaccines lost their effectiveness 2 to 10 years after being given. What this means is that at least half the population, that is the baby boomers, have had no vaccine-induced immunity against any of these diseases for which they had been vaccinated very early in life. In essence, at least 50% or more of the population was unprotected for decades.*[2]

Today the science is clear that all vaccines wane in four to ten years.[3] With the adult population less than 50 percent up to date on vaccines, we're nowhere near herd immunity and never have been.[4] "Herd immunity" is one of the many sophisticated PR strategies designed to compel parents into vaccinating their children through emotional manipulation.

In the fall of 2004, I returned to work, but I was often holed up in my office researching autism, biomedical intervention, and vaccines. It felt like there was so much to learn, Jamison's future was in our hands, and we were racing against the clock.

Managing my own anger was a challenge. The more I learned, the stronger I felt that greed, ignorance, and spineless bureaucrats had contributed to a situation that injured my son and put a normal life for him out of reach. When you learn what I learned and when you step back and really think about the scale of destruction and when you see that people in positions of authority know and yet refuse to act, it's hard to bear. Every time we'd see Jamison's health improve, it reminded us how avoidable this was, and that made us madder still.

Eight months after Jamison's diagnosis, Lisa and I channeled our energy and anger to create an organization and a website called Generation Rescue. It allowed parents with newly diagnosed children to quickly get all the information they needed about biomedical intervention, connect with other parents, and find a doctor in their state. It had taken us weeks on the computer to find all this information; why not make it easier for the next family by putting it all in one place? We launched in May 2005, and the organization has helped tens of thousands of families begin the journey to recovery. Today the number of stories of recovery and improvement by families that found our website number in the thousands.

A few years after we launched, Jenny McCarthy happened on Generation Rescue's website, used the guidance it provided, and fully recovered her own son. Out of gratitude, she found us and said she wanted to help, and she's been the leader ever since. Jenny and Executive Director Candace McDonald have spearheaded a Rescue Grant program, so that families without the money to start biomedical treatment are now supported. They also run the annual Autism Education Summit, the leading conference to feature doctors and scientists discussing cutting-edge developments in biomedical research.

Discussing vaccinations and autism isn't an explosive topic, it's thermonuclear. Both sides of the argument feel, with great passion, that the health and welfare of our children are at stake. Much of that passion is the product of several lies told repeatedly. These lies form a foundation for self-interested parties to deny, obscure, and misdirect the truth about what's happening to millions of children. They pit well-meaning parents against well-meaning parents. Remove the lies, and you're left with a deeply disturbing explanation for why so many children have autism, seemingly out of the blue.

Interestingly, the belief that vaccines can cause autism isn't the fringe topic many mainstream media articles make it out to be. In the 2016 election of the 128 million people who voted for either Hillary Clinton or Donald Trump, 24.3 percent of them believe this statement is true: "Vaccines have been shown to cause autism." That's 31.3 million people.[5] It's not a conspiracy theory, as I hope this book will show you through sound logic, data, and scientific studies.

That said, what you're about to read may challenge many things you believe to be true. I know how that feels. I trusted my doctors. I listened to authorities. I struggled to accept that people would lie. Yes, I'm incredibly angry about what happened to my son, and about the ridiculous number of children now affected by autism, but I'm not angry because I need someone to blame. I'm angry because after fifteen years of immersing myself in the scientific literature, beating down the doors of the most knowledgeable doctors and scientists in the country, weighing every argument I encountered, and witnessing the experiences of so many families, including my own—essentially eating, breathing, and living autism—I know that autism is preventable and recoverable, but we'll never end this epidemic until we reckon with the lies and obfuscation that enable it.

So the first step to ending the autism epidemic is to be honest about how it started, and expose the lies told, time and again, to distract and confuse the issue. We need to name names and hold people and institutions accountable. We need to look at common arguments—that the rate of autism isn't actually increasing and that the science is settled, for example—and intellectually dismantle them in a logical, fact-based way. We need to look at the role of the media, Big Pharma, and trusted institutions such as the Centers for Disease Control and Prevention (CDC) and the AAP. We need to follow the money. This is what I cover in part one.

The second step is to understand the clear and compelling scientific evidence that supports the connection between vaccines and autism. What many people don't know (because the mainstream media doesn't report this) is that since 2004 there has been a revolution in the understanding of the cause of autism, based on the rapid-fire publication of a number of biological studies that point to an "immune activation event" in the brain—immune activation being the whole point, by the way, of vaccination. Does that mean vaccines are the only cause of autism? No. Other things can cause immune activation events; it just appears that vaccines do it most consistently and devastatingly.

What many people also don't know is that recently some highly respected scientists—experts who were relied on to testify against parents in the

National Vaccine Injury Compensation Program's "vaccine court"—have recently switched sides and now support the view of so many parents that vaccines can indeed cause autism. They have amended their views based on evolving science. Their words carry tremendous weight, and I hope this book helps put their comments, many of which have never before seen the light of day, into proper context. This is what I cover in part two.

The third step to ending the autism epidemic is to develop a constructive plan for how we protect future generations from a devastating epidemic now impacting one in thirty-six American children based on what we understand about the cause of autism and where families and doctors have experienced success in recovery. This is what I cover in part three.

The autism epidemic is ultimately a failing of our public health officials. In the United States the Centers for Disease Control and Prevention—a federal agency within the Department of Health and Human Services—is not only responsible for implementing our national vaccination program but, in a twist of bitter irony, is also responsible for tracking the number of children with autism. It's as if the expression, "the fox guarding the henhouse" had been waiting its whole life for this moment. Sadly, the CDC's failings are further enabled by scientists, doctors, and many members of the media willing to parrot the same old lies that obscure an honest discourse about the epidemic and how to end it.

I know some people will label me or this book as "anti-vaccine." This is a slur used to quell debate and a waste of my time and yours. People for safer cars are not "anti-car." As Professor Christopher Exley of Keele University, a pioneer in establishing the biological relationship between vaccine aluminum and autism, explains:

> How do you express a legitimate concern about aluminium adjuvants in vaccines without being labelled as 'anti-vaccine'? . . . The answer appears to be that you cannot.[6]

We don't have time for these kinds of oversimplified attacks and binary labels. Our kids desperately need us to rise to the occasion of an informed, intellectual, and fact-based debate that examines arguments on their merits. I'm not saying I'm not angry—you'll see plenty of anger throughout this book directed at the people and institutions I have learned are responsible for the current unprecedented crisis in our kids' health—but simplistic ad hominem attacks that a person is anti-vaccine for expressing a legitimate and informed concern get us no closer to ending this devastating epidemic.

What I genuinely believe is that each vaccine needs to be evaluated on its own merits. While I acknowledge that vaccines provide some benefit to society in reducing cases of certain acute illness, they also cause brain damage in some of the vulnerable kids who receive them. Parents have a right to all the information they need—this is called "informed consent"—to make an informed risk/reward decision on behalf of their kids. The public health establishment in this country has not been forthcoming with us. They exaggerate the overall benefits from vaccination and severely downplay the risks, either through improper monitoring and testing or through blatant misrepresentations. And while we have the capacity to do it, we don't systematically assess the children who are more vulnerable to vaccination before they receive any. I believe the public's trust in the very institutions whose charge it is to protect our health has been severely compromised.

Thank you for reading this book, thank you for being willing to consider that what I'm about to tell you is true, and thank you, if you so choose, for sharing it with others.

PART ONE

The Lies about Vaccines and Autism

CHAPTER 1

"There Is No Autism Epidemic"

The question is stark: Is autism an ancient and genetic variation that demands acceptance and celebration, or is it new and disabling, triggered by something in the environment that is damaging more children every day?

—Dan Olmsted and Mark Blaxill,
coauthors of *Denial*[1]

In 2015 Steven Silberman published *NeuroTribes: The Legacy of Autism and the Future of Neurodiversity*. Silberman, a former record producer, restaurant critic, and teaching assistant to the poet Allen Ginsberg, created a stir in the autism world and brought the tortured idea that autism has always been with us at exactly the same rate back into the public debate. He described a world in which autism is a "naturally occurring form of cognitive difference akin to certain forms of genius." The geeks of Silicon Valley? Nikola Tesla? All "blessed" with autism. "Whatever autism is, it is not a unique product of modern civilization. It is a strange gift from our deep past passed down through millions of years of evolution," Mr. Silberman writes, attempting to erase an epidemic with the stroke of a pen.[2]

The term *neurodiversity* first appeared in the late 1990s, coined by sociologist Judy Singer. She likened acceptance of diverse ways of thinking to other social acceptance movements taking shape and hoped "to do for neurologically different people what feminism and gay rights had done for their constituencies."[3] On the surface this appears to be a noble pursuit—what could possibly be wrong with advocating for acceptance? In *Wired* magazine, Mr. Silberman examined the social revolution he believed was taking shape, as advocates with autism and "others who think differently are raising the rainbow banner of neurodiversity to encourage society to appreciate and celebrate cognitive differences, while demanding reasonable accommodations in schools, housing, and the workplace."[4]

Mr. Silberman's message met the needs of the media's social agenda to make autism normal and resonated both in elite circles and with vaccine injury deniers. Featured in many prominent publications (*Forbes*, the *Washington Post*, the *New York Times*, *The Economist*, and the *New Yorker*, to name a few), Silberman won the Samuel Johnson Prize for nonfiction in 2015. A glowing review in *The Atlantic* praised Mr. Silberman's book and noted that autism self-advocates "make space for anyone who feels not quite normal."[5]

Mr. Silberman took it a step further, pinning the survival of our species on our ability to accept neurological diversity, explaining that "the value of biological diversity is resilience: the ability to withstand shifting conditions and resist attacks from predators. In a world changing faster than ever, honoring and nurturing neurodiversity is civilization's best chance to thrive in an uncertain future."[6]

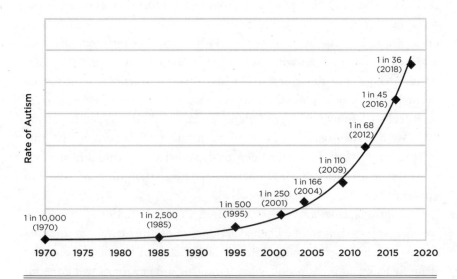

Figure 1.1. Change in the Rate of Autism Since 1970 (Up 277-fold). Data from Treffert et al., 1970, the Centers for Disease Control and Prevention.

I'm approaching fifty years old, and as a child I'd never seen or heard of even one peer with autism. Ask any teacher, doctor, nurse, or coach who has been working for three decades or more and you'll always hear the same thing: something new and very different is happening with children today. My teenage children know dozens of kids with autism, and schools are bursting at the seams with special education classes. When you look at a graph of the change in the rate of autism over time, it's breathtaking (see figure 1.1). When I first heard that there were researchers, spokespeople, and experts claiming that the growth in the number of kids with autism was all a big mirage and that these children had always been here, I really couldn't take it seriously.

A simple question refutes this narrative: "Where are all the adults with autism?" If Mr. Silberman's version of history is plausible, you'd need almost 3 percent of American adults to be exhibiting clear signs of autism. Let's do the quick math: Fifty-four percent of the US population is over the age of thirty-five. That's roughly 174 million people. If one in thirty-six of those adults had autism, that's 4.8 million American adults with autism—4.8 million adults over the age of thirty-five who have a disabling condition that makes independent living a challenge for all but the mildest of cases.

Robert F. Kennedy Jr., an environmental activist and lawyer, has often discussed the lack of adults with autism, citing his family's decades-long involvement with the Special Olympics, which he asserts never used to have participants with autism. He asked (in 2017 when the autism rate was one in forty-five), "Why isn't one in forty-five older people you see walking around the mall, why isn't one in forty-five wearing diapers and wearing a football helmet, and having seizures, head banging and stimming?"[7]

There is no data anywhere that supports an adult autism number anywhere close to 4.8 million. To accommodate that many individuals, you'd have nursing homes, group homes, and mental institutions overrun with adults with autism. The best data I could find about housing for adults with disabilities was in Canada, where a federal health system makes data more trackable. In Canada's largest province, Ontario, there are 13.6 million people. Adults over thirty-five make up 7.34 million people, which at a rate of one in thirty-six would mean 204,000 adults with autism. And how many group home spaces does Ontario offer for adults with all forms of developmental disabilities? Eighteen thousand.[8] Keep in mind, autism is only one form of developmental disability and represents well under half of all cases. Ontario doesn't have more beds, because they don't need more beds (yet)—there are nowhere near that many adults with autism. In fact, forty-two thousand adults are being serviced in Ontario for all disabilities, and if the rough math says that if autism is half that number, there are 90 percent of the adults with autism in Mr. Silberman's world "missing" from Ontario (twenty thousand actually there versus two hundred thousand). Because they don't exist.

If that simple math isn't enough to convince you, a book was published in 2017 that I believe will do for "epidemic denial" what Rachel Carson's *Silent Spring* did for DDT. *Denial: How refusing to face the facts about our autism epidemic hurts children, families, and our future*, was written by former UPI investigative journalist Dan Olmsted and Harvard MBA and autism parent Mark Blaxill. Apparently, the authors had similar misgivings about writing an entire book dedicated to a topic that one would hope most people consider to be poppycock, noting that "part of our personal challenge as an autism parent and a health journalist becomes taking the 'idea' [that there is no real autism epidemic] seriously enough to debunk it thoroughly, not just wait for history to stomp all over nonsense as it is eventually wont to do."[9]

Olmsted and Blaxill's book is so incisive and so clear, and so specifically destructive of Mr. Silberman's entire thesis (they dedicate many chapters to refuting *NeuroTribes*), that I will struggle to do the book justice in a lone chapter. What I can do is offer you a few select passages from the book that I think stand alone in painting epidemic denial in the absurd light it deserves:

> *Epidemic denial doesn't add up. Take the US population of 124 million in 1931—the year the eldest child in that first report on autism was born. Divide that number by the current autism prevalence of one in sixty-eight children* [Note: it's now one in thirty-six]. *There should have been 1.8 million Americans with autism in 1931. There weren't. We have scoured the medical literature for cases before then, and there are essentially none to be found.*[10]

They also provide "since the beginning of time" math, which makes Mr. Silberman's and other's claims even harder to accept:

> *Back up a bit more: how many people have ever lived on earth? About 100 billion by 1931. Again, simple math yields about*

one-and-a-half-billion autistic individuals who have lived before 1930. Now we begin to glimpse the emptiness behind the Epidemic Denier's claims. There may have been scattered individuals with enough traits to qualify for an autism diagnosis, but 1.5 billion would have been far more visible. Someone would have said something. Given the distinctive profile of autistic children, it's impossible that no doctor or social observer commented on their markedly different behavior.[11]

Romanticizing a Devastating Disability

As an autism parent, if I immerse myself in Mr. Silberman's fictional version of autism and its history for long enough, it all starts to sound sort of fine, if not even a little great. Autism is just a different way of thinking. It's always been here. People with autism are gifted and have so much to offer the world. Heck, a new TV series on ABC, *The Good Doctor*, brings autism even further into the mainstream—the central character is a doctor with autism who has extraordinary powers to heal.

Unfortunately, the Good Doctor is like a guy with a small limp and a cane representing paraplegics to the world. His story is fascinating and compelling but bears little resemblance to the autism most parents, myself included, actually deal with every single day. And on a personal level I resent the way Mr. Silberman, *The Good Doctor*, and many neurodiversity advocates are romanticizing a devastating disability. If you "discovered you have autism in college," you don't have the autism now afflicting more than one million American children. Including my own son.

Despite what you may have read, the definition of autism has remained remarkably consistent over time. Because autism can't be diagnosed with a blood test, it's diagnosed through observation, and anyone possessing enough qualities of autism has autism. The hallmarks of an autism diagnosis include early onset of symptoms (typically before thirty months), an inability to relate to others (called "social-emotional reciprocity"), "gross deficits" in language development, peculiar speech patterns, and unusual relationships with the environment (attachment to inanimate objects, rigidity, etc.)

As Olmsted and Blaxill explain, "Most with an autism diagnosis will never be employed, pay taxes, fall in love, get married, have children, or be responsible for their health and welfare."[12] In fact, upward of 50 percent of children with an autism diagnosis are unable to speak at all, according to the

California Department of Education.[13] A study in the *Journal of Autism and Developmental Disorders* showed that 28 percent of eight-year-old children with autism spectrum disorder (ASD) exhibit self-injurious behavior (they physically hurt themselves).[14] *Maternal and Child Health Journal* published a study showing that kids with autism are twice as likely to be obese.[15] A study in *Pediatrics* showed 35 percent of young adults with autism have never had a job or received any education after high school.[16] The average cost to support an individual with autism over his or her lifetime? $2.4 million.[17]

If those figures aren't bad enough, a study published in the journal *Research in Developmental Disabilities* showed that children with autism are also considerably sicker than their non-autism peers.[18] Asthma, skin allergies, food allergies, ear infections, severe headaches, and diarrhea or colitis are all far more likely to be present in a child with autism. In fact, the gastrointestinal problems of children with autism were so much worse than any other group that the study authors thought it deserved special attention, noting "one finding stood out in particular when we compared the developmental disability groups to each other: Children with autism were twice as likely as children with ADHD, learning disability or other developmental delay to have had frequent diarrhea or colitis during the past year. They were seven times more likely to have experienced these gastrointestinal problems than were children without any developmental disability." Recently, National Public Radio reported that people with developmental disabilities are seven times more like to be sexually assaulted and that the assaults typically "happen in places where they are supposed to be protected and safe"—a nightmare scenario for every autism parent.[19]

Finally, and tragically, the organization Autism Speaks estimates that fully one-third of children with autism also have epilepsy, "a brain disorder marked by recurring seizures, or convulsions."[20] And a European study in 2016 found that people on the autism spectrum "are dying younger than the average person—by 12 to 30 years" with the leading cause of early death being epilepsy.[21] Is this the same happy world Mr. Silberman depicts? Not on your life. Or theirs.

Even Congress Thinks We Have an Epidemic

In 2012 the US House's Committee on Oversight and Government Reform held a hearing about autism. The name of the hearing? "1 in 88 children [the autism rate at the time]: A look into the federal response to rising autism rates." Chairman of the Committee Darrell Issa opened the hearing and said, "But right now, if the numbers are accurate, and if they continue to grow from the now 1 in 88 that in some way are ASD affected, we, in fact, have an epidemic. It could be that some of the 1 in 150 at the start of the previous century was too low; that, in fact, people were simply not diagnosed. But few people believe that." Dan Burton, a congressman from Indiana, added, "we've gone from 1 in 10,000 children to be autistic to 1 in 88. It is worse than an epidemic; it is an absolute disaster."[22]

Carolyn Maloney, a congresswoman from New York, was even more emphatic:

> *Autism is becoming a growing epidemic in the United States, and it definitely needs to be addressed. . . . Now, the numbers that he pointed out earlier, that it used to be 1 in 10,000 kids got autism, it's now 1 in 88, and I'd like to ask Dr. Boyle [a CDC employee], why? And I don't want to hear that we have better detection. We have better detection, but detection would not account for a jump from 1 in 10,000 to 1 in 88. That is a huge, huge, huge jump. What other factors could be part of making that happen besides better detection? Take better detection off the table. I agree we have better detection, but it doesn't account for those numbers.*

Our own elected representatives seem to know the truth, and yet people like Mr. Silberman continue to be featured all over the media.

No Epidemic, No Responsibility

Robert F. Kennedy Jr. delivered a compelling take on why he thinks epidemic denialism remains in the public conversation. In a pointed essay discussing Mr. Silberman's book in 2015, Mr. Kennedy stated:

> *A threadworm tactic employed for a decade by Big Pharma and the Center[s] for Disease Control (CDC) and their allies to combat the scientific evidence that the autism explosion is a manmade epidemic of recent origins has been to hint that there is no autism epidemic at all. Public health agencies maintain a disciplined refusal to call*

the disease's sudden explosion an "epidemic" or "crisis" and actively discourage scientific investigations of environmental triggers. "You will never ever hear CDC characterizing the autism explosion as a crisis or an epidemic," Dr. Brian Hooker, Simpson University epidemiologist, said. "So long as there is no epidemic, no one needs to look for the environmental trigger." All this accounts for the giddy excitement among Big Pharma funded media outlets at the debut of Steve Silberman's book, NeuroTribes: The Legacy of Autism and the Future of Neurodiversity. *Parroting Pharma's old propaganda canard, Silberman suggests that autism is a wholly genetic psychological ailment that has always been with us in prevalences similar to those found today. Silberman argues that we never noticed autism until recently, because affected persons with the illness were formerly stashed in mental institutions or misdiagnosed.*[23]

Mr. Kennedy concludes that "Silberman's overarching message is that we should stop investigating the environmental cause of the autism epidemic—and potential cures—and simply celebrate humanity's neurodiversity mosaic. This, of course, is all crackpot stuff."

Olmsted and Blaxill offer up their own take on why by asking, "Who benefits?"

The first question we need to ask is the inevitable one of self-interest: Cui bono? Who benefits from this unconscionable failure to admit and address the simple truth? Given the magnitude of the autism problem, it's not surprising that powerful interests would look for ways to avoid being blamed for the problem and, even worse, being held accountable in some fashion—financial or otherwise. As we wrote in the book's first sentence, trillions of dollars are at stake, including billions in profit, stock prices, bonuses, and liability. The dollar signs associated with the epidemic are so large that it's worth billions for the prime suspects to evade accountability.[24]

The Epidemic Denial Food Chain

Sitting atop the epidemic denial food chain is one man—Dr. Paul Offit. On the surface there's no reason Dr. Offit should have much of an opinion about autism, or ever be quoted about autism by the mainstream press, given that his area of expertise is . . . vaccines. Dr. Offit is a professor of "Vaccinology" at the Children's Hospital of Philadelphia and personally made tens of millions of dollars when one of his inventions—a rotavirus vaccine—was accepted onto the US recommended vaccine schedule.[25] Dr. Offit has no formal training in anything to do with autism, but that hasn't kept him from writing books about autism (*Autism's False Prophets: Bad Science, Risky Medicine, and the Search for a Cure*), and he's often quoted in the media discussing autism. In 2010 the *Age of Autism* blog voted Dr. Offit "Denialist of the Decade" for the 2000s.[26] Here's a typical quote from Dr. Offit about autism's rate:

> *It's not an actual epidemic. In the mid-1990s, the definition of autism was broadened to what is now called autism spectrum disorder. Much milder parts of the spectrum—problems with speech, social interaction—were brought into the spectrum. We also have more awareness, so we see it more often. And there is a financial impetus to include children in the wider definition so that their treatment will be covered by insurance. People say if you took the current criteria and went back 50 years, you'd see about as many children with autism then.[27]*

In Dr. Offit's world there is no problem here. Things are as they always were; we just understand it better. And if there's no epidemic, there is no environmental trigger, because why have a trigger if something hasn't actually grown? Said differently: Denying the autism epidemic is to deny the suffering of millions of children and their families and also to deny the exploration into the true cause so the epidemic might end. But what is Dr. Offit's real motivation? In my opinion, the autism epidemic is the single biggest threat to the vaccine program in its current form. As I mentioned earlier, if vaccinations are triggering autism in one in thirty-six children, the risk/reward equation for the vaccine program is destroyed. On the other hand, if autism has always been with us, vaccines couldn't possibly be playing a role.

Dr. Offit is a public mouthpiece with deep financial ties to one company in particular: Merck, the largest vaccine maker in the world. In fact, Dr. Offit is the Maurice R. Hilleman (the same Maurice Hilleman who invented the MMR vaccine) Professor of Vaccinology at the University of Pennsylvania's Perelman School of Medicine, a chair endowed by Merck.

Is it really that hard to understand why he is the go-to media contact for epidemic denial quotes?

Dr. Offit isn't alone in providing convenient sound bites, commentary on studies, and, at times, primary research to maintain doubt about autism's increase. Dr. Peter Hotez, Dr. Eric Fombonne, and Dr. Paul Shattuck are three other media-friendly mouthpieces with deep ties to the vaccine industry who are typically treated in the mainstream press like objective, expert witnesses on any stories dealing with autism.

In the case of Dr. Hotez, perhaps the most quoted "expert" on vaccines and autism in recent years, he's actually a patent holder of several experimental vaccines.[28] Dr. Fombonne, in addition to authoring one of the most mystifyingly poor studies on the measles-mumps-rubella (MMR) vaccine (which I discuss in chapter 3), has also served as an expert witness for vaccine makers, testifying against the parents of vaccine-injured children in court.[29] Dr. Shattuck was a Merck Scholar and has received grants from the CDC of more than $500,000 to fund his research.[30] Objective experts? Not even close. Do they "benefit" from denying an epidemic? Of course they do, as Blaxill and Olmsted so eloquently explain:

> *The People who benefit most from Autism Epidemic Denial are those who make the toxins and orchestrate the exposures that, however inadvertently, have caused the epidemic. They benefit, it should not be necessary to say, first by making money and then by avoiding culpability in the forms of legal, financial, and possibly even criminal liability.*[31]

The World's Autism Authority

In *NeuroTribes* Mr. Silberman praised the work of Dr. Bernard Rimland, a pioneering psychologist whose famous 1964 book, *Infantile Autism*, destroyed the idea forever that autism was the result of emotionally distant parents. Mr. Silberman's choice to lionize Dr. Rimland, while completely appropriate given his immense contributions to the field of autism, is also devastatingly ironic, given that Dr. Rimland was also the earliest and most public voice to challenge a creeping dynamic in the autism debate that first appeared in the mid-1990s: epidemic denialism.

Dr. Rimland, who founded both the Autism Society of America and the Autism Research Institute, was the foremost authority on autism during the decades of the 1980s and '90s, and until his passing in 2006. In fact, he was the pioneer of biomedical intervention, which many parents have used to recover their children. By the mid-1990s he was seeing incontrovertible evidence of a massive uptick in the number of children with autism, writing as early as 1995 an essay titled, "Is there an autism epidemic?"[32] Dr. Rimland's response was simple and straightforward: "Yes! There clearly has been a sharp increase in the number of autistic children." By 2000 Dr. Rimland could hardly keep up with an ever-increasing number of children with autism, as well as an ongoing attempt by some to muddy the waters. In that year he published a now famous essay in the *Journal of Nutritional & Environmental Medicine*, in which he stated:

> *While there are a few Flat-Earthers who insist that there is no real epidemic of autism, only an increased awareness, it is obvious to everyone else that the number of young children with autism spectrum disorders (ASD) has risen, and continues to rise, dramatically. . . . The evidence was compelling in 1995, and is overwhelming in 2000. Nevertheless, I read and hear daily about professionals, including many regarded as authorities on autism, who assert that there is no real increase in the autism population. . . . I saw the word autism for the first time in the spring of 1958, five years after I had earned my PhD in psychology. . . . I have heard similar tales from many physicians as well as special education teachers and school administrators whose experience dates back to the early 1970s and before. Autism was truly rare in those days.*[33]

Three Main Arguments by Deniers

While Dr. Rimland was arguably the most well-known researcher in the autism community when epidemic denialism first emerged in the mid-1990s, his words alone may not be enough to convince everyone. It's important to look at the actual data, details, and published studies, of which there are plenty.

Epidemic deniers offer up three separate but related explanations for why they believe autism has always been with us at the same rate: that

diagnosis has improved, that autism is a reclassification of mental retardation, and that the definition of autism has expanded. Each explanation
sounds plausible on the surface but is decimated by facts and published
science. And each of the three commonly used explanations is easily
testable, so let's see what the evidence shows. But first, let's establish
a baseline.

Establishing a Baseline in Wisconsin

In 1970, in the *Archives of General Psychiatry*, a baseline for autism's prevalence was established.[34] Using data from Wisconsin, Dr. Darold Treffert and
colleagues sought to "identify the incidence and prevalence of childhood
schizophrenia and infantile autism in an entire state population age 12 and
under." This was the first time a thorough process had been undertaken to
identify the autism rate, and Dr. Treffert and his team looked at roughly
899,000 kids. His finding: 0.7 children per 10,000 "fit the definition of
classic early infantile autism." This is the study where the widely used "1 in
10,000" figure comes from.

It's worth noting that Dr. Treffert reported the qualities utilized to cate-
gorize a Wisconsin child as having autism:

> *Classic infantile autism which excludes organicity and is charac-
> terized by early onset, withdrawal and inability to relate, speech
> problems, suspected deafness, and need for sameness.* [My son would
> have met all these criteria].

Dr. Treffert's study also correctly identified a wide disparity in the gender
ratio of autism, noting that boys outnumbered girls 3.4 to 1, and also found
that parents of children with autism had achieved "high educational attain-
ment" and had "low incidence of mental illness." The study was exceptionally thorough and had access to the entire mental health infrastructure of
Wisconsin, including any facility where a child exhibiting symptoms of a
mental disorder would be seen.

Dr. Treffert felt "because of the complex nature of the disorder, the
difficult differential diagnosis, and complicated disposition planning, that
in a five-year period it was highly unlikely that any case of childhood
schizophrenia or infantile autism in the 12-and-under age group would not
have been seen in one of the above settings." If Mr. Silberman's view of the

world were accurate, there should have been more than eighteen thousand children with autism found in Wisconsin. Dr. Treffert and his team found just over sixty.

Fast-forward forty-five years, and Dr. Treffert commented on the autism epidemic for the Wisconsin Medical Society in a blog post in 2015. While he felt that some of the increase in autism might be due to widening criteria (see "Denialist Argument #3" section, page 36), he also made it clear that he is "convinced there is an actual increase in the disorder . . . And in my view, part of the increase is actually due to some environmental factors (pollutants of various sorts that may contribute as well to a rise in other congenital abnormalities and premature births)."[35]

Let me spell this out, because it's a really big deal: The very first epidemiologist to analyze the autism rate in Wisconsin in 1970 feels there's an actual increase in the rate of autism, due at least in part to environmental factors.

Denialist Argument #1: Diagnosis Has Improved

Most people have a hard time internalizing the difference between an autism rate of 3.3 per 10,000 and an autism rate of 277 per 10,000. They know the second number is a lot bigger, but perhaps don't appreciate the practical application of this difference, so let's consider a real-world example: In 1987, just before the 1989 inflection point of the autism epidemic, a peer-reviewed study was published called "A Prevalence Study of Pervasive Developmental Disorders in North Dakota," which aimed to count how many kids had a PDD/autism diagnosis in the entire state.[36] The researchers looked at all 180,000 children under the age of eighteen and determined that North Dakota's rate of autism was 3.3 per 10,000.

Here's how the authors summarized their findings:

Of North Dakota's 180,986 children, ages 2 through 18, 21 met DSM-III criteria for infantile autism (IA), two met criteria for childhood onset pervasive developmental disorder (COPDD), and 36 were diagnosed as having atypical pervasive developmental disorder (APDD) because they met behavioral criteria for COPDD before age 30 months but never met criteria for IA. The prevalence rates were estimated at 1.16 per 10,000 for IA, 0.11 per 10,000 for COPDD, and 1.99 per 10,000 for APDD. The combined rate for all PDD was 3.26 per 10,000 with a male to female ratio of 2.7 to 1.

This was an exceptionally thorough study. The children with an autism diagnosis were assessed in person by a doctor. The data was published in a journal. It was peer reviewed. It was replicable. They found 3.3 per 10,000 kids had autism. Could the researchers have been wrong? Was the real number actually very different? Maybe. Perhaps the real rate was as high as 5 per 10,000 or as low as 2 per 10,000. But ballpark, we are talking about 3.3 out of 10,000 kids with autism or roughly 1 in 3,300.

We now know autism impacts 1 in 36, that's eighty-three times more kids than the North Dakota study found in 1987. But it's worse than that if you think about it a different way: In 1987 if you had 1 million kids, 330 would have autism. Today if you have 1 million kids, 27,777 have autism. Let me say that again. In 1987 the rate of autism prevalence meant for every 1 million kids, 330 had autism. With today's number, about eighty-three times higher, you'd have almost 28,000 with autism.

If you're to believe Mr. Silberman and other epidemic deniers, you have to believe that the research on autism prevalence done in 1987 was simply wrong. The researchers in North Dakota missed a ton of kids and wildly underreported the actual number of autism cases. How many kids did they miss? Well, if the North Dakota researchers found 3.3 kids per 10,000 when they should have found 277 per 10,000 kids with autism, they missed 98.8 percent of autism cases in North Dakota. That means in 1987 the pediatricians, psychologists, and all of the screeners (not to mention all the parents) in North Dakota were missing 98.8 percent of kids with autism and just letting them slip through the cracks. These kids, all 98.8 percent of them, were sitting right next to you in class, and you, and their parents and doctors, never knew it. It's an impossible world, but it's the one that Mr. Silberman, Dr. Offit, and others want us to believe in.

Back to North Dakota for a second. The scientists and doctors who did that study in 1987, the one showing 3.3 kids per 10,000 with autism, they were damn serious about making sure they were accurate in their count. You see, they followed the same birth cohort, the almost 200,000 kids who made up their original study in 1987, for twelve years. They published a second study, thirteen years later in January of 2000, called, "A Prevalence Methodology for Mental Illness and Developmental Disorders in Rural and Frontier Settings."[37] The authors concluded:

The results of the prevalence study [the original study in 1987] *were compared with the results of a 12-year ongoing surveillance of the cohort. The 12-year ongoing surveillance identified one case missed by the original prevalence study. Thus the original prevalence study methodology identified 98% of the cases of autism-pervasive developmental disorder in the population. This methodology may also be useful for studies of other developmental disorders in rural and frontier settings.*

So these researchers went back twelve years later and checked their work. With a couple of hundred thousand kids, they found they had undercounted their original estimate of prevalence of autism in North Dakota by exactly one child. One child! This study alone should silence anyone claiming "better diagnosis," but there's more.

The National Collaborative Perinatal Project

Olmsted and Blaxill wrote extensively about this 1975 study in their book, *Denial*:

It would be awfully convenient to our own argument if the relevant authorities had spent the time and money to create a more modern survey of the autism rate, one that deployed the gold standard of surveillance methods, a prospective study of the autism rate. Such a prospective study would follow a large group of children from birth through childhood, monitoring their development at regular intervals with rigorous consistency to see how they progressed and whether or not they had developmental problems like autism. A prospective study that included autism would tell us what the real autism rate was by carefully tracking a defined population, not by looking back retrospectively trying to identify cases in a population defined after their onset had already occurred. Ideally, to make a compelling case for low rates of autism before the onset of any purported "epidemic," such a study should have been done somewhere between the recognition of autism in the 1930s and its explosion in the 1990s. Another ideal feature of such a study would be a large sample size—tens of thousands of children tracked from birth to see what percent were diagnosed with autism. This dream study would cull data from computerized medical records and also from neurological, psychological, speech, and hearing exams at every stage in child development. Top medical centers, leading researchers, and strict government supervision would ensure no conflicts of interest. Compare this mythical study to today's rates and you'd really know if there is an autism epidemic, a mild tick upward, or nothing at all but a change in the gestalt—in the way we describe the varieties of human disability. Oh, wait. That study was done.[38]

Researchers from fourteen different hospitals associated with major universities followed a group of newborns (thirty thousand of them) born between 1959 and 1965.[39] Children received highly structured evaluations on a defined interval from the day they were born until they turned eight years old. The National Institutes of Health (the federal agency responsible for medical research) was clear in explaining why the data from this study was so valuable:

The data were collected as part of a prospective study [following children from birth and reevaluating them continuously], *unique in its design and magnitude. The data constitute a repository of information of great value. Books and monographs based on analyses of these data and other publications number in the hundreds. Even so, the possibilities for the development of further knowledge based on this study are immense. It is unlikely that such a study will be undertaken again and it is thus of particular importance that the data be utilized as fully as possible.*[40]

To put this in further context, the original name for this study was the "Collaborative Study of Cerebral Palsy, Mental Retardation, and Other Neurological and Sensory Disorders of Infancy and Childhood." I mention this only to make sure it's clear to everyone that this study's primary purpose was to find any aberration in childhood development, of which autism would have stuck out like a sore thumb. As Robert F. Kennedy Jr. has said, missing autism "is like missing a train wreck."[41]

The National Collaborative Perinatal Project (NCPP) was a momentous undertaking and received its funding directly from the Committee on Appropriations of the US House of Representatives. According to a summary of the study, many mental health professionals testified before Congress on the importance of this study, and the need for scale:

> *The need for prospective data, systematically recorded, coupled with the rarity of neurological deficits in childhood, made the availability of a large group of pregnant women imperative. . . . The crux of the research effort was to study a large number of cases in great detail in order to evaluate the effects of perinatal factors on the health of the individual child.*[42]

"Prospective data, systematically recorded" looking exactly for things like autism; thirty thousand children, a project so big that the "size and complexity of the NCPP required a highly developed and integrated staff to conduct the research developed and directed by the above referenced committees." Children were screened nine separate times between birth and eight years old; the screenings included pediatrics; psychology; neurology; speech, language, and hearing; and visual screening. At three years old all children were tested for language reception, language expression, auditory memory for digits and nonsense syllables, speech mechanism, speech production, and additional observations—which brings up an obvious question: "What are the chances that a study this thorough would miss autism?" The answer is pretty easy: zero.

Dr. E. Fuller Torrey and his colleagues independently combed the NCPP's data for their own separate study to examine the impact that maternal uterine bleeding could have on mental disorders. The authors noted that "approximately 4,000 separate pieces of information have been collected on each pregnancy and its outcome." One of the outcomes they were looking for—autism—was therefore closely analyzed. The results of Dr. Torrey's study, published in the *Journal of Autism and Childhood Schizophrenia* in 1975, found fourteen children meeting the criteria for autism from the NCPP data.[43]

Fourteen children with autism were found in the most comprehensive study of children that's ever been done in the United States, in a study looking specifically for "neurological and sensory disorders of infancy and childhood," which is the definition of autism: a neurological and sensory disorder. Those 14 children equate to 4.7 children per 10,000, versus today's rate of 277 per 10,000, which is fifty-nine times more kids. The NCPP's rate of 4.7 per 10,000 is consistent with the North Dakota study's rate of 3.3 kids per 10,000.

If the real rate of autism had been 1 in 36 during the time of the NCPP, the researchers would have missed 98.4 percent, or 819 of the children with autism. They didn't.

Today Dr. Torrey remains an active scientific researcher. His area of specialization is schizophrenia. I asked him in an interview about this study from 1975, and he told me, "I find it very hard to believe that the people involved with the study missed that many children [with autism]. They were very thorough." I asked him what he felt could account for so many children with autism today. Dr. Torrey was quick to point out that his area of expertise is schizophrenia but that he "suspects that autism, multiple sclerosis, and schizophrenia are the results of an infectious agent in the brain."[44]

The better diagnosis argument doesn't work. The facts don't support it, studies don't support it, and common sense doesn't support it. Even our congresspersons know it's ridiculous. Remember Congresswoman Carolyn Maloney? She knew better diagnosis was absurd, and the question she was asking in the 2012 congressional hearing was directed at Dr. Coleen Boyle, who happens to be the person at the CDC in charge of tracking autism numbers. Dr. Boyle was under oath, which meant she needed to choose her words carefully. Ms. Maloney wanted to know what—besides "better detection"—could possibly account for all this autism? Here's the back and forth between Congresswoman Maloney and Dr. Boyle:

> **Congresswoman Maloney: What other factors could be part of making that happen besides better detection? Take better detection off the table. I agree we have better detection, but it doesn't account for those numbers.**
>
> Ms. Boyle: So just to put it in context, better detection is accounting for some of it.
>
> **Maloney: I know some, but what other factors? I don't want to hear—**
>
> Boyle: Our surveillance program counts cases of autism and establishes the prevalence. It doesn't tell us all the answers to the questions as to why.

Maloney: Okay.

Boyle: So we are doing a number of studies to try to understand the "why," and one of the things that we've looked at, we've tried to look at what's changed in the environment, things we know are risk factors for autism, things like preterm birth and birth weight.

Maloney: Well, are you looking at vaccinations? Is that part of your studies?

Boyle: Let me just finish this.

Maloney: I have a question. Are you looking at vaccinations? Is that part—pardon me?

Boyle: So there is a large literature, as I mentioned.

Maloney: Are you having a study on vaccinations and the fact that they're cramming them down and having kids have nine at one time? Is that a cause? Do you have any studies on vaccinations?

Boyle: There have been a number of studies done by CDC on vaccinations of—

Maloney: Could you send them to the ranking member and the chairman here?

Boyle: Yes.

I think it's fair to conclude from reading Dr. Boyle's response, where she discusses "what's changed in the environment," that even the CDC understands that better diagnosis is a losing explanation for autism's stratospheric rise. Unfortunately, spokespeople like Mr. Silberman and Dr. Offit, who continually make their epidemic denial arguments to the press, are never making their comments under oath. Olmsted and Blaxill provide a great eulogy to the better diagnosis argument:

> *Against the idea of this hidden horde of autistic adults we'd like to repeat the commonsense test that Kanner's eldest case was born in 1931 [for his work published in 1943], and that despite his frequent writing about the condition there is no evidence of any older person ever being referred to him or his associates. . . . We believe Kanner's report should have generated a flood of people of all ages. A hidden*

horde should have spilled out into the open, with rediagnoses and recognition—and not just of children.[45]

And they never did, because they didn't exist.

Denialist Argument #2:
Autism Is a Reclassification of Mental Retardation

The autism epidemic appears to have begun in the late 1980s. The recognition of the epidemic didn't emerge until the mid-1990s, and the "shot heard around the world" about autism came from a 1999 report issued by the California Department of Developmental Services (CDDS) titled "Changes in the Population of Persons with Autism and Pervasive Developmental Disorders in California's Developmental Services System: 1987 through 1998."[46] The report confirmed what many felt they were seeing: Autism cases in the California system had nearly quadrupled in just ten years, while all other mental disorders had remained flat. This was hard evidence from California, the state that was viewed as the most precise on tracking autism cases. Olmsted and Blaxill explain what a shock this report really was to conventional thinking about autism:

> *A credible report from a large state that found the rate of severe autism almost quadrupling in a decade with no obvious explanation made a big splash. That was in part because it confirmed what many were feeling—that there were simply lots more cases of autism. This was a direct challenge to autism orthodoxy—that autism was a genetic disorder that was not susceptible to the kind of sudden increase the California numbers showed. Not surprisingly, an orthodox response to this challenge popped up quickly.*[47]

Olmsted and Blaxill are referring to a report published in 2002 in the *Journal of Autism and Developmental Disorder* that allowed the flawed theory of diagnostic substitution to take flight, before it quickly crashed and burned forever.[48] Researchers from Kaiser Permanente reanalyzed the California numbers from the CDDS's 1999 report, and claimed the data showed "changes in diagnosis account for the observed increase in autism." Said differently, the researchers concluded there was no real autism epidemic, nothing for anyone to worry about.

Diagnostic substitution as a credible explanation for the rise in autism cases experienced a very short shelf life. Data from California, Minnesota, and the US Department of Education quickly repudiated the diagnostic substitution argument, but first the authors of the 2002 study had to retract their results, after a methodological flaw was pointed out to them by Harvard MBA and coauthor of *Denial* Mark Blaxill. Dr. Lisa Croen, the lead author of the 2002 study implying no autism epidemic, reevaluated her data and concluded that, after taking into account Mr. Blaxill's criticisms (which he published in a scientific journal), "diagnostic substitution does not appear to account for the increased trend in autism prevalence we observed in our original analysis."[49]

Let me highlight this important development: The one published article that supported the "diagnostic substitution" article was dead on arrival. In the meantime, researchers at the UC Davis MIND Institute published a report in 2003 (funded by a one million dollar emergency grant from the California legislature) titled, *Report to the Legislature on the Principal Findings from the Epidemiology of Autism in California*, and their conclusions left no room for interpretation:

> *Prior to 1985, autism was believed to be a rare condition with an estimated prevalence of 4–5 per 10,000. . . . One of the most controversial aspects of the DDS Report is whether the significant increase in numbers of Regional Center individuals with autism is due to increased rates of autism or to some other factor. . . . Has there been a loosening in the criteria used to diagnose autism, qualifying more children for Regional Center services and increasing the number of autism cases? We did not find this to be the case. . . . Has the increase in cases of autism been created artificially by having "missed" the diagnosis in the past, and instead reporting autistic children as "mentally retarded"? This explanation was not supported by our data. . . . The Autism Epidemiology Study did not find evidence that the rise in autism cases can be attributed to artificial factors, such as loosening of the diagnostic criteria for autism; more misclassification of autism cases as mentally retarded in the past; or an increase in in-migration of children with autism to California. Without evidence for an artificial increase in autism cases, we conclude that some, if not all, of the observed increase represents a true increase in cases of autism in California, and the*

number of cases presenting to the Regional Center system is not an overestimation of the number of children with autism in California.[50]

It's shocking to reread this report more than a dozen years later, because the conclusions from the UC Davis researchers are so clear and stark: The rise in autism cases is a real rise. Period.

Also in 2003 University of Minnesota researchers analyzed state data and shared their results in a study titled, "Analysis of Prevalence Trends of Autism Spectrum Disorder in Minnesota."[51] Their conclusions were equally stark:

> *We observed dramatic increases in the prevalence of autism spectrum disorder as a primary special educational disability starting in the 1991–1992 school year, and the trends show no sign of abatement. We found no corresponding decrease in any special educational disability category to suggest diagnostic substitution as an explanation for the autism trends in Minnesota.*

Finally, in 2005 in the journal *Pediatrics*, Dr. Craig Newschaffer and colleagues published an analysis of autism rates using US Department of Education data and reached a similar conclusion:

> *Cohort curves suggest that autism prevalence has been increasing with time, as evidenced by higher prevalences among younger birth cohorts. . . . No concomitant decreases in categories of mental retardation or speech/language impairment were seen.*[52]

California, Minnesota, and the US Department of Education all analyzed autism data, and all clearly concluded: Diagnostic substitution is not responsible for the rise in autism rates. If you hear people make the opposite argument in public, they're uninformed, repeating a lie they heard, or lying themselves.

Denialist Argument #3: The Definition of Autism Has Expanded

To make a potentially confusing series of events simple, let's just discuss the final outcome. The *Diagnostic and Statistical Manual of Mental Disorders*

(DSM), in their fourth edition in 1994, added Asperger's syndrome to the list of autism spectrum disorders. This was an expansion in the definition of autism and created what's commonly called the "DSM-IV" criteria for autism. In the most generous of analyses, the addition of Asperger's to the definition of autism in the DSM-IV expanded the number of children by just under 10 percent. A change in numbers? Yes. Enough to explain the mind-numbing increase of eighty times or more in the number of children with autism? Not even close. Blaxill and Olmsted explain:

> Adding Asperger's expanded the effective diagnostic reach of the DSM-IV by roughly 10 percent—enough for an arithmetic increase proportionate to the category expansion but not an exponential one—ten, twenty, one hundred times—that kept rising every year. . . . In all respects, when assessing the impact of adding Asperger's, all one has to do is make sure to know whether or not Asperger's cases are added to the numbers one is considering. In most cases, the scary autism numbers we hear aren't affected very much by Asperger's cases.[53]

Interestingly, "diagnostic expansion" is the least used explanation for the lack of a "real" increase in the rate of autism, despite the fact that it holds some validity. What the addition of Asperger's didn't do to the autism numbers was materially impact their rise. In 2009 a critical study corroborated the limited impact of adding Asperger's to the criteria for an autism diagnosis, while also sounding a global alarm. A study done by Dr. Irva Hertz-Picciotto of UC Davis's MIND Institute and her colleagues titled "The Rise in Autism and the Role of Age at Diagnosis" made it clear that the rise in the number of children with autism was very real, and the increase "cannot be explained by either changes in how the condition is diagnosed or counted."[54] In an interview Dr. Hertz-Picciotto was even more emphatic:

> There is no evidence that a loosening in the diagnostic criteria has contributed to increased number of autism clients. . . . We conclude that some, if not all, of the observed increase represents a true increase in cases of autism in California. . . . A purely genetic basis for autism does not fully explain the increasing autism prevalence.

Dr. Hertz-Picciotto even called for a renewed focus on studying environmental factors that may be playing a role in autism:

> *It's time to start looking for the environmental culprits responsible for the remarkable increase in the rate of autism in California. We're looking at the possible effects of metals, pesticides and infectious agents on neurodevelopment. If we're going to stop the rise in autism in California, we need to keep these studies going and expand them to the extent possible. . . . Right now, about 10 to 20 times more research dollars are spent on studies of the genetic causes of autism than on environmental ones. We need to even out the funding.*[55]

In 2014 Dr. Cynthia Nevison published what many view as the most recent seminal and definitive work on autism rates, "A Comparison of Temporal Trends in United States Autism Prevalence to Trends in Suspected Environmental Factors," in the peer-reviewed journal *Environmental Health*.[56] Dr. Nevison also used data from the California Department of Developmental Services and the US Department of Education Individuals with Disabilities Education Act (IDEA), and her study concluded:

> *The CDDS and IDEA data sets are qualitatively consistent in suggesting a strong increase in autism prevalence over recent decades. The quantitative comparison of IDEA snapshot and constant-age tracking trend slopes suggests that ~75–80% of the tracked increase in autism since 1988 is due to an actual increase in the disorder rather than to changing diagnostic criteria.*

In an interview Dr. Nevison expanded on the results of her study:

> *Diagnosed autism prevalence has risen dramatically in the U.S. over the last several decades and continued to trend upward as of birth year 2005. The increase in autism is mainly real, with only about 20–25 percent attributable to increased autism awareness/ diagnoses, and has occurred mostly since the late 1980s.*

She also compared the rise in autism to certain environmental exposures:

The environmental factors with time trends that correlate positively to autism include 2 vaccine-related indices: cumulative aluminum adjuvant exposure and cumulative total number of disease-doses by 18 months; polybrominated diphenyl ethers (used as flame retardants); the herbicide glyphosate (used on GM crops); and maternal obesity.[57]

Framing Autism as a Genetic Condition

I've never seen more tortured explanations than the ones used to try to frame autism as a genetic condition, despite no evidence to support the claim. Literally hundreds of millions of dollars have been spent on the genetics of autism. Scientists have produced endless studies, all of them entirely theoretical. There is no "autism gene," and according to geneticist Dr. James Lyons-Weiler, "Studies of genetics have revealed 850 genes associated with autism, but no single gene explains more than 1% of ASD."[58] What's more likely is there are genes for things like mitochondrial dysfunction, impaired detoxification, and so on that predispose certain children to reacting more strongly to environmental insults, but the science has yet to be done to prove that conclusively.

In March 2016 the CDC published data showing that the rate of autism in the United States had "stabilized" because the data was "largely unchanged" from two years before.[59] The data came from eleven separate regional sites where autism data is collected, including Utah, where, one month after the data was published, researcher Dr. Judith Pinborough-Zimmerman filed a whistleblower lawsuit against the CDC.[60] Ms. Pinborough-Zimmerman wasn't just a researcher; she'd been the principal investigator for the CDC's Autism and Developmental Disabilities Monitoring (ADDM) Network in Utah. Her allegations were serious, claiming that she had felt pressure to moderate the autism numbers, helping to make a case that autism numbers were plateauing:

Depositions from Zimmerman and her former colleagues suggest that the alleged data errors were serious and have the potential to produce major differences in reported Utah autism rates.[61]

In December 2017 the CDC quietly released new autism numbers, showing that the number had in fact risen to one in thirty-six. In her

Facebook account Ms. Pinborough-Zimmerman made her position on how the CDC has "managed" autism numbers very clear:

> *Ten years of my research was spent doing ASD prevalence research. We documented staggering changes in prevalence only to be downplayed by the same government who had funded the research. . . . The world is crazy.*[62]

When I explain epidemic denialism to close friends of mine who aren't particularly familiar with autism, they struggle to believe this is actually a thing. "People say there's not more autism?" Autism's massive increase is self-evident to most adults who grew up in the 1950s, '60s, '70s, '80s, or even '90s. Dr. Michael Merzenich has published more than 150 articles in peer-reviewed journals and even won the Kavli Prize (one of the world's most prestigious prizes in neuroscience) for his work on brain plasticity. He says,

> *It irritates me to no end that we still argue over whether there is an increase in incidence* [of autism]. *I think there is lots of evidence for increased incidence. Overwhelmingly it supports that there are things in the environment that are contributing to the rate of incidence. But people still argue.*[63]

I concur with Dr. Merzenich; it "irritates me to no end" that we are still fighting in the public about whether there's been a real rise in the number of children with autism. In my opinion, it shows that vested interests have been effective in doing exactly what they want to do: sow doubt and confusion.

Pouring cold water on the severity of the autism epidemic inhibits the call to action we all need to find causation. It gives scientists on the fence an "out" where they can describe the autism epidemic as "up for debate." It denies the suffering of so many impacted children, and it's prevented a redirection of research dollars to find environmental causes. In the end, saying the autism epidemic isn't real is simply a lie, and it's a lie that extends the suffering of so many children.

CHAPTER 2

"Vaccines Are Safe and Effective"

Men of science have made abundant mistakes of every kind; their knowledge has improved only because of their gradual abandonment of ancient errors, poor approximations, and premature conclusions.
—George Sarton, founder,
History of Science Society

The message that vaccines are safe and effective made perfect sense to my wife Lisa and me. Our beautiful boys would be fully vaccinated. I'd been vaccinated, and my wife had been vaccinated. It was the easiest decision two parents could make. You even get to kill two birds with one stone: protect your babies from infectious disease and contribute to herd immunity, and so protect others. What was the risk of something bad happening from a vaccine? The number thrown around—and still in wide use today—was "one in a million."

Losing faith in my pediatrician and ultimately the entire medical establishment triggered a massive case of cognitive dissonance for me, as it does for so many parents who trusted their pediatricians with their children's lives. Could my pediatrician be leading me astray? Could these vaccines really be harming my son? Are those crazy parents actually right? It's an alienating, disturbing, troubling path that many autism parents must walk. In many cases the parents of children with autism were the most compliant when it came to mainstream medical care—our children typically received every vaccine and medical intervention recommended to us by our trusted doctors. We're not "anti-vaxxers"; we're mostly "ex-vaxxers," the compliant parents who learned the hard way.

Few parents know how recent our high-volume vaccine program really is (I certainly didn't), how different the US vaccine schedule is from many other developed countries, how low US vaccination rates for children were as late as the 1980s (without any deadly epidemics), the wide range of side effects ("vaccine injury") vaccines can create, the straightforward published science that shows vaccines are the culprit of an epidemic of autoimmune conditions (asthma, food allergies, etc.), or the fact that public health officials are well aware that clean water, sanitation, plumbing, and refrigeration had a much larger impact on infectious disease prevention than vaccines. There were so many things I didn't know when I let my boys get all their vaccines; it's hard to shake feelings of guilt for not doing my homework.

I've personally studied the US vaccination program for more than ten years, looking for clues that might help me better understand what exactly happened to my son. After all, how can I help him get better if I don't know what hurt him? Mind you, even saying that confuses some people; there's just not a lot of awareness of the extreme and long-term side effects vaccines can cause in certain children. Much of what you hear in the mainstream media is actually public relations and spin expertly placed there by vaccine makers.

The "safe and effective" message repeated over and over again is a marketing message, but is not fully fact based. Consider the American Academy of Pediatrics (AAP), an organization typically quoted anytime a discussion of vaccines takes place. Is the AAP a benevolent, objective advocate for your baby? No, they are a trade union for pediatricians, and pediatricians generate the majority of their income from, you guessed it, vaccines.[1] What about the nation's keeper of the vaccine program, the CDC? Do they give parents objective information about the risks and benefits of vaccines? Or do they feel entitled to scare the heck out of the public to induce them to get vaccinated?

Most people have at least a little bit of cynicism when it comes to the pharmaceutical industry. Approval ratings for "Big Pharma" aren't much higher than for members of Congress. A journal study published in 2013 titled "Undue Industry Influences that Distort Healthcare Research, Strategy, Expenditure and Practice: A Review" by University College London researchers looked carefully at how the pharmaceutical industry influences medical research, policy, and practice.[2] What they found won't surprise you too much:

To serve its interests, the industry masterfully influences evidence base production, evidence synthesis, understanding of harms issues, cost-effectiveness evaluations, clinical practice guidelines and healthcare professional education and also exerts direct influences on professional decisions and health consumers. . . . As a result of these interferences, the benefits of drugs and other products are often exaggerated and their potential harms are downplayed, and clinical guidelines, medical practice, and healthcare expenditure decisions are biased.

Some people mistakenly think vaccines don't produce the same profit motivation as other products for pharmaceutical companies, but they do.[3] What if I told you that the market for vaccines is expected to be worth $60 billion in 2020,[4] up from $170 million in the early 1980s?[5] That's a 350-fold increase in revenues for vaccine makers in the last thirty years! (See figure 2.2.) And it's not just vaccine makers who will manipulate the

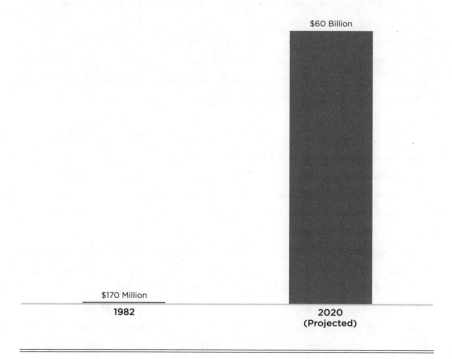

Figure 2.1. Vaccine Revenues by Year (up 350-Fold). Data from Sanford et al., 1985, and Zion Research, 2016.

facts to serve their interests; they are joined by a federal agency that Robert F. Kennedy Jr. has described as a "captive agency" of the pharmaceutical industry, the CDC.

Inducing Fear, Anxiety, and Worry

On April 14, 2004, Glen Nowak, an employee of the CDC, addressed his public health colleagues at the National Influenza Vaccine Summit in Atlanta, Georgia. The conference, cosponsored by the CDC and the American Medical Association, was filled to capacity in the Noble Ballroom of the tony Crowne Plaza Buckhead with public health officials, doctors, and representatives of the world's largest vaccine makers.

Mr. Nowak's presentation, titled "Increasing Awareness and Uptake of Influenza Immunization," provided insight into the mind-set of American public health officials.[6] As the director of media relations for the CDC, Mr. Nowak told the crowd he considered his job to be to promote "concern, anxiety, and worry" amongst the general population, especially with people who "don't routinely receive an annual influenza vaccination." Want more people to get vaccinated? Demand will come from a "perception or sense of vulnerability to contracting or experiencing bad illness," Mr. Nowak explained. During his speech Mr. Nowak made it clear that without provoking anxiety you won't get the behavior you want:

> *The belief that you can inform and warn people, and get them to take appropriate actions or precautions with respect to a health threat or risk without actually making them anxious or concerned. This is not possible. . . . This is like breaking up with your boyfriend without hurting his feelings. It can't be done.*

Mr. Nowak's presentation included a "recipe" for creating high vaccine demand. Step #3 of Mr. Nowak's seven-step recipe stressed the importance of medical experts and public health officials stating "concern and alarm" and predicting "dire outcomes" if people don't get vaccinated. It's critical spokespeople frame the flu season in ways that motivate behavior, Mr. Nowak explained, like "very severe" and "deadly." References to "pandemic influenza" from the early 1900s might also help scare the populace into acting, he noted.

A few years later GlaxoSmithKline (GSK), a London-based vaccine maker, would brag to this same crowd that they had invested more than $2 billion in flu vaccine manufacturing for the US market. Mitch Johnson, executive director of the Influenza Franchise for GSK, told the crowd that GSK is "committed to working with the government, public health agencies and healthcare providers to raise awareness surrounding the importance of flu vaccination."[7]

Lost in Mr. Nowak's seventeen-slide presentation that day was the acknowledgment that some of the messaging Mr. Nowak was encouraging, and that GSK would later sponsor, looked a lot like lying. Just nine months after Mr. Nowak's presentation, in an article published in the *British Medical Journal* (*BMJ*), Dr. Peter Doshi asked (and answered) a question that put Mr. Nowak's recommendations under intense scrutiny. Dr. Doshi's article, "Are US Flu Death Figures More PR Than Science?" explained that the CDC's claims of thirty-six thousand annual deaths from flu were "surely exaggerated" and that "until corrected and until unbiased statistics are developed, the chances for sound discussion and public health policy are limited."[8] In an unusually tough critique, Dr. Doshi (who today serves as editor of the *BMJ*) even called Mr. Nowak out by name and cited his seven-step recipe as proof of the willingness of the CDC to cite figures and outcomes that science can't support, all in the name of getting more people vaccinated.

In 2006, a year after Dr. Doshi's critique, Dr. Tom Jefferson of the highly esteemed and independent Cochrane Collaboration issued a blistering report about the flu vaccine, again in the *BMJ*.[9] Cochrane's goal as an organization is to provide consumers with "health information that is free from commercial sponsorship and other conflicts of interest," and Dr. Jefferson's article, "Influenza Vaccination: Policy Versus Evidence," not only supported Dr. Doshi's arguments but also challenged the entirety of Mr. Nowak's messaging (and therefore the CDC's).

Dr. Jefferson found a "large gap between policy and what the data tell us" and "a gross overestimation of the impact of influenza" and also felt that "the optimistic and confident tone of some predictions of viral circulation and of the impact of inactivated vaccines, which are at odds with the evidence, is striking." Said differently, he was astonished by how much public health officials were lying, and he urged that a "re-evaluation [of the entire use of flu vaccine] should be urgently undertaken." It's rare to see a scientific beat down administered in such striking tones, but neither Dr. Doshi nor Dr.

Jefferson held back in their critique that the evidence supporting the flu vaccine recommendations was grossly inadequate.

Dr. Doshi, by now a postdoctoral fellow at Johns Hopkins, took another swing at the flu vaccine in 2013. His essay (once again in the *BMJ*), "Influenza: Marketing Vaccine by Marketing Disease," should make the CEO of Walgreens, Rite Aid, and any of the other drug stores pushing flu shots every winter season blush with embarrassment.[10] His words were incisive:

> *Promotion of influenza vaccines is one of the most visible and aggressive public health policies today. Twenty years ago, in 1990, 32 million doses of influenza vaccine were available in the United States. Today around 135 million doses of influenza vaccine annually enter the US market, with vaccinations administered in drug stores, supermarkets—even some drive-throughs. This enormous growth has not been fueled by popular demand but instead by a public health campaign that delivers a straightforward, who-in-their-right-mind-could-possibly-disagree message: influenza is a serious disease, we are all at risk of complications from influenza, the flu shot is virtually risk free, and vaccination saves lives. Through this lens, the lack of influenza vaccine availability for all 315 million US citizens seems to border on the unethical. Yet across the country, mandatory influenza vaccination policies have cropped up, particularly in healthcare facilities, precisely because not everyone wants the vaccination, and compulsion appears the only way to achieve high vaccination rates. Closer examination of influenza vaccine policies shows that although proponents employ the rhetoric of science, the studies underlying the policy are often of low quality, and do not substantiate officials' claims. The vaccine might be less beneficial and less safe than has been claimed, and the threat of influenza appears overstated.*

A reasonable question to ask if you read Dr. Doshi's essay from start to finish would be, "How does the flu vaccine survive such pointed criticism?" Yet look around today, and nothing has changed. The "36,000 flu deaths per year" unsupportable statistic is still routinely cited, and marketing for the flu shot remains driven by doctors and public health officials predicting dire outcomes that never come to pass, with much of the marketing funded by vaccine makers. Head over to the CDC's website in the fall and winter, and you'll be greeted with encouragement to get your flu vaccine today, to "protect" both you and your family. When it comes to the flu vaccine, or really any vaccine, the CDC serves as both judge and jury. There is no check, there is no balance. There's one agency. Many CDC employees end up on the payroll of Big Pharma, like Dr. Julie Gerberding, who parlayed her position as head of the CDC into president of Merck's vaccine division.

In late 2017 *Science Magazine* further exposed the limitations and false assumptions behind the flu vaccine in an article titled "Why Flu Vaccines So Often Fail."[11] It turns out the reason is more complicated than the oft-repeated claim that it's hard to guess what the primary strain of flu will be next season:

> *For many decades, researchers believed the flu vaccine offered solid protection if it was a good match to the circulating strains; studies from the 1940s through the 1960s routinely showed an efficacy of 70% to 90%. But those studies relied on a misleading methodology. Without a simple way to detect the virus in the blood, researchers measured antibody levels, looking for a spike that occurs after infection. Then in the 1990s, sensitive polymerase chain reaction tests enabled researchers to actually measure viral levels, and they told a different story. It turned out that some people who did not have the big antibody spike after exposure—and were therefore counted as a vaccine success—actually did show a jump in viral levels, signaling infection. Earlier assessments had exaggerated vaccine efficacy. What's more, efficacy was sometimes low even when the vaccine and circulating strains appeared well matched.*

In 2012 the news got worse for the flu vaccine with the publication of a study in *Clinical Infectious Diseases* that found that children who had received the flu vaccine didn't have a lower risk of getting the flu, but they had a more than four times higher risk of getting other respiratory infections, causing the researchers to conclude that "the protection against influenza virus infection conferred by TIV [flu vaccine] was offset by an increased risk of other respiratory virus infection," which they attributed to the flu vaccine's "viral interference" with the natural immune system.

How come the public is never told about all this new information? We can learn a lot from the unwillingness of public health officials to amend their story when called out in esteemed medical journals. From Mr. Nowak's "recipe" we know that public health officials are willing to exaggerate, spin, and lie when appropriate as a matter of policy.

Vaccines Didn't Save Humanity

Hiding in plain sight and published in the AAP's own journal, *Pediatrics*, is a study from 2000 by public health scientists from both the CDC and the Johns Hopkins School of Public Health that singularly refutes the oft-told lie that vaccines saved humanity. As anyone who studies public health can tell you, clean water, sanitation, plumbing, refrigeration, and proper food handling are far more important to reducing the spread of infectious disease, and it was the gains in these standards of living in the United States that lead to a dramatic drop in death from infectious disease. How big a drop? In the study "Annual Summary of Vital Statistics: Trends in the Health of Americans During the 20th Century," the scientists explain that "vaccination does not account for the impressive declines in mortality seen in the first half of the century. . . . Nearly 90% of the decline in infectious disease mortality among US children occurred before 1940, when few antibiotics or vaccine were available.[12] (See figure 2.2.)

What did contribute to a massive decline in child mortality from the early 1900s to the end of the twentieth century? The study cites a number of things, including local health departments being created in every state, water treatment, food safety, waste disposal, decreased crowding in urban housing, and "public education about hygienic practices." What's particularly odd is that many other infectious diseases also declined precipitously, despite the fact that no vaccine ever existed for them—how can both be true? As Dr. Jayne Donegan explains:

> *It was a received "article of faith" for me and my contemporaries, that vaccination was the single most useful health intervention that had ever been introduced. . . . I was taught that vaccines were the reason children and adults stopped dying from diseases for which there are vaccines. . . . We were told that other diseases, such as scarlet fever, rheumatic fever, typhus, typhoid, cholera, and so on,*

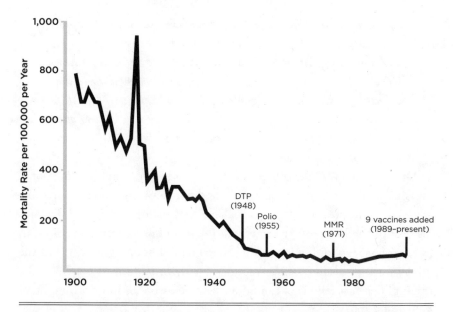

Figure 2.2. Infectious Diseases Mortality and Vaccine Introduction in the 20th Century. Note: Infectious disease data extends through 1996 only. Data from Centers for Disease Control and Prevention. Graph adapted from "Trends in Infectious Disease Mortality," *Journal of the American Medical Association, JAMA.* Gregory L. Armstrong, MD; Laura A. Conn, MPH; Robert W. Pinner, MD, 1999; 281(1): 61–66.

> *for which there were no vaccines at the time, diminished both in incidence and mortality due to better social conditions. You would think that some of us would have asked, "But if deaths from these diseases decreased due to improved social condition, why mightn't the ones for which there are vaccines also have decreased at the same time for the same reason?"*[13]

Well ahead of his time, Englishman John Thomas Biggs was the sanitary engineer for his town of Leicester and had to actively respond to outbreaks of smallpox. He quickly learned that the public health outcomes from sanitation vastly outweighed the impact of vaccination (where he saw dramatic vaccine injury and ineffectiveness). He wrote a definitive work in 1912, *Leicester: Sanitation versus Vaccination.*[14] More than one hundred years ago, Mr. Biggs had discovered what the CDC reaffirmed in 2000: Nothing protects from infectious disease like proper sanitation. He explained:

Leicester has furnished, both by precept and example, irrefutable proof of the capability and influence of Sanitation, not only in combating and controlling, but also in practically banishing infectious diseases from its midst. . . . A town newly planned on the most up-to-date principles of space and air, and adopting the "Leicester Method" of Sanitation, could bid defiance not to small-pox only, but to other infectious, if not to nearly all zymotic, diseases.

Dr. Andrew Weil, the oft-quoted celebrity doctor, reenforces the point, explaining that "medicine has taken credit it does not deserve for some advances in health. Most people believe that victory over the infectious diseases of the last century came with the invention of immunizations. In fact, cholera, typhoid, tetanus, diphtheria, and whooping cough, and the others were in decline before vaccines for them became available — the result of better methods of sanitation, sewage disposal, and distribution of food and water."[15]

Vaccines didn't save humanity. Improvement in sanitation and standards of living really did. Did vaccines contribute to a small decrease of certain acute illnesses? Yes, but their relative benefit is often exaggerated to an extreme. Consider this: In late 2017 it was reported that Emory University scientists were developing a common cold vaccine. Professor Martin Moore bragged that his research "takes 50 strains of the common cold and puts it into one shot" and that the monkeys who served as test subjects "responded very well." You should expect to see this vaccine at your pediatrician's office in the next five years, which will likely be rolled out soon after the stories start to appear in the media about the common cold causing childhood deaths.

The Myth of Herd Immunity

If you still need more convincing that public health officials and vaccine makers will mislead the public, consider the fable of "herd immunity," the oft-cited reason that everyone needs to be vaccinated. If most people ("the herd") are vaccinated against an illness, the story goes, then the herd is protected from that disease. In many cases pediatricians and talking heads will get very specific about herd immunity, citing important-sounding statistics that say vaccination rates on certain diseases must stay above a certain percentage of people to have herd immunity. Drop below that threshold?

It's a recipe for disaster. When there was an "epidemic" of measles (it wasn't actually an epidemic, just a minor and typical outbreak) at Disneyland a few years ago, experts were quoted on TV saying the herd immunity threshold for measles vaccine was 95 percent, meaning 95 percent of the population needed to be vaccinated against measles to prevent "epidemics."

Perhaps no one has beaten the herd immunity drum more loudly than California State Senator Richard Pan, the author and sponsor of SB 277, a bill that made California the third state in the union (Mississippi and West Virginia are the other two) to make vaccinations mandatory for children's school attendance. In fact, he used the Disneyland measles outbreak as the reason his bill needed to be passed. In a recent missive to his constituents, Senator Pan noted that his 2015 bill was raising kindergarten vaccination rates and bragged, "This success is a first step toward reducing the number of unimmunized people putting our families at-risk for preventable diseases, thereby restoring community immunity throughout our state in the coming years."[16]

Let's look at Senator Pan's words carefully. "Restoring community immunity" has several implications. Firstly, it implies that California had somehow "lost" community immunity (which is a nonscientific synonym for herd immunity) at some point. Secondly, "restoring" community immunity implies that until vaccination rates hit a certain threshold, grave risks will be present—restoration of safety is a top priority! The absurdity of Senator Pan's convictions about the importance of herd immunity and of hitting certain vaccination targets is that the United States has never been close to achieving herd immunity for any vaccine-preventable disease for two simple reasons: (1) The overwhelming majority of adults in the United States are not up to date on their vaccines, and (2) The efficacy of vaccines to prevent disease wanes over time, meaning protection from a vaccine "wears off," typically in ten years or less.[17] (It's called "protection waning.")

To put this in perspective, there are roughly 150 million adults in the United States walking around with no vaccine-provided protection from many diseases that we are supposed to have met herd immunity thresholds for. The CDC surveys adults every year, so it's easy enough to find vaccination coverage rates. Here are just a few: hepatitis A (9 percent), hepatitis B (24.5 percent), pneumococcal (20.4 percent), and influenza (43.2 percent).[18] These adults work in schools (where they don't have the same immunization requirements as children), work in restaurants, work in stores, and are in every community, which means we are nowhere close to herd immunity and never have been. In fact, I don't think most adults even realize the CDC maintains an adult immunization schedule. When people like Senator Pan pat themselves on the back for protecting society by reestablishing herd immunity, it has no basis in fact. With so many people unvaccinated, where are all the crippling epidemics?

A recent article in the congressional newspaper *The Hill* titled "If Only Half of America Is Properly Vaccinated, Where Are the Epidemics?" and written by Gretchen DuBeau, the executive director of the Alliance for Natural Health, explains this logic gap:

> *While herd immunity may not exist, herd mentality most definitely does. Health authorities, media commentators, and schools and their parent–teacher associations waste no opportunity in perpetuating this myth. Proponents have done such a thorough job of convincing the public that a parent who questions it is treated like someone who thinks the earth is flat or believes climate change is a conspiracy. On*

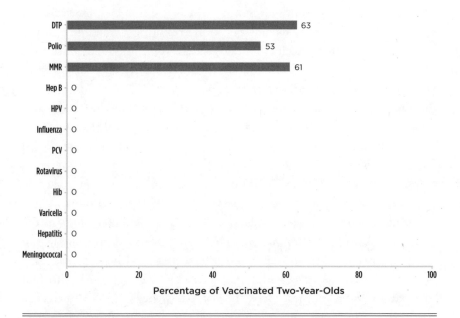

Figure 2.3. US Vaccination Rates in 1985. Note: Vaccines with a rate of 0 percent had not been added to the schedule by 1985. Data from Centers for Disease Control and Prevention.

*the contrary: an unprejudiced view of the science about vaccines,
and an examination of history, clearly show that the herd immunity
theory is—and always has been—flawed.[19]*

Vaccination rates among American children for the three primary
vaccines given in the 1960s and 1970s were far lower than today's vaccination rates. For example, in 1973, the first year the CDC tracked national
vaccination rates, the vaccination rates for DTP (diphtheria, tetanus, and
pertussis or whooping cough), polio, and MMR were 72 percent, 59 percent,
and 61 percent, respectively. In 1985 those numbers were 63 percent, 53
percent, and 61 percent.[20] Much as the question is asked of adults today,
where were all the childhood epidemics in 1973 and 1985 with such "low"
vaccination rates? They didn't exist (see figure 2.3).

Politicians stand up in front of their colleagues, pound the table, and advocate
passing mandatory vaccination laws to "preserve herd immunity." Pediatricians
get on TV and explain how critical it is that we all "maintain herd immunity."

The notion of herd immunity is nonsense. The truth is out there for any
parent willing to look at the facts.

Vaccine Makers Are Indemnified

On October 20, 1986, the *Los Angeles Times* ran a story regarding a
controversial bill making its way through Congress. The headline shouted,
"Vaccine Injury Fund Bill Approved but Faces Veto."[21] The story went on
to explain the divisive nature of the bill, intended to shield vaccine makers
from liability if their product caused harm, and the Reagan administration
was speaking out to express their opposition:

> *In a strongly worded letter to House Speaker Tip O'Neill, the then
> secretary of the Department of Health and Human Services, Otis R.
> Bowen said, "The bill is likely to do little to assure the vaccine supply
> or to improve our childhood immunization efforts." Assistant Attorney
> General John R. Bolton, writing to the head of the House Judiciary
> Committee on behalf of the Department of Justice, said the White
> House opposed the legislation because it was creating, "a major new
> entitlement program for which no legitimate need has been demon-
> strated." President Reagan was troubled by the vaccine compensation*

bill and was quoted as saying, "Although the goal of compensating those persons is a worthy one, the program has . . . serious deficiencies."

The Reagan administration seemed to be particularly concerned with two issues: who was going to pay for the compensation required for vaccine injury and the precedent of the federal government indemnifying private companies from liability. As the *New York Times* reported, "The program would be 'administered not by the executive branch, but by the Federal judiciary,' Mr. Reagan said, calling it an 'unprecedented arrangement' that was inconsistent with the constitutional requirement for separation of powers among the branches of the Federal Government.'"[22]

The National Childhood Vaccine Injury Act was actually part of a larger bill, the Omnibus Health Bill (S. 1744), that was introduced in the waning days of the Ninety-Ninth Congress in late 1986. Leading a four-year effort to pass the controversial legislation on vaccine liability was a congressman from California, Henry Waxman. Waxman's bill was supported by vaccine manufacturers, who were lobbying hard on its behalf, and the American Academy of Pediatrics.

To be fair, like many pieces of legislation, the bill had some reasonable intentions. Unbeknownst to most parents today, an older version of the DTP shot was causing severe brain damage in many children, and parental lawsuits against vaccine makers were mounting.[23] There was genuine fear that pharmaceutical companies might get out of the vaccine business altogether, because the risks were too high (not very comforting). And the bill proposed the establishment of VAERS—today's Vaccine Adverse Event Reporting System—which beat the nonexistent safety monitoring system in place at the time.

With only days to go before the congressional recess, the bill's passage was up in the air, with the White House declaring plans to veto the entire omnibus package, due almost exclusively to the provisions in the National Childhood Vaccine Injury Act. Congressman Waxman, the bill's author, was unyielding and worked the press to his advantage in the final days, declaring:

This bill is the first step to taking care of children hurt in the process of protecting society from epidemics, and to ensure an adequate supply of vaccines. . . . If the President vetoes it, he will leave these children to fend for themselves and leave the country with risks or shortages or skyrocketing prices. . . . If he vetoes it, I hope he has some emergency plans to start making vaccines himself because the manufacturers tell us they may very well stop.[24]

Worried by the threat of losing the entire manufacturing base of vaccine makers coming from Henry Waxman and the AAP, Ronald Reagan made the bill law on November 15, 1986, "with mixed feelings" and "serious reservations."[25] He gave vaccine makers an early holiday gift when it came to vaccines, as the new law made clear:

No vaccine manufacturer shall be liable in a civil action for damages arising from a vaccine-related injury or death associated with the administration of a vaccine after October 1, 1988, if the injury or death resulted from side effects that were unavoidable even though the vaccine was properly prepared and was accompanied by proper directions and warnings.

What happened next should surprise no one who understands how capitalism works. The same industry that brought you Vioxx, thalidomide, fen-phen, Prozac, and the opioid epidemic had just had product liability removed and handed over to a newly established "vaccine court" that would be funded with a surtax on every vaccine purchased (yes, Americans fund the vaccine injury compensation program when they pay for a vaccine for themselves or their child) and ultimately managed and backstopped by the federal government. Remember, when this bill was passed in late 1986, it was viewed as a way to keep vaccine makers in the vaccine business. I'm not sure anyone (except perhaps pharmaceutical company executives and their lobbyists) could have predicted how vastly things would change. Consider the following:*

In 1962 a child following the CDC's recommended schedule would have received three vaccines by age five.

In 1983 a child following the CDC's recommended schedule would have received ten vaccines by age five.

---

* Counting vaccines can be confusing. To keep numbers consistent, every vaccine is just counted as one. So even though the MMR contains three separate antigens, it's counted as one vaccine, just like the hepatitis B vaccine (with only one antigen).

Table 2.1. CDC's Recommended Immunization Schedule for children (age 0 to 5) for 1962, 1983, and 2018

1962	1983		2018	
Polio	DTP	(2)	Flu	Pregnancy
Smallpox	Polio	(2)	DTaP	Pregnancy
DTP	DTP	(4)	Hep B	Birth
3 vaccines	Polio	(4)	Hep B	(2)
	DTP	(6)	Rotavirus	(2)
	MMR	(15)	DTaP	(2)
	DTP	(18)	Hib	(2)
	Polio	(18)	PCV	(2)
	DTP	(48)	IPV	(2)
	Polio	(48)	Hep B	(4)
	10 vaccines		Rotavirus	(4)
			DTaP	(4)
			Hib	(4)
			PCV	(4)
			IPV	(4)
			Hep B	(6)
			Rotavirus	(6)
			DTaP	(6)
			Hib	(6)
			PCV	(6)

In 2017 a child following the CDC's recommended schedule received thirty-eight vaccines by age five, *nearly quadruple* what a child received in the 1980s and more than *twelve times* what a child received in the 1960s. (See table 2.1.)

When I was a child in the 1980s, there were just three vaccines that children received: DTP, polio, and MMR (administered several times to "boost" immunity). Today, influenza (Flu), hepatitis B, hepatitis A, haemophilus influenzae type B (Hib), pneumococcal conjugate (PCV), rotavirus, meningitis, and varicella (chickenpox) vaccines have all been

Table 2.1 (continued)

1962	1983	2018	
		IPV	(6)
		Flu	(6)
		Flu	(12)
		Hib	(12)
		PCV	(12)
		MMR	(12)
		Varicella	(12)
		Hep A	(12)
		DTaP	(18)
		Flu	(18)
		Hep A	(18)
		Flu	(30)
		Flu	(42)
		DTaP	(48)
		Polio	(48)
		MMR	(48)
		Varicella	(48)
		Flu	(60)
		38 vaccines	

Note: Number in parentheses indicates age in months at which a child is given the vaccine. Bold numbers indicate total number of vaccines given.

added to the childhood schedule (and been given multiple times through booster shots). When someone asks you if your child is "fully vaccinated," perhaps the right reply is, "Based on which decade?" It's worth noting that children were not "dying in the streets" during the 1980s, when we gave far fewer vaccines (and had one in ten thousand children with autism).

Let me pause for a moment and draw your attention to the words "recommended schedule." If as a parent you are wondering about what vaccinations your child will receive at her next "well baby" visit, you might visit the CDC's website and find the "recommended schedule." Be aware that this schedule is not "recommended" to parents, as if you have agency (though the CDC wants you to believe you do). This schedule is recommended to the AAP, which instantly adopts it, and pediatricians, who often receive bonuses for full vaccine compliance in their practice. For parents it is a de facto mandated schedule because in most states your child can't attend school without being vaccinated. While you might seek out an exemption—religious, philosophical, medical—these are getting harder and harder to come by. In fact, there is a movement by many state legislatures to remove vaccine exemptions altogether, as California did in 2015 with the passage of SB 277 (becoming the third state with only a medical exemption).

As of today, the vaccine court created in 1986 has paid out more than $3.7 billion for vaccine injury claims—remember, funded by American taxpayers. The majority of those claims are filed by the families of vaccine-injured children.[26] Meanwhile, the market for vaccines is expected to be worth $60 billion in 2020,[27] up from $170 million in the early 1980s,[28] just as the 1986 act was put in place. As the *New York Times* reported in 2014, "Once a loss leader for manufacturers, because they are often more expensive to produce than conventional drugs, vaccines now can be very profitable. . . . Since 1986, they have pushed up the average cost to fully vaccinate a child with private insurance to the age of 18 to $2,192 from $100, according to data from the Centers for Disease Control and Prevention."[29]

It's hard to believe. The one thing that could slow the party down on the way to $60 billion is consumer doubt. If parents don't question vaccines, just as my wife Lisa and I did not, the juggernaut steams forward to more profits. But if parents begin to doubt vaccine safety, Big Pharma could be looking at a titanic loss. That's where autism comes into play. At a rate of one in thirty-six, this is not an acceptable trade-off. It's not that hard to imagine why there is so much suppression of the truth, and such vicious fighting.

Other Countries Give Far Fewer Vaccines

Even the definition of "vaccinated" is hard to pin down. Not only did being vaccinated mean something very different twenty years ago, being vaccinated today varies depending on where you are born in the world. Take, for example, the vaccination schedule of Denmark, which is managed and monitored by the Danish Health and Medicines Authority.[30] It provides parents with a scheduled childhood vaccination program, similar to that of

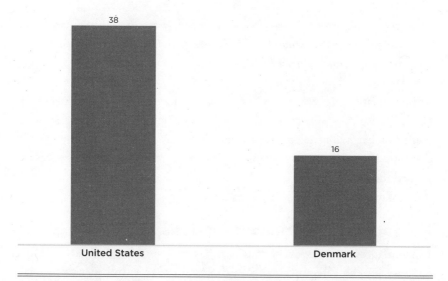

Figure 2.4. Number of Vaccines a "Fully Vaccinated" Child Receives by Age Five. Data from Centers for Disease Control and Prevention and the Danish Childhood Vaccination Program.

the United States, but missing from the Danish schedule are the following five vaccines that American children get: hepatitis B, hepatitis A, influenza (flu), rotavirus, and varicella (chickenpox).

A "fully vaccinated" American child and a fully vaccinated Danish child are not the same. A Danish child gets far fewer vaccines (sixteen total vaccines in Denmark versus thirty-eight in the United States) (see figure 2.4). If these vaccines are vitally important, why would a country that serves as an entry point for many to travel to Europe exclude the vaccinations on the American schedule? Hepatitis B vaccine is only given in most European countries to the offspring of mothers who have hepatitis B themselves. Most European countries do not routinely give hepatitis A, rotavirus, varicella (chickenpox), or the flu shot.

Digging a little deeper, we find that the United Kingdom doesn't give children the chickenpox vaccine. In the UK the National Health Service (NHS) manages the vaccine program, and they explain why they have chosen not to give the varicella (chickenpox) vaccine to children:

> *The chickenpox vaccine is not part of the routine UK childhood vaccination programme because chickenpox is usually a mild illness,*

particularly in children. There's also a worry that introducing chickenpox vaccination for all children could increase the risk of chickenpox and shingles in adults.[31]

In England chickenpox is not a recommended vaccine, but a parent in the United States who chooses to avoid the chickenpox vaccine might be chided by her pediatrician for "undervaccinating" her child or have trouble enrolling that child in daycare or school. Welcome to the land of vaccination confusion.

No Vaccines for Many Infectious Diseases

I live in Oregon. Like every state, we have a state health department. In our case it's the Oregon Health Authority, or OHA. In order to manage the monitoring of infectious disease, the state has laws about how quickly a health-care provider must report the presence of certain infectious diseases in a patient to the OHA. Diseases are classified into three categories: report immediately, report within twenty-four hours, and report within one working day—it's a ranking system for how concerned the OHA is about various infectious diseases.

There are sixty-seven total diseases that are "reportable" in my state. Of those sixty-seven, we have vaccines for only ten. The other fifty-seven reportable diseases have no vaccine available. Of the seventeen diseases that require immediate reporting, we vaccinate for four of them, leaving 100 percent of children "unprotected" against the other thirteen diseases.[32]

Vaccines don't form a protective ring around anyone; our immune system remains our primary defense against disease, at least for the fifty-seven reportable ones here in Oregon for which we have no vaccine. As best-selling author Dr. Bob Sears explains:

> *A healthy immune system is the key to preventing infectious diseases. We are all exposed to millions of germs every day, and vaccines only cover a tiny fraction of one percent of these germs. So we must rely on our own immune system to fight off most potential infections.*[33]

In fact, I'd argue most people's understanding of what a vaccine does and how it works is cartoonishly simple and goes something like this: You get a perfectly safe vaccine, it boosts your immune system, and then you're protected from whatever disease you were vaccinated for, perhaps forever. Except no part of that simple explanation is true.

There Will Always Be Outbreaks

Every year there are reported outbreaks of pertussis, mumps, and measles. There's a simple explanation for this consistency, and it's not what you think. Put simply: The vaccines don't work that well. As the Associated Press reported in 2013: "A government study offers a new theory on why the whooping cough vaccine doesn't seem to be working as well as expected. The research suggests that while the vaccine may keep people from getting sick, it doesn't prevent them from spreading whooping cough—also known as pertussis—to others. 'It could explain the increase in pertussis that we're seeing in the U.S.,' said one of the researchers, Tod Merkel of the Food and Drug Administration."[34]

In 2017 public health researchers at Boston University argued that the resurgence of whooping cough cases "can largely be attributed to the immunological failures of acellular vaccines," as lead researcher Dr. Christopher J. Gill explained:

> *This disease is back because we didn't really understand how our immune defenses against whooping cough worked, and did not understand how the vaccines needed to work to prevent it. Instead we layered assumptions upon assumptions, and now find ourselves in the uncomfortable position of admitting that we may [have] made some crucial errors. This is definitely not where we thought we'd be in 2017.*[35]

And the media reporting on measles and other outbreaks rarely explains that the majority of people infected with pertussis or measles or mumps have been vaccinated. There was a mumps outbreak at Harvard University just a few years ago. It turns out "the infected students had all been vaccinated against mumps, as required by law. It's possible the vaccine didn't work in some people, or that the virus mutated in ways that made the shot less effective. The mumps vaccine fails to induce immunity in about 12 percent of people who receive it, so mumps outbreaks occur occasionally even in highly vaccinated populations."[36]

In 2017 the CDC's own Advisory Committee on Immunization Practices held an October meeting to discuss the issue of vaccine effectiveness, explaining that "research suggests that 10 or more years after the second childhood dose [of mumps], protection against the virus fades enough to help outbreaks take hold."[37] It's worth noting there is a whistle-blower lawsuit against Merck in Pennsylvania, the maker of the mumps vaccine, with former Merck employees claiming Merck hid the efficacy data on mumps, because it was showing that the vaccine often didn't work. The whistle-blowers charge that "the drug maker knew its vaccine was less effective than the purported 95% level, and alleged senior management was aware and also oversaw testing that concealed the actual effectiveness."[38]

Vaccine Safety Testing Is Inadequate

Vaccines aren't required to undergo double-blind trials before they are given to babies. When a pharmaceutical company tests vaccines, they don't have a "control group" receiving a placebo vaccine to see if there is a difference in adverse outcomes from getting a new vaccine. Worse, the safety testing during a new vaccine trial evaluates adverse reactions after participants received a vaccine for somewhere between two and five days. As one example, the only stand-alone polio vaccine in the United States was monitored for only forty-eight hours after administration.[39] That's it. Autism, which takes time to manifest, would never be captured in these safety trails. In fact, many of the known adverse events from vaccines with names like Guillain-Barré syndrome, chronic inflammatory demyelinating polyneuropathy, and rheumatoid arthritis may take weeks, months, or even years to manifest, so safety testing wouldn't capture any of them.

As another example, the safety study from Recombivax, one of the most widely used hepatitis B vaccines in the world, and given to many American babies on day one of life, included "434 doses of RECOMBIVAX HB, 5 mcg . . . administered to 147 healthy infants and children (up to 10 years of age) who were monitored for 5 days after each dose."[40] The entire safety profile for this vaccine, given to millions of children, was based on 147 infants who were monitored for five days. And the infants were not given any other vaccines, despite the fact that at two months, four months, six months, and twelve months of age, babies simultaneously receive at least four other vaccines: rotavirus, DTP, Hib, and PCV. As pediatrician Dr. Harold E. Buttram explains in a letter to the *BMJ*:

> *In order to meet the criteria of scientific proof, a vaccine safety study would need to perform before-and-after human studies designed to screen for possible adverse effects on the neurological, immunologic, and hematological systems, comparing vaccinated with unvaccinated subjects, both in sufficient numbers and followed for sufficient periods of time to be meaningful. There have never been any studies of this nature, and apparently none have been attempted. Based on personal observation, it appears that before-and-after testing has been studiously avoided by government health agencies for fear that the results would discourage public confidence in vaccine programs. Until this level of safety testing is done, it is a virtual certainty that many adverse vaccine reactions are taking place unrecognized and will continue to take place. By the same token, until meaningful, objective vaccine safety testings are done, in my opinion the NIH, CDC, FDA can justifiably be accused of negligence in protecting the health and welfare of the American public, especially the children.*[41]

Because of how limited safety testing is for vaccines prior to rolling them out to more than seventy million American children, the CDC relies on safety monitoring once vaccines are being given in the real world, which is where things get even more problematic.

Adverse Events Are Closer to One in Fifty

The 1986 law that indemnified vaccine makers from harm also created VAERS, which is a passive reporting system for vaccine adverse events. What this means is that VAERS only works to the extent doctors or parents decide to report a vaccine injury to the VAERS online system. Since most parents have no idea what a vaccine injury looks like and most doctors aren't trained to recognize a vaccine injury, and the general stance is that vaccines are completely benign, you can imagine the limitations of this system, and science has born that out. In 2007 the CDC funded a study by Harvard Pilgrim Health Care for three years involving 715,000 patients that found "fewer than 1% of vaccine adverse events are reported."[42]

In 2016 VAERS received 59,117 reports of vaccine adverse events, including 432 deaths and 10,284 emergency room visits.[43] If those 59,117 reports were 1 percent of the actual total, that would imply there had actually been 5.9 million reportable adverse events from vaccines in a single year.

The CDC-funded Harvard Pilgrim study's purpose was to automate the reporting of vaccine injuries by programming known vaccine reactions into medical charts of patients experiencing certain reactions near the time of vaccination. The pilot study yielded troubling results, because of 715,000 individuals, 35,570 possible vaccine reactions were identified.[44] That's 2.6 percent of vaccine recipients—a far cry from the "one in a million" figure tossed around by vaccine marketers! The Harvard Pilgrim researchers stood ready to integrate this new reporting system with VAERS but reported instead that the CDC went radio silent on a study that cost more than $1 million, as principal investigator Ross Lazarus reported:

> *Unfortunately, there was never an opportunity to perform system performance assessments because the necessary CDC contacts were no longer available and the CDC consultants responsible for receiving data were no longer responsive to our multiple requests to proceed with testing and evaluation.*

A three-year study produced results so potentially devastating to the CDC—because the adverse event rate was so much higher than anything the CDC could share with the public—that the program was shut down.

Adverse Events Are Poorly Understood

What harm, exactly, can a vaccine cause? In 1991 the prestigious Institute of Medicine (IOM) looked at side effects from just one vaccine, the DTP, and concluded that science supported a causal relationship with the following six vaccine injuries: acute encephalopathy, chronic arthritis, acute arthritis, shock and unusual shock-like state, anaphylaxis, and protracted inconsolable crying.[45] In 2012 the IOM looked at the 158 most common vaccine injuries reported to VAERS and found that science "convincingly supports a causal relationship" with 18 of those injuries but found that there wasn't any science to either confirm or deny

135 additional injuries.[46] Here's the list of injuries that might be caused by vaccines, except no one has looked:

Encephalitis, encephalopathy, infantile spasms, afebrile seizures, seizures, cerebellar ataxia, acute disseminated encephalomyelitis, transverse myelitis, optic neuritis, neuromyelitis optica, multiple sclerosis, Guillain-Barré syndrome, chronic inflammatory demyelinating polyneuropathy, brachial neuritis, amyotrophic lateral sclerosis, small fiber neuropathy, chronic urticaria, erythema nodosum, systemic lupus erythematosus, polyarteritis nodosa, psoriatic arthritis, reactive arthritis, rheumatoid arthritis, juvenile idiopathic arthritis, arthralgia, autoimmune hepatitis, stroke, chronic headache, fibromyalgia, sudden infant death syndrome, hearing loss, thrombocytopenia, immune thrombocytopenic purpura.

In 86 percent of the vaccine injuries reported to VAERS, no one has any idea whether they are related to vaccines.

No One Knows the True Impact of Multiple Doses

In 2012 a study looking at data from the aforementioned VAERS database noted several disturbing patterns. The more vaccines a child received in a single setting, the more likely she was to be hospitalized or die.[47] In the study, published in *Human and Experimental Toxicology*, Dr. Gary Goldman and Neil Miller found a "a positive correlation between hospitalization rates and the number of vaccine doses" and also "younger infants were significantly more likely than older infants to be hospitalized or die after receiving vaccines." The authors also affirmed the inadequacies of current vaccine testing:

> *Studies have not been conducted to determine the safety (or efficacy) of administering multiple vaccine doses in a variety of combinations as recommended by CDC guidelines.*

Frustrating for parents is the contradictory, and scientifically unsupported, perspective the American Academy of Pediatrics provides on their website about vaccinating a child with multiple vaccines at once, which states: "Vaccines are well-studied to make sure that it is safe to give them all at once."[48] Parents are understandably confused.

The DTP Vaccine: More Harm than Good in Africa

There is little science comparing health outcomes of vaccinated children versus completely unvaccinated children; that is until 2017, when arguably the most disturbing science ever done on this topic produced an outcome that reflects very poorly on global vaccination efforts and asks and answers the ultimate question about vaccines: Are they really "safe and effective"? Published in the peer-reviewed journal *EBioMedicine*, the study is titled, "The Introduction of Diphtheria-Tetanus-Pertussis and Oral Polio Vaccine Among Young Infants in an Urban African Community: A Natural Experiment."[49]

Researchers from the Research Center for Vitamins and Vaccines, Statens Serum Institut (Denmark), and Bandim Health Project looked closely at data from the West African nation of Guinea-Bissau. The scientists in this study closely explored the concept of NSEs, "nonspecific effects" of vaccines, which is a fancy way of saying vaccines may make a child more susceptible to other infections. They found that the data for children who had been vaccinated with the DTP vaccine "was associated with 5-fold higher mortality than being unvaccinated. No prospective study has shown beneficial survival effects of DTP. . . . DTP is the most widely used vaccine. . . . All currently available evidence suggests that DTP vaccine may kill more children from other causes than it saves from diphtheria, tetanus, or pertussis. Though a vaccine protects children against the target disease, it may simultaneously increase susceptibility to unrelated infections."

In lay terms, this means that giving a child the DTP vaccine may make the child sick from other infections. Life is about risk and reward. As a venture capital expert throughout my career, I used risk/reward to analyze every deal I ever made. Parents should have all the information they need, so that they too can make a risk/reward decision on behalf of their kids; in other words, informed consent. You and I and every other parent in the world want safety and health for our kids.

Perhaps no scientist has been more eloquent or public in discussing this issue than Dr. Tetyana Obukhanych, who wrote a book, *Vaccine Illusion: How Vaccination Compromises Our Natural Immunity and What We Can Do to Regain Our Health*, that discusses the issue of NSEs from vaccines. Dr. Obukhanych testified before the California State Assembly, just before they voted to make vaccines mandatory for school attendance in California. Her training is in immunology, and she herself would tell you that she began her education "very enthusiastic about the concept of vaccination, just like any typical immunologist."[50] However, Dr. Obukhanych quickly lost her enthusiasm for vaccinations, noting that

> *despite the fact that the biological basis of naturally acquired immunity is not understood, present day medical practices insist upon artificial manipulation of the immune response (a.k.a. immunization or vaccination) to secure "immunity" without going through the actual disease process. The vaccine-induced process, although not resembling a natural disease, is nevertheless still a disease process with its own risks. And it is not immunity that we gain via vaccination but a puny surrogate of immunity. For this reason, vaccination at its core is neither a safe nor an effective method of disease prevention.*

What we learn from the African study, and that is perfectly explained by Dr. Obukhanych, is that children going through the artificial disease process triggered by a vaccine are actually more susceptible to suffer (and sometimes die) from other diseases, because their immune system is weakened and compromised in ways we really don't yet understand.

The Dengue Fever Vaccine

Another real-world example of the unanticipated NSEs from vaccines emerged from a scandal in the Philippines in late 2017. The dengue fever vaccine, administered to more than seven hundred thousand children, actually made dengue fever worse (and often deadly) for any vaccine recipients who hadn't previously had dengue fever. The scandal engulfed the nation and prompted scathing condemnations of pharmaceutical industry influence by the president of the Philippines, Rodrigo Duterte, who stated through his spokesperson, "We will leave no stone unturned in making those responsible for this shameless public health scam which puts hundreds of thousands of young lives at risk accountable."[51] National Public Radio covered the scandal and reported:

> *The world's only vaccine against dengue has hit a roadblock, and this complication is causing some countries to restrict use of the vaccine. Sanofi Pasteur, the French company that manufactures the shot,*

raised new safety concerns last week about the vaccine. In response, the Philippines suspended a mass immunization campaign, which has already given one dose of the vaccine to more than 700,000 children. And the Brazilian government has tightened restrictions on the shot. The vaccine—called Dengvaxia—raises the risk of a deadly form of dengue for people who have never been exposed to the virus, Sanofi Pasteur wrote Wednesday in a statement. The company says it discovered the complication after analyzing data from a six-year study. . .[52]

The *Manila Times* was highly critical of the dengue fever vaccine fiasco, blaming former Philippine president Aquino (who ordered the mass vaccination against dengue fever) and quoting dengue fever researcher Dr. Scott Halstead, who provided some dark irony: "It's happened. We have a vaccine that enhances dengue."[53]

The Flu Vaccine Made Canadians More Vulnerable

It's unlikely many Americans heard about the dengue fever vaccine scandal, and probably fewer still knew that a similar study in Canada had noted the phenomenon of a weakened immune response after being vaccinated back in 2015, this time involving the flu vaccine. University of Calgary researchers, profiled in an article in *Global News* titled "Canadian study finds flu shot could increase risk of getting sick" discovered that the 2014–15 flu vaccine worked far better for people who hadn't received a flu vaccine in the previous year.[54] Said differently, the more vaccines for flu you received, the less well it worked.

In the *Global News* article, University of Calgary researcher Dr. Jim Dickinson explained: "A negative effectiveness suggests the vaccine made people more susceptible to the flu. We need to do further research to understand why this has happened."

Bolstering the case that repeated flu vaccines may alter the immune system in unpredictable ways, in 2018 University of Maryland scientists discovered that receiving a flu vaccine made your risk of infecting others far more likely, because the volume of flu vaccine you shed through breathing and sneezing was six times higher than for those who hadn't received a flu vaccine:

[We found] 6.3 (95% CI 1.9–21.5) times more aerosol shedding among cases with vaccination in the current and previous season compared with having no vaccination in those two seasons.[55]

Parents Are Concerned about Gardasil

Gardasil, a vaccine intended to prevent the spread of the human papilloma virus (HPV), is the most important new vaccine for Merck, the largest vaccine maker in the world. Gardasil alone accounted for more than $2 billion in revenues in 2016, making Gardasil Merck's single largest vaccine.[56]

Gardasil is typically administered to healthy teenage girls, and the devastating stories of chronically ill and injured girls following Gardasil administration has crept up in every country where the vaccine is administered. In Japan, a country with a robust history of honesty about vaccine side effects, the stories of Gardasil injuries became such a public scandal that uptake rates for the vaccine are now under 1 percent (current rate in the United States is over 60 percent for teenage girls).[57] In late 2016 a Japanese industry watchdog group—Medwatcher Japan—issued a scathing letter criticizing, among others, the World Health Organization, which they felt was endorsing the Gardasil vaccine without acknowledging the growing body of science demonstrating high rates of devastating side effects:

Countries other than Japan have also indicated major problems with the safety of HPV vaccines. Ignoring these "inconvenient" facts in an effort to promote HPV vaccination contradicts the primary responsibility of WHO, which is to dispassionately assess risks and benefits. . . . Reported serious AEs [adverse events] include diverse, complex, multi-system symptoms such as seizures; disturbance of consciousness; systemic pain including headache, myalgia, arthralgia, back pain and other pain; motor dysfunction such as paralysis, muscular weakness, exhaustion, and involuntary movements; numbness and sensory disturbance; autonomic symptoms including dizziness, hypotension, tachycardia, nausea, vomiting, and diarrhea; respiratory dysfunction including dyspnea and asthma; endocrine disorders such as menstrual disorder and hypermenorrhea; hypersensitivity to light

and sound; psychological symptoms including anxiety, frustration,
hallucinations, and overeating; higher brain dysfunction and cogni-
tive impairments including memory impairment, disorientation,
and loss of concentration; and sleep disorders, hypersomnia and
sudden sleep attacks. In some cases, these symptoms impair learning
and result in extreme fatigue and decreased motivation, negatively
impacting everyday life.[58]

Meanwhile, in Ireland the furious debate about Gardasil was frequently front page news throughout 2017 as a well-organized group of parents—calling themselves "Regret"—turned the debate about Gardasil into a national issue. In the late fall of 2017, the *Irish Times* reported that "uptake for the vaccine has plummeted from a high of 87 per cent to 50 per cent. Any further decline is likely to call into question the economic, medical and political rationale of the programme" and that "almost 650 girls in Ireland reported requiring medical intervention or treatment after receiving the HPV vaccine, according to data collected by the State's medicines watchdog."[59]

In 2017 a published meta-analysis of Gardasil clinical trials stated that "two of the largest randomized trials found significantly more severe adverse events in the tested HPV vaccine arm of the study." The study, "Serious Adverse Events After HPV Vaccination: A Critical Review of Randomized Trials and Post-marketing Case Series," concluded, "These findings raise further doubt on HPV vaccine safety."[60]

Merck's most important vaccine receiving withering, worldwide criticism may serve to accelerate a reckoning about vaccines in general and perhaps shed the light more fully on autism, too. Gardasil shares something in common with most of the vaccines given to infants: a very high level of aluminum adjuvant.

Vaccines Are Linked to Autoimmune Disease

While this book is specifically about autism, it's important to point out that autism may just be the tip of the iceberg for a host of neurological and physical disorders impacting our children at epidemic levels. Conditions of autoimmunity—asthma, diabetes, food allergies, eczema, and so on—are growing at rates similar to autism. Could vaccines also be behind their explosion? According to many scientists, absolutely.

As one example, scientists at the University of Virginia have drawn a direct line between the aluminum (referred to as "alum") used in vaccines to stimulate the immune system and the explosion in food allergies, stating "the era of food allergy began with the post-millennial generation, the same faction who received new immunizations during early childhood. Many of these vaccines contain alum, an adjuvant known to induce allergic phenotypes."[61] (As you will soon learn, aluminum adjuvant may explain much, much more.)

Allergy scientists know that if they want to create a food allergy in rats, the quickest way to do it is by injecting them with vaccine ingredients. In a study from Norway—"Development and Characterization of an Effective Food Allergy Model in Brown Norway Rats"—scientists wanted to figure out the quickest way to give lab rats a food allergy so they could study various food allergy suppression drugs on them.[62] Since rats aren't born with food allergies, the most effective method was clear: inject the rats with egg protein and aluminum adjuvant, and they will soon be allergic to eggs.

There's even a textbook from one of the largest textbook companies in the world (Wiley & Sons) titled *Vaccines and Autoimmunity*, a book that "explores the role of adjuvants—specifically aluminum in different vaccines—and how they can induce diverse autoimmune clinical manifestations in genetically prone individuals."[63] The book's coauthor, Dr. Yehuda Shoenfeld, is viewed as the world's foremost authority on autoimmunity, and he is very direct in raising the alarm bell about vaccine side effects: "Due to the adverse effects exerted by adjuvants, there is no controversy over the need for safer adjuvants for incorporation into future vaccines."

Vaccines Didn't Cause the Decline in Measles

The idea that vaccines saved humanity is unsupportable by the facts. But it's worth addressing the two diseases that everyone talks about whenever a vaccine debate takes place: measles and polio. I'll start with measles.

Just before the first rollout of a nationwide measles vaccine program, the three leading scientists at what was then called the Public Health Service (today's CDC) made a presentation in San Francisco at the American Public Health Association's annual meeting. The date was November 1, 1966. The presentation was led by Dr. David J. Sencer, who at the time held the title of chief of the PHS's National Communicable Disease Center.

He was joined by his assistant chief, Dr. H. Bruce Dull, as well as the PHS's chief of epidemiology, Dr. Alexander Langmuir. It's fair to say that at this point in history no one knew more about the measles virus than these three scientists. The PHS scientists used the APHA's annual meeting to announce plans for their ambitious national launch, with the hopes of eradicating measles by the end of 1967.

The doctors also turned their presentation into a report titled "Epidemiological Basis for Eradication of Measles in 1967," and some of the matter-of-fact statements they made might get a doctor banned from the mainstream media today as even a single case of measles is a cause for panic and outbreak stories that often make the national news.[64] In fact, a new parent might think measles was just like Ebola, except it's not, as the PHS scientists made very clear in 1966, stating, "For centuries the measles virus has maintained a remarkably stable ecological relationship with man. The clinical disease is a characteristic syndrome of notable constancy and only moderate severity. Complications are infrequent, and, with adequate medical care, fatality is rare."

In the 1950s and '60s, even without vaccines, measles outbreaks only happened every few years, on a somewhat dependable cycle; they noted that "in large population centers, as in cities or whole metropolitan areas, measles epidemics recur in 2-to-3-year cycles." They also established a vaccination threshold to eradicate measles well below the 95 percent number public health officials use today, noting that "it is evident that when the level of immunity was higher than 55 percent, epidemics did not develop." Before the vaccine had been introduced, it's worth noting that the death rate from measles in the United States had already declined by approximately 99.96 percent from its peak in the mid-1800s. In 1960 the death rate from measles was 0.23 per 100,000 people.[65] Asthma, by comparison, had a mortality rate more than ten times higher for the same year.[66]

In 2013 "Measles Vaccination Before the Measles-Mumps-Rubella Vaccine" was published in the *American Journal of Public Health*, looking at the history of the measles vaccine, and it had many similar observations about the history of measles, including the view from parents and doctors that measles was "unpleasant but inevitable":

> *At the beginning of the 1960s, it was clear that a vaccine against measles would soon be available. Although measles was (and*

remains) a killer disease in the developing world, in the United States and Western Europe this was no longer so. Many parents and many medical practitioners considered measles an inevitable stage of a child's development. . . . By 1960, thanks to the use of antibiotics and improvements in living conditions, measles mortality was declining steadily in industrialized countries. . . . Parents largely came to see measles as an unpleasant, although more or less inevitable, part of childhood. Many primary care physicians shared this view.[67]

"So what?" some might argue, even if measles was considered a mild and inevitable illness of childhood, aren't we better off as a society by having even less measles around? But I think we should all be suspicious of the extreme fear-mongering generated in the press every time even a single case of measles surfaces and ask the question, "Who is generating all the panic?" Also, we have to be honest about the adverse events from the MMR vaccine and decide if they outweigh the benefits of reducing the incidence of a mild childhood illness. According to Physicians for Informed Consent, a large group of doctors in California:

There is no evidence that the measles vaccine causes less death or permanent disability than measles. The vaccine package insert raises questions about safety testing for cancer, genetic mutations, and impaired fertility. Although VAERS tracks some adverse events, it is too inaccurate to measure against the risk of measles. Clinical trials do not have the ability to detect less common adverse reactions, and epidemiological studies are limited by the effects of chance and possible confounders. Safety studies of the measles vaccine are particularly lacking in statistical power. A review of more than 60 measles vaccine studies conducted for the Cochrane Library states, "The design and reporting of safety outcomes in MMR vaccine studies, both pre- and post-marketing, are largely inadequate." Because permanent sequalae (after effects) from measles, especially in individuals with normal levels of vitamin A, are so rare, the level of accuracy of the research studies available is insufficient to prove that the vaccine causes less death or permanent injury than measles.[68]

That's quite a statement from a group of doctors. They're saying the risk/reward equation to have the measles vaccine isn't there.

What about Polio?

It wouldn't be an exaggeration to say that the modern vaccine industry was built on the reputation the polio vaccine carries forth to this day for having saved the children of the world from the scourge of polio. Nothing stirs the emotions quite like polio, especially for anyone who lived through the polio scares of the 1940s and '50s. The images of children in iron lungs, casts, and using crutches to walk is the most chilling imagery we have of any infectious disease in the modern era, and polio is always referenced whenever debates about vaccines erupt.

Ending the polio epidemic is the iconic achievement of vaccines, and maintaining the purity and simplicity of the narrative that vaccines ended the polio epidemic is critical to maintaining the image of vaccines as infallible and essential. That being said, there are several unanswered questions about polio that deeply challenge the narrative that the polio vaccine saved the world:

Why did poliovirus, a well-known and fairly mild enterovirus, suddenly provoke a devastating epidemic in the late 1940s and early 1950s? For most, a bout with poliovirus is a minor event, but for a small number (perhaps 1 to 2 percent), the virus somehow makes its way into the nervous system, where it can be far more dangerous, and sometimes deadly poliomyelitis. The outbreaks were confined largely to warm-weather months. They had higher prevalence in agricultural areas. Do any of these facts relate to each other?

Did DDT escort poliovirus into the nervous system? In November 1953 Dr. Morton S. Biskind published a pretty clear answer in the *American Journal of Digestive Diseases*.[69] His famous paper, "Public Health Aspects of the New Insecticides," minced absolutely no words in making it clear what was causing mild poliovirus to morph into paralytic poliomyelitis: DDT. The insecticide, utilized for the first time in 1945, had become ubiquitous in the United States, even though the public health service warned in 1951 how risky its use was: "DDT is a delayed-action poison. Due to the fact that it accumulates in the body

74

tissues, especially in females, the repeated inhalation or ingestion of DDT constitutes a distinct health hazard. The deleterious effects are manifested principally in the liver, spleen, kidneys, and spinal cord. . . . Children and infants especially are much more susceptible to poisoning than adults."

Can DDT use explain the trends in polio outbreaks? DDT spraying was much more prevalent in the warm-weather months. Many of the first cases of polio took place in agricultural areas. There were many case examples to compare and contrast: Israel, which was late in introducing DDT (in the early 1950s), was late in having a polio epidemic.[70] In the Philippines, American troops used DDT on the military bases and had high poliomyelitis outbreaks, but natives living outside the base didn't.[71]

Most importantly, Dr. Biskind explained in his article that the biological science published in 1944 and 1947 showed that DDT did the very thing that made the nervous system susceptible to poliovirus's becoming poliomyelitis: It produced "degeneration of the anterior horn cells of the spinal cord in animals." These cells at the top of the spinal column are the key entry point to the spinal column, where the poliovirus then creates inflammation of the myelin sheath, creating, you got it, poliomyelitis.

Once biological plausibility was firmly established, Dr. Biskind then asked in his article the most important question about the polio epidemic you've never heard before: "When the population is exposed to a chemical agent known to produce in animals lesions in the spinal cord resembling those in human polio, and thereafter the latter disease increases sharply in incidence and maintains its epidemic character year after year, is it unreasonable to suspect an etiologic relationship?"

Why does polio stubbornly persist in countries like India, even though many Indian children are vaccinated fifteen or more times before the age of five? Perhaps it also won't surprise you that in India, where polio stubbornly persists even with children receiving as many as two dozen polio vaccines each, DDT remains in wide use.[72]

Did polio decline in near lockstep with the decline and ultimate ban of DDT in the United States? Yes, it did. The United States, in fact, hasn't had a case of polio since 1979. DDT was banned by the EPA in 1972.[73]

Could "polio provocation" also explain the rise in polio? What's clear about poliovirus's becoming poliomyelitis is that somehow the virus needs to be able to jump into the nervous system. DDT appears to be a potent escort, given its capacity to degenerate the spinal cord. Another potential escort is what's known as "polio provocation," a theory that recently moved from hypothesis to biological fact. An article from Cambridge University explains: "In 1998 scientists Drs. Matthias Gromeier and Eckard Wimmer were able to show that tissue injury caused by certain injections gives the polio virus easy access to nerve channels, thereby increasing its ability to cause paralysis."[74]

The study, "Mechanism of Injury-Provoked Poliomyelitis," explained:

> Using a mouse model developed for the study of poliomyelitis, we have shown that muscular trauma induced by multiple injections can lead to rapid progression of PV–induced paralysis, upregulation of viral replication in certain tissues, and acceleration of the progression of histopathological lesions. Thus, our data provide direct experimental evidence for the concept of PPM [provocation poliomyelitis].

The study authors raised a very concerning question:

> What if the very act of repeated vaccination was the thing leading to poliomyelitis in the developing world? "Skeletal muscle injury is known to predispose its sufferers to neurological complications of concurrent poliovirus infections. This phenomenon, labeled 'provocation poliomyelitis,' continues to cause numerous cases of childhood paralysis due to the administration of unnecessary injections to children in areas where poliovirus is endemic. Recently, it has been reported that intramuscular injections may also increase the likelihood of vaccine-associated paralytic poliomyelitis in recipients of live attenuated poliovirus vaccines."[75]

During the 1950s, tonsillectomy surgeries on children also exploded, and children who had received the operation were three times likelier to develop polio. Could any tissue injury increase the risk that poliovirus might jump into the nervous system?

The elimination of DDT may have had as much, if not more, to do with the reduction of polio cases in the United States as the vaccine did. A blog post titled "The Age of Polio" by journalist Dan Olmsted and autism father Mark Blaxill considered this very issue, wondering if the narrative we've been fed about polio is too simplistic, the authors arguing "that a single-minded focus on germs—and an unwillingness to explore novel and potentially uncomfortable ideas from outside medical orthodoxy [such as DDT's being a trigger for poliomyelitis]—is an inadequate strategy when it comes to modern diseases." Worse, the simplistic view that epidemics such as polio's can be conquered solely with a vaccine might inhibit a more holistic understanding of how to fight disease:

> But the victory over the epidemics of poliomyelitis means our understanding of polio is essentially frozen in amber, circa 1955. Few diseases have been so completely conquered, at least at home, while being so incompletely understood, and that is not a good outcome. In leaving so many important topics on the table—why outbreaks occurred, why the pattern of contagion was so atypical for an infectious disease—scientists allowed some weak ideas to become conventional wisdom and some important ones to be missed. . . . And the connection of other illnesses to pesticides, and environmental toxins in general, has been slow in dawning. . . . The suffering of polio's victims is honored by learning all of its lessons, including the danger of environmental toxins and the perils of ignoring their role in modern disease; the risk of focusing all of our energy on vaccinations as magic bullets, and the fundamental ethical obligation to search for the truth without fear or favor. Only then can we work out the real nature of illnesses that confront us here and now, ranging from autism to Parkinson's to the persistence of poliomyelitis itself. Only then can we begin to prevent such disasters as The Age of Polio.[76]

I'm sure some are wondering, if I can even criticize the polio vaccine, am I really just saying that no vaccines are worth it? I think each vaccine needs to be evaluated on its own merits. As Physicians for Informed Consent showed with their analysis of the measles data, sometimes the risks from a vaccine outweigh the potential benefits, but these facts are very hard for the average parent to ascertain. And the history of vaccination needs to be accounted for in a more honest and transparent manner. Finally, the relationship between man and infectious disease is likely far more complicated and intertwined than we all appreciate.

What if there was a synergistic component to having certain illnesses, meaning they actually made your immune system more robust in the long term? That may sound esoteric to you, but scientists are aggressively pursuing just this angle, and the results are thought-provoking. A 2010 study, "Mumps and Ovarian Cancer: Modern Interpretation of an Historic Association," found that having had mumps (the other "M" of the MMR vaccine) might make someone less susceptible to ovarian cancer.[77] A 1998 study found that children who had measles and other "febrile infectious childhood diseases" had lower cancer risk as adults.[78] A 2000 *British Journal of Cancer* study found that measles in childhood led to a lower risk of Hodgkin's disease and that having childhood illnesses in general created lower cancer rates: "These results support previous evidence that early exposure to infection protects against HD [Hodgkin's Disease]."[79] A 2005 study by scientists from Canada examined many studies and found, "infections may play a paradoxical role in cancer development with chronic infections often being tumorigenic and acute infections being antagonistic to cancer," meaning exposure to infectious childhood diseases lowers cancer risk.[80] And in 2016 Baylor scientists "reported an inverse relationship between a history of chicken pox and glioma, a type of brain cancer, meaning that children who have had the chicken pox may be less likely to develop brain cancer."[81] What if certain illnesses and our immune system really do have a synergistic relationship? What if nature is actually more complicated than we think?

There may be many parents who feel, even after understanding the true history of polio, compelled to get the polio vaccine for their child. I have no personal problem with that. My problem is with the exaggerated, one-sided, fault-free history of vaccines that parents are presented with, one that hits parents over the head with the "safe and effective" mantra and discourages critical thinking. And if we can't talk honestly about vaccines, we really can't talk about how to end the autism epidemic. And that's my real beef.

A Perfect Circle of Denial

Vaccine injury, in my opinion, hides in plain sight, largely due to the way vaccines are tested and monitored, which is compounded by how poorly

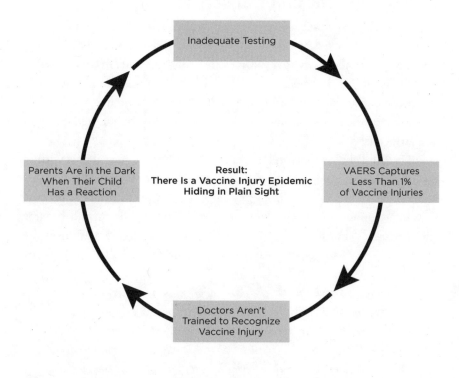

Figure 2.5. The Vaccine Injury Circle of Denial.

understood vaccine injuries are by the typical first line of defense when problems happen: pediatricians. Let's think through this perfect "circle of denial" for a moment:

Vaccines are tested, as single doses, by observing side effects for just a few days after they are given. This ensures that any conditions that take time to manifest, which would be most autoimmune and neurological conditions, will never be captured through safety testing. Next, the postadministration form of capturing adverse events, VAERS, has been shown to capture less than 1 percent of all vaccine injuries. Add to this that pediatricians are never taught how to identify vaccine injuries, partially because the safety testing and reporting are so inadequate. And finally, parents are left completely in the dark about what's happening when their child has a reaction. When you think about this circle of denial (see figure 2.5), you can see how an epidemic of vaccine injuries could be hiding in plain sight.

Doctors Are Raising Concerns

When I started to closely research vaccines after I watched my son's health decline, I was shocked by how many doctors and scientists had raised very public concerns about whether vaccines are really "safe and effective" and had been doing so for decades. Dr. Robert Mendelsohn was the most famous American pediatrician of the 1970s and '80s. He made over five hundred TV and radio appearances, authored six best-selling books about medicine and pediatrics that sold over a million copies, and wrote a nationally syndicated column, The People's Doctor, for twelve years. Over those years his writing on the topic increased accordingly, and he told his readers that "although I administered them myself during my early years of practice, I have become a steadfast opponent of mass inoculations because of the myriad hazards they present."[82] He also realized that railing against the false narratives the vaccine industry had helped create would be hard for many to understand:

> I know, as I write about the dangers of mass immunization, that it is a concept that you may find difficult to accept. Immunizations have been so artfully and aggressively marketed that most parents believe them to be the "miracle" that has eliminated many once-feared diseases. Consequently, for anyone to oppose them borders on the foolhardy. For a pediatrician to attack what has become the "bread and butter" of pediatric practice is equivalent to a priest's denying the infallibility of the pope.[83]

Dr. Mendelsohn passed away in 1988, just as the United States was embarking on a massive campaign to increase the total number of vaccines given to children. He was the first nationally known pediatrician to express public concern about the growing hazards vaccines were creating, but he was far from the last. Perhaps the most well-known pediatrician today is California's Dr. Robert Sears, whose 2008 book, The Vaccine Book: Making the Right Decision for Your Child, has sold more than 250,000 copies, and he provides some perspective on why he speaks out about the risks of vaccines:

> I got interested in the topic of vaccines way back in medical school. A friend of mine convinced me to read a book about vaccines, and it ended up being a very anti-vaccine book. It was all about an old

vaccine called the DTP vaccine that we don't use anymore. But the book talked a lot about the risks and the dangers of that vaccine. The author of that book was calling for that vaccine to no longer be used. A number of years later, it turns out that they did discover that vaccine was causing a lot of very severe, life-threatening, even fatal side effects, so they did end up taking that vaccine off the market. So it kind of opened my eyes to the fact that there are some very severe, fortunately very rare, side effects to vaccines, and I wanted to learn more about this issue. I started reading a lot more books.[84]

Dr. Sears is joined by many other pediatricians, including pediatrician Dr. Lawrence Palevsky of New York, who provides some insight into what he learned about vaccines during medical school:

When I went through medical school, I was taught that vaccines were completely safe and completely effective, and I had no reason to believe otherwise. All the information that I was taught was pretty standard in all the medical schools and the teachings and scientific literature throughout the country. . . . Over the years, I kept practicing medicine and using vaccines and thinking that my approach to vaccines was completely onboard with everything else I was taught. But more and more, I kept seeing that my experience of the world, my experience in using and reading about vaccines, and hearing what parents were saying about vaccines were very different from what I was taught in medical school and my residency training . . . and it became clearer to me as I read the research, listened to more and more parents, and found other practitioners who also shared the same concern that vaccines had not been completely proven safe or even completely effective, based on the literature that we have today. . . . It didn't appear that the scientific studies that we were given were actually appropriately designed to prove and test the safety and efficacy.[85]

Dr. Suzanne Humphries, a board-certified nephrologist turned activist and the author of *Dissolving Illusions*, shared some perspective on her journey:

Do you know how much doctors learn about vaccines in medical school? When we participate in pediatrics training, we learn that vaccines need to be given on schedule. We learn that smallpox and polio were eliminated by vaccines. We learn that there's no need to know how to treat diphtheria, because we won't see it again anyway. We are indoctrinated with the mantra that "vaccines are safe and effective"—neither of which is true. Doctors today are given extensive training on how to talk to "hesitant" parents—how to frighten them by vastly inflating the risks during natural infection. They are trained on the necessity of twisting parents' arms to conform, or fire them from their practices. Doctors are trained that nothing bad should be said about any vaccine, period.[86]

Dr. Rachael Ross spent three seasons cohosting the Emmy Award–winning and nationally syndicated TV Show, *The Doctors.* When she wasn't hosting the show, Dr. Ross was commuting home to run her family practice in Gary, Indiana, alongside her father and brother, both physicians. When Dr. Ross changed her tune about using vaccines in her practice, the mainstream media met her announcement with silence, but her words were powerful and clear. In 2016 Dr. Ross explained her change of heart in a widely read blog post titled, "Vaccines, Vaccine Injury, & My Perspective as a Doctor & Mom."

I have witnessed the vaccine schedule grow from 16 doses of 4 vaccines from birth to six years old when I was a child, to the current recommendation of 49 doses of 14 vaccines between birth and age six, and 69 doses of 16 vaccines between birth and the age of eighteen . . . and we've been giving them on–time, sometimes five shots a day to help kids "catch–up," and all without question. Medical school and residency taught us all to do so. I guess I can't help but wonder if there's a connection between the fact that when we had to give fewer vaccines we had fewer childhood diseases. It is only human to wonder. We had fewer learning disabilities, less asthma, less autism, and less diabetes. Autism in particular was 1 in 500 in the late seventies and it has now skyrocketed to 1 in 50. Why so many? Why so soon?[87]

Dr. Ross's concern, when you look at a chart of the data, is deeply disturbing; the linear relationship between the rise in vaccines and the rise in autism is hard to miss (see figure 2.6).

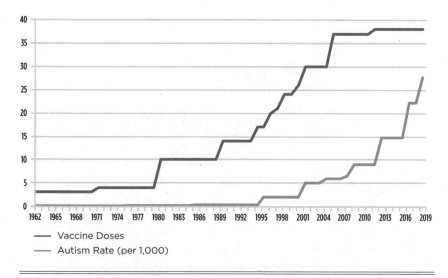

Figure 2.6. The Corresponding Growth in the Number of Vaccines American Children Receive and Growth in the Rate of Autism (per 1,000 Children). Data from Treffert et al., the Centers for Disease Control and Prevention.

In early 2017 Dr. Daniel Neides, the medical director of Cleveland Clinic Wellness Institute caused a controversy when he wrote an article for the Cleveland *Plain Dealer* titled, "Make 2017 the year to avoid toxins (good luck) and master your domain: Words on Wellness."[88] He specifically addressed whether the risk/reward of the current vaccination program was worth it: "Some of the vaccines have helped reduce the incidence of childhood communicable diseases. That is great news. But not at the expense of neurologic diseases like autism and ADHD increasing at alarming rates."

I agree with Dr. Neides. In many cases I don't think the vaccine trade-off is worth it. I think we're swapping a minor reduction in a handful of acute illnesses for an explosion in lifelong chronic illness, including some as devastating as autism. But worst of all, I deeply resent the people in positions of authority and power who endlessly repeat the lie that vaccines are "safe and effective," which serves to not only shame parents, but also to shut down an open debate. If we can't honestly look at the facts about vaccines and recognize that they have real risks as well as some benefits, we will never be able to openly and honestly discuss the autism epidemic.

CHAPTER 3

"The Science Is Settled"

Let's be clear: the work of science has nothing whatever to do with consensus. Consensus is the business of politics. Science, on the contrary, requires only one investigator who happens to be right, which means that he or she has results that are verifiable by reference to the real world. In science consensus is irrelevant. What is relevant is reproducible results. The greatest scientists in history are great precisely because they broke with the consensus.

—Michael Crichton,
MD, best-selling author

Very few people in the world have read every single published study purporting to show that vaccines don't cause autism. I happen to be one of them. Not since President George W. Bush stood on the aircraft carrier USS *Abraham Lincoln* in 2003 to declare "mission accomplished" about the war in Iraq (right before it descended into a decade of chaotic hell) has so little evidence actually been marshaled to support a declaration that a critical question has been asked and answered—or, in this case, that the science is settled.

The "Tobacco Playbook"—more on this shortly—is alive and well, and it's been both perfected and expanded in the fight to obfuscate the truth about vaccines and autism through the propagation of what's called "distracting research" and, whenever necessary, outright lies about the science that's been published exploring this topic. What's actually true? Almost no science has actually been done, and what little has been completed has been done with a singular focus: exonerate vaccines.

Feigned Exasperation by Vaccine Spokespeople

Perhaps not surprising, but still a bit breathtaking, are the backgrounds of the two most public spokespeople for the "science is settled" side of the vaccine-autism debate. The aforementioned Dr. Paul Offit of the Children's Hospital of Philadelphia ("CHOP") and Dr. Peter Hotez of Baylor University share something else besides their exuberance that vaccines are innocent: They're both patent holders for vaccines and owe their careers to the vaccine industry. In Dr. Offit's case, his rotavirus vaccine patent has already been parlayed into a small fortune.[1]

When it comes to any discussion of vaccine-autism science, Drs. Offit and Hotez both take the tone in public interviews that it's silly to even ask the question, because the science has been done so many times, you must be sort of stupid if you still feel the need to talk about it. As one example, in early 2017 actor Robert De Niro publicly raised the question about vaccines triggering his own son's autism, and Dr. Offit was there to quickly admonish him, stating on NBC News, "It's been answered again and again and again."[2]

Soon after, Robert F. Kennedy Jr. held a press conference alongside Robert De Niro, and Dr. Hotez was immediately quoted on the pharma-friendly newsite Vox, saying, "I'm a bit baffled as to why Bobby Kennedy focuses on vaccines and autism, which has been debunked, instead of focusing on the known risks and demanding more research and studies."[3] Again and again and again. Baffled. Debunked. Exasperated. This is the strategy for how the vaccine industry is now approaching the vaccine-autism link, by feigning extreme exasperation, despite the fact that very little relevant science has ever taken an honest look into the possible role of vaccines in the explosion of autism.

One Vaccine and One Ingredient Studied

The most shocking thing about all these studies that make Drs. Offit and Hotez so exasperated is that for all the griping that vaccines have been studied, in fact only one vaccine and one vaccine ingredient have actually ever been scientifically explored. Let me explain.

Remember that in 1962 the maximum number of vaccines a child would receive by age five was three.[4] In 1983 the maximum number of vaccines a child would receive by age five was ten.[5] Today that number is thirty-eight, which is nearly quadruple what it was in 1983 and more than twelve times what it was in 1962.

Today by the time a child is five years old, if his parents follow the CDC's recommended schedule, he will have received the following vaccines, with most being given three to four separate times: (1) hepatitis B, (2) rotavirus, (3) DTP, (4) Hib, (5) pneumococcal, (6) polio, (7) flu, (8) MMR, (9) varicella, (10) hepatitis A, (11) meningococcal (only for certain groups), and (12) HPV (teenagers).[6]

Today at his two-month-old "well baby" visit, the average American infant will receive six separate vaccines in about fifteen minutes: hepatitis B, rotavirus, DTaP, Hib, pneumococcal, and polio. Two months later, at four months of age, most American children will again receive the same six vaccines, all administered at the same time: hepatitis B, rotavirus, DTaP, Hib, pneumococcal, and polio. Two months later, at six months of age, most American children then receive seven vaccines, all administered at the same time: hepatitis B, rotavirus, DTaP, Hib, pneumococcal, polio, and flu. By six months of age most American children receive nineteen vaccines in three visits to the doctor. Many kids also receive a birth dose of hepatitis B, boosting this number to twenty vaccines.

So of the first twenty vaccines given to American babies, how many have been studied for their relationship to autism? None. That's right, because only one vaccine, the MMR, has ever been studied for its relationship to autism. The MMR is a vaccine first administered to American children at thirteen months of age. But what about the two-month, four-month, and six-month "well baby" visits during which children receive so many vaccines? The truth is none of those vaccines have ever been studied or considered for their relationship to autism, so no one has any idea. This would be like trying to identify the source of a plane crash, suspecting mechanical failure, solely analyzing one of the wings, and then declaring the entire airplane free of culpability.

Separate from looking at one vaccine (the MMR), studies have also been published looking at a single ingredient within vaccines—thimerosal—a vaccine preservative comprised of ethylmercury. According to the CDC, there are thirty-eight separate ingredients present in two or more vaccines on the American schedule. While it certainly made sense to start the search by looking at thimerosal, given that it contains a known neurotoxin, that still leaves thirty-seven ingredients that have never been analyzed. David

Vaccine Ingredients (Present in 2 or more vaccines)	Vaccines: 0–18 months (United States)	
2-Phenoxyethanol	Pregnancy	Flu
Aluminum potassium sulfate		DTaP
Aluminum hydroxide		
Amino acids	Birth	Hep B
Ammonium sulfate		
Antibiotics	2 months	Hep B
Bovine components		Rotavirus
Bovine serum albumin		DTaP
Chick embryo cell culture		Hib
Culture, human embryonic		PCV
Detergent		IPV
Dextrose		
Enzymes	4 months	Hep B
Ethanol		Rotavirus
Formaldehyde		DTaP
Gelatin, hydrolyzed gelatin		Hib
Glutaraldehyde		PCV
Human components		IPV
Lactalbumin hydrolysate		
Medium 199	6 months	Hep B
Mineral salts		Rotavirus
Monosodium l-glutamate		DTaP
Phenol		Hib
Phosphate		PCV
Polymyxin B sulfate		IPV
Polysorbate-80		Flu
Potassium aluminum sulfate		
Potassium chloride	12–18 months	Flu
Potassium phosphate monobasic		Hib
Sodium borate		PCV
Sodium chloride		MMR
Sodium phosphate dibasic		Varicella
Sorbitol		Hep A
Soy peptone		DTaP
Sucrose		Flu
Thimerosal		Hep A
Vero (monkey kidney) cells		

> If I'm looking for scientific evidence of what happened to my son, I only have the science of one ingredient (thimerosal) and one vaccine (MMR) to consider.

Figure 3.1. Vaccine–Autism Science: What's Been Studied? Data from Centers for Disease Control and Prevention.

Kirby, former *New York Times* investigative journalist and the award-winning author of *Evidence of Harm*, is the only journalist I have seen who actually understands the extreme limitations of the completed science, and here's how he explains it:

> *To begin with, it is unscientific and perilously misleading for anyone to assert that "vaccines and autism" have been studied and that no link has been found. That's because the 16 or so studies constantly*

cited by critics of the hypothesis have examined just one vaccine and one vaccine ingredient. . . . It is illogical to exonerate all vaccines, all vaccine ingredients, and the total US vaccine program as a whole, based solely on a handful of epidemiological studies of just one vaccine and one vaccine ingredient. It is akin to claiming that every form of animal protein is beneficial to people, when all you have studied is fish.[7]

Here's a complete list of every vaccine American children receive. I've underlined the one that has been studied for its relationship to autism: hepatitis B, rotavirus, DTaP, Hib, pneumococcal, polio, flu, <u>MMR</u>, varicella, hepatitis A, meningococcal, and HPV (teenagers).

And here are all thirty-eight vaccine ingredients. Once again I've underlined the one that has been studied for its relationship to autism: 2-Phenoxyethanol, albumin, aluminum hydroxide, aluminum potassium sulfate, amino acids, ammonium sulfate, antibiotics, bovine components, bovine serum, chick embryo cell culture, culture, detergent, dextrose, enzymes, formaldehyde, gelatin, glutaraldehyde, human components, human embryonic cells, lactalbumin hydrolysate, medium 199, mineral salts, monosodium l-glutamate, phenol, phosphate, polymixin B sulfate, polysorbate-80, potassium aluminum sulfate, potassium chloride, potassium phosphate monobasic, sodium borate, sodium chloride, sodium phosphate dibasic, sorbitol, soy peptone, sucrose, <u>thimerosal</u>, vero (monkey kidney) cells, and yeast protein.[8]

Do you think it's reasonable to say, "Case closed; we've studied vaccines and autism"? (See figure 3.1.)

Twenty-Seven Studies and All the Wrong Questions

The Autism Science Foundation (ASF) serves as a repository for the "asked and answered" question about vaccines and autism and also as a platform for Dr. Offit of CHOP, who sits on the board of the organization and speaks on their behalf. The organization's website cites twenty-seven studies that they assert prove that "vaccines and autism" are unrelated. Thirteen of the studies look at the thimerosal-autism relationship. Ten of the studies look at the MMR-autism relationship. And four of the studies are "meta-analyses" of the aforementioned twenty-three thimerosal and MMR studies. That's it. One vaccine, one ingredient.

None of the twenty-seven studies cited by the ASF used to "prove" vaccines don't cause autism have come close to asking the right questions about cause and effect or have even considered the proper control group (fully unvaccinated children) to get to an answer. Having spent the time to critically read every study produced to "prove" vaccines don't cause autism, I'm dumbfounded by their inadequacy. And the comments public officials make about these studies are even more absurd and unsupportable. To help you understand what I mean, let's review the actual questions asked by three of the most common studies cited to "prove" that "vaccines don't cause autism."

Wrong Question #1: Do children who received more thimerosal in their vaccines have different neurological outcomes from children who received less thimerosal in their vaccines? This study, published in *Pediatrics* in 2000 and commonly called the "Verstraeten study," effectively compared two-pack-a-day smokers to one-pack-a-day smokers, looking at children who received more mercury in their vaccines to children who received slightly less mercury in their vaccines, to see if there were any differences in a variety of neurological disorders.[9] This is arguably the signature study of the "vaccines don't cause autism" crowd, which makes a careful reading of the study so bewildering. The study, "Safety of Thimerosal-Containing Vaccines: A Two-Phased Study of Computerized Health Maintenance Organization Databases," reached a conclusion that everyone seems to have forgotten; namely, the study authors could neither prove nor disprove an association between mercury and vaccines, stating: "The biological plausibility of the small doses of ethylmercury present in vaccines leading to increased risks of neurodevelopmental disorders is uncertain."

This is a very instructive and important study to scrutinize for many reasons. First, this was the first study ever done to explore any link between vaccines and autism, albeit the exploration was solely to see whether more or less mercury might impact the autism rate. When the study was published, the vaccine industry PR machine went into overdrive, declaring that a new study in *Pediatrics* had proven vaccines don't cause autism. In fact, the study author was so irked by the way his findings were being misinterpreted that he took the extraordinary step of penning a letter to *Pediatrics* to complain. Dr. Thomas Verstraeten, the study author, wrote this letter right before he left his position at the CDC to take a job with vaccine maker GlaxoSmithKline in Belgium:

> *Surprisingly, however, the study is being interpreted now as negative* [where "negative" implies no association was shown between thimerosal and autism] *by many. . . . The article does not state that we found evidence against an association, as a negative study would. It does state, on the contrary, that additional study is recommended, which is the conclusion to which a neutral study must come. . . . A neutral study carries a very distinct message: the investigators could neither confirm nor exclude an association, and therefore more study is required.*[10]

It's hard to understate how irresponsible and inaccurate it is that people like Dr. Paul Offit and Dr. Peter Hotez still routinely cite this study as "proof" vaccines don't cause autism, since the study only considered mercury level exposure in fully vaccinated kids, reached a neutral outcome, and recommended more work needed to be done. Even crazier, the study did find that "tics" (a motor disorder) are in fact correlated to mercury levels, writing that "cumulative exposure at 3 months resulted in a significant positive association with tics."

Wrong Question #2: Are autism rates different for children who received 62.5 mcg or 137.5 mcg of ethylmercury? Published in 2009, also in *Pediatrics*, this study from Italy was released with great fanfare[11] and is commonly called the "Tozzi study." The Associated Press headline shouted, "Study Adds to Evidence of Vaccine Safety"[12] and the editor-in-chief of *Pediatrics*, Dr. Lewis First, included a note to pediatricians advising that "you'll want to know this information when talking with parents of your patients about the safety and benefits of vaccines."[13]

What's bizarre is that eight years after the Verstraeten study above, the Tozzi study utilized the exact same trick, looking at children who received more mercury in their shots and less mercury in their shots to see if there was any difference in neurological outcomes. Even more mystifying, the Tozzi study had a sample of children with a miniscule autism rate; as the study authors explained, "We detected, through the telephone interviews with parents and reviews of medical charts, 1 case of autism among the 856 children in the lower thimerosal intake group and no cases among the 848 children in the higher thimerosal intake group." So in their sample the rate of autism of the children analyzed was 1 in 1,704 (the US rate is 1 in 36, approximately 47 times higher than the sample rate) meaning this data is both suspect and useless. Another Italian doctor, Dr. Vincenzo Miranda, offered up a stunning rebuke of the Tozzi study, agreeing with the abject uselessness of the data:

> *This study is not methodologically correct. The study by Tozzi and others has many limitations. No comparison is done with children not exposed to thimerosal and neuropsychological disturbances are studied in recruiting voluntary* [sic] *all children even healthy ones, without assessing the sensitivity individual mercury. With this background this study cannot lead to any conclusion.*[14]

Let's pause here for one moment. I have just walked you through two of the signature studies held up by the spokespeople for the vaccine industry who claim "vaccines don't cause autism," despite the fact that neither study gets anywhere near exploring that actual topic of whether vaccines are causing autism. The PR machine for these studies is something to behold. *Pediatrics*, the scientific journal of the American Academy of Pediatrics, publishes these studies, and on the day they are released, every major news organization in the country reports on the studies, and every article sends the same basic message: Vaccines are safe, and they don't cause autism.

By the way, guess who funded these first two studies? If you guessed the CDC, you're right. The federal agency that's responsible for implementing the vaccine program is also responsible for safety monitoring, and they also sponsor studies that don't look at the vaccine-autism connection in any honest way, and then they support the promotion of the studies where doctors and scientists lie about what the studies actually did and what conclusions they actually reached.

Wrong Question #3: Are autism rates higher among the younger siblings of children with autism if they receive the MMR vaccine? It's no exaggeration to say that this 2015 study—"Autism Occurrence by MMR Vaccine Status among US Children with Older Siblings with and without Autism"—is the most hyped study I've ever seen, with every mainstream media outlet running a story to say that the MMR-autism hypothesis had been conclusively disproven.[15] In a novel approach, the study authors focused their analysis on children who had an older sibling with autism or without. In a more novel approach, the study authors chose to use the word "unvaccinated" to describe any child in the study who hadn't received the MMR vaccine. What they failed to clarify for anyone not reading the details was that "unvaccinated" could also mean, and often did mean, that the child had gotten every vaccine except the MMR. In other words, the authors blatantly misused the word "unvaccinated," and the press ate it up. Even more shocking was the prerelease publicity page from the *Journal of the American Medical Association*, where the study was published. To help reporters get ready to write a story, they included some quotes from some "third parties" discussing the findings. Here's an important quote they provide from Dr. Bryan King of the University of Washington:

> *Taken together, some dozen studies have now shown that the age of onset of ASD does not differ between vaccinated and unvaccinated children, the severity or course of ASD does not differ between vaccinated and unvaccinated children, and now the risk of ASD recurrence in families does not differ between vaccinated and unvaccinated children.*[16]

What's absolutely, positively mystifying about this quote, a quote you can find on the website of the journal that published this study, is that it's 100 percent false. There have never been any studies comparing vaccinated to unvaccinated kids until very recently, which is the holy grail study that needs to be done, and which I will discuss at length in one moment. Furthermore, it was never mentioned that this study was actually written by researchers imbedded inside a large PR/consulting firm called The Lewin Group, which counts the largest vaccine makers in the world as its clients.

I'm not going to bore you with too many more details about this study, but I will with one, which is the number of total kids in the study, a number that's been bandied about impressively. This study was heralded as being a "large" study of "unvaccinated" kids. I've already shown you that the "unvaccinated" part of that claim was untrue, and so was the "large" part. Yes, the study authors started with over ninety-five thousand kids, and this was certainly the number used everywhere in the media. But the power of this study was in looking at younger siblings who had an older sibling with autism. This group is considerably more "at risk" for autism, and it's therefore their outcome that was of interest to the study authors.

The real "gem" in the study would be a child who met three separate criteria: (1) had an older sibling with autism, (2) had autism themselves, and (3) had not received the MMR vaccine. You see, if you met all three criteria, you were the proof the study authors were looking for, that MMR had not caused your autism. How many kids in this large study met the three criteria that mattered? How many had an older sibling with autism, had autism themselves, and had never received the MMR? Twenty-three kids. That's it. Twenty-three kids is not very much to slam the door on whether or not "vaccines cause autism," much less the actual question the study considered about MMR's potential role in autism. And yet these twenty-three kids were the "proof" that MMR doesn't cause autism, because they had a sibling with autism, had autism themselves, and had never received the MMR vaccine. And the rest of their vaccination status was completely unknown and never discussed.

And remember, for all the different ways I can find fault with this study, particularly its misappropriation of the word "unvaccinated," it still only looked at a single vaccine: the MMR.

Even the Head of the NIMH Doesn't Get It

In mid-2017 Dr. Joshua Gordon, the newly appointed head of the National Institute of Mental Health (NIMH), met with a number of parents from the autism community. As Dr. Gordon's biography explains, he sits in a position to have a huge impact on autism science, as he now directs the agency that is the "largest funder of research into mental illness":

> *He oversees an extensive research portfolio of basic and clinical research that seeks to transform the understanding and treatment of mental illnesses, paving the way for prevention, recovery, and cure.*[17]

The parents pressed Dr. Gordon on the very issue I have raised in this chapter: What science was he relying on to dismiss the vaccine-autism connection? Dr. Gordon felt confident that vaccinated children had been studied versus unvaccinated children and promised he would follow up by providing evidence, and indeed he did, by sending an email on May 31[18] with a link to a single study titled, "Vaccines Are Not Associated with Autism: An Evidence-Based Meta-analysis of Case-Control and Cohort Studies."[19]

When I saw the email, I was dumbfounded. Dr. Gordon, aside from chairing the NIMH, is also the chair of the Interagency Autism Coordinating Committee (IACC), a "Federal advisory committee that coordinates Federal efforts and provides advice to the Secretary of Health and Human Services on issues related to autism spectrum disorder (ASD)." In short, he's the single most important person in the US government to try to resolve the autism epidemic, and the study he provided that convinced him vaccines and autism were unrelated was based on the very trick I have already explained to you:

Every study in the meta-analysis (which is basically a study looking at a larger sample of other studies) Dr. Gordon provided to support his view that vaccines don't cause autism was either a thimerosal study or an MMR study, in all cases comparing heavily vaccinated children to heavily vaccinated children. More specifically, six of the studies looked at MMR vaccine and four of the studies looked at thimerosal. Did any studies look at any other vaccine or in any way consider the mounting biological evidence implicating vaccine adjuvants in autism that I will discuss in chapter 5? Did any of the studies have any sample of children who had received no vaccines? No, not even a little. One of the parents to whom Dr. Gordon sent the email responded swiftly, making many of the same points I have made in this chapter:

> *The abstract/review article you sent me below highlights the concern raised that there has never been a study assessing the relative risk of autism between vaccinated and unvaccinated child. To be sure, this review (and its abstract) leave the impression that the studies it relies upon compare "unvaccinated" children (no vaccines) with vaccinated children. Unfortunately, this is misleading since all 10 of the underlying studies relied upon*

for this review compared highly vaccinated children with highly vaccinated children. The only difference typically between the study and control groups was a single MMR vaccine or thimerosal vs. non-thimerosal vaccines. (I would be happy to provide you with a breakdown of each of the 10 studies reflecting same.) Meaning, what this review considers "unvaccinated" are vaccinated children typically only missing the MMR vaccine. Assuming the control children in these studies followed the current CDC recommended vaccination schedule, they would each have received 21 vaccine injections during the first 12 months of life excluding the MMR vaccine. Hence, these studies tell us virtually nothing about the relationship of vaccines to autism because they are not comparing vaccinated and unvaccinated children.[20]

How did Dr. Gordon respond to a pointed email, effectively dismantling his understanding of vaccine-autism science? With this curt reply:

I appreciate you following up with me, and apologize for the delay in my response. I think the information you are seeking would be best obtained from the CDC.[21]

I have seen this time and again, even with experts like Dr. Gordon, whom I hold—reasonably, I think—to a high standard of professionalism and curiosity. They're quick to send a link to a study reinforcing their belief that vaccines and autism are unrelated but one that doesn't hold up to even a minor amount of scrutiny. And when pressed, Dr. Gordon simply chose to kick the can. This is a person who, if he wanted, could fund enough science to end the autism epidemic! It's disappointing, and disturbing. My own opinion is that people like Dr. Gordon are too scared to consider the truth and too worried about what looking for it (by funding true vaccine-autism science) might do to their careers and reputations.

What's the *Right* Question?

The three questions and three studies I shared with you above come from three of the most commonly listed studies cited as "proof" that "vaccines do not cause autism." Yet not one of them comes close to answering the question parents of children with autism really care about, which goes something like this:

> *My child received thirty-eight vaccines by the time he was five, including twenty vaccines by his first birthday. Is the administration of so many vaccines causing autism in certain children?*

That question, so important to the health of our children and our nation, has never been asked, so how could it be answered? Well, I should probably clarify that question, especially the part where I say "never been asked," because the question has been asked, several times, in fact, but the answers don't suit the Dr. Offits and Dr. Hotezes of the world, so you never hear about them, but you will in a moment, after a quick digression. I want to walk you through three simple but important concepts that will help put vaccine-autism science in proper perspective:

Biological plausibility "refers to the proposal of a causal association—a relationship between a putative cause and an outcome—that is consistent with existing biological and medical knowledge."[22]

Encephalopathy "means disorder or disease of the brain. In modern usage, encephalopathy does not refer to a single disease, but rather to a syndrome of overall brain dysfunction; this syndrome can have many different organic and inorganic causes."[23]

Wisdom of crowds is the notion that "large groups of people are smarter than an elite few, no matter how brilliant—better at solving problems, fostering innovation, coming to wise decisions, even predicting the future."[24]

No one wants to blame the childhood vaccine schedule for the autism epidemic. Vaccines were invented to save the lives of children, not harm them, and I believe most people on both sides of this debate believe they are helping children by either fighting for more vaccines or fighting for the recognition that vaccines are causing autism in a subset of children.

But blaming vaccines for the autism epidemic is the most "biologically plausible" hypothesis. Sorry, vaccines, but it's just true. You provide some benefits to society in reducing a portion of certain acute illnesses, but you also have a very nasty underbelly: You cause brain damage in some of the kids who receive you.

Don't take my word for it—our federal government could not be clearer that vaccines cause brain damage in some children. Time and again on their own website, the Department of Health and Human Services' National Vaccine Injury Compensation Program makes it clear that "encephalopathy" is a vaccine injury, and they define "chronic encephalopathy" in the following way: "Chronic Encephalopathy occurs when a change in mental or neurologic status, first manifested during the applicable time period, persists for a period of at least 6 months from the date of vaccination."[25] Like many children with autism, my son is suffering from a chronic encephalopathy that occurred after his vaccine appointments.

I don't really have to use that many of my IQ points to think that there may be a correlation between a product that causes brain damage (vaccines) and my son's brain damage. It would be enough, frankly, that brain damage is known to be a side effect of vaccines in some children to assert how biologically plausible the vaccine-autism connection is, but the argument is bolstered by two additional points: (1) As you now know, the number of vaccines given to children has nearly quadrupled since the early 1980s, and the autism rate is up more than 30,000 percent during the same time period. (2) There are tens of thousands (or more) of parental reports of regression into autism after vaccination. These reports are worldwide, in every socioeconomic level and every race. The stories are remarkably consistent. The "wisdom of crowds" is taken to an extreme when it comes to the vaccine-autism connection, according to the parents, and many of their doctors, who witnessed the regression of their children firsthand.

An Embezzler and a Whistle-Blower

Two authors, both affiliated with the CDC, have either led or been coauthors on a total of eight of the studies that are cited by spokespeople as "proof" that vaccines don't cause autism. One is an embezzler listed as a "Most Wanted" fugitive, and one became a whistle-blower due to scientific fraud he and his colleagues committed in one of the studies.

Poul Thorsen, a Danish researcher, has been the lead or coauthor of four of the studies routinely cited as proof vaccines don't cause autism. Mr. Thorsen is wanted by the Office of Inspector General (OIG) for embezzling funds from the CDC.[26] According to the OIG, Mr. Thorsen "executed a scheme to steal grant money awarded by the Centers for Disease Control and Prevention (CDC)." They claim he "diverted over $1 million of the CDC grant money to his own personal bank account. Thorsen submitted fraudulent invoices on CDC letterhead to medical facilities assisting in the research for reimbursement of work allegedly covered by the grants."

In 2011 Mr. Thorsen was indicted "on 22 counts of wire fraud and money laundering" and "according to bank account records, Thorsen purchased a home in Atlanta, a Harley Davidson motorcycle, an Audi automobile, and a Honda SUV with funds that he received from the CDC grants." The subject of all the grant money he stole? Vaccines and autism.

Dr. William Thompson, a CDC researcher, has led or coauthored four papers as well, and he issued a statement through a whistle-blower attorney that the findings in one of the MMR-autism studies for which he served as the lead author were fraudulent:

> *I regret that my coauthors and I omitted statistically significant information in our 2004 article published in the journal* Pediatrics. *The omitted data suggested that African American males who received the MMR vaccine before age 36 months were at increased risk for autism. Decisions were made regarding which findings to report after the data were collected, and I believe that the final study protocol was not followed.*[27]

Congressman Bill Posey, who privately met with Dr. Thompson, said in a congressional briefing that CDC scientists met in a private room and resolved to destroy all the primary data and notes from Dr. Thompson's MMR-autism study, which was published in *Pediatrics* and still quoted by many. Dr. Thompson issued the following statement about the meeting:

> *The co-authors scheduled a meeting to destroy documents related to the study. The remaining four co-authors all met and brought a big garbage can into the meeting room, and reviewed and went through all the hardcopy documents that we had thought we should discard, and put them into a huge garbage can. However, because I assumed it was illegal and would violate both FOIA and DOJ requests, I kept hardcopies of all documents in my office, and I retain all associated computer files. I believe we intentionally withheld controversial findings from the final draft of the* Pediatrics *paper.*[28]

An embezzler and a whistle-blower involved with eight of the crucial studies proving no link between vaccine and autism? It's hard to believe things are this shady, but they are.

Epidemiological Science versus Biological Science

While embezzlers and whistle-blowers are fascinating, the purpose of this chapter is to explain that the science on the connection between vaccines and autism has barely scratched the surface, and anyone saying it's settled is lying. Noteworthy is that the most public liars are, of course, economically intertwined with the vaccine industry; namely, Drs. Paul Offit and Peter Hotez, who are the primary spokespeople for any mainstream media you read about vaccines and autism these days. But I'd be remiss not to mention that there is science, compelling science, that has looked at vaccinated children versus unvaccinated children. This science has shown a devastatingly strong link between vaccines and autism, which is why you've never heard of these studies. Before I share that science with you, I want to explain two really important points.

First, all the science I have talked about so far is epidemiology. Scientists are looking at data, in this case medical records and vaccination records of children, and they're analyzing them to look for patterns and relationships. This is what they did with tobacco. They looked at smokers. They looked at nonsmokers. They looked at lung cancer rates. At some point the correlation between being a smoker and having lung cancer was so high that the connection was undeniable. Epidemiology takes all that data, finds relationships and correlations, and concludes whether any two things might be connected; for example, being vaccinated and having autism.

But there's a different kind of science that's even more revealing. It's biological science. It's science looking at living things and how they actually respond to other things. This was also done with tobacco when researchers painted mice with tobacco tar in the 1950s and proved, biologically, that tobacco tar can cause cancer (see chapter 5). That biological science was devastating for tobacco, and it began the process of revealing the truth about tobacco and lung cancer.

In the vaccine-autism debate, we have a growing body of biological science. It's compelling, and it's all very recent. We have mice studies in which the mice are injected with vaccine ingredients, producing devastating results. And we have clear biological plausibility for how, exactly, a vaccine can cause autism in a child. That's not the point of this chapter, to discuss all the biological science that has been done, but that is the point of chapter 5, which will show you that scientists are actually very close to identifying how, exactly, a vaccine can cause autism.

Second, I want you to appreciate that most published science goes unnoticed by the public. Most scientists have no PR firm behind them, alerting the media in advance whenever a new study comes out. Most scientists don't know the first thing about PR; they have no PR budget, and that's not why they are publishing research. They do their research to advance science, and their audience is really other scientists.

Vaccine-autism science is uniquely different. The vaccine makers do have PR budgets and PR firms, and any vaccine-autism study that shows "vaccines don't cause autism" makes national news. Every single one, every single time. The studies that actually compare vaccinated versus unvaccinated children? They don't make the news, because their answers implicate vaccines. They hide in plain sight, are shared widely in the autism community, and are ignored by the mainstream press.

Five Studies of Unvaccinated Children

The first study that compared children who had received a vaccine with children who hadn't was published in 2000. Although autism wasn't something the study considered, it was still revealing. Titled "Effects of Diphtheria-Tetanus-Pertussis or Tetanus Vaccination on Allergies and Allergy-Related Respiratory Symptoms among Children and Adolescents in the United States," this study from the UCLA school of public health did look specifically at the DTP vaccine to see if it might be responsible for allergies and allergy-related symptoms, such as asthma.[29] Looking at more than thirteen thousand children, the study found that:

> *DTP or tetanus vaccination in US children is associated with life-time history of asthma or other allergies and allergy-related symptoms. . . . Assuming that the estimated vaccination effect is unbiased, 50% of diagnosed asthma cases (2.93 million) in US children and*

adolescents would be prevented if the DTP or tetanus vaccination was not administered.

So the first study to ever compare a group that received a vaccine with a group that didn't found a dramatic difference in rates of asthma and allergies among the vaccinated group, so much so that they thought not getting the DTP vaccine might reduce cases of asthma by 50 percent! Note that many children with autism suffer from what are known as comorbid conditions, such as asthma, allergies, and other autoimmune conditions.

In 2008 in the second study ever looking at a group of children who didn't receive a vaccine, public health researchers Carolyn Gallagher and Melody Goodman from SUNY Stony Brook looked at the possible relationship between the hepatitis B vaccine and special education.[30] Were children who received the full series of hepatitis B vaccines (three separate vaccines, the first one often given on day one of life) more likely to end up in special education classes than children who didn't receive any hepatitis B vaccines? The study, "Hepatitis B Triple Series Vaccine and Developmental Disability in US Children Aged 1–9 Years," was published in the journal *Toxicological and Environmental Chemistry*, and the results were pretty clear: The full series of hepatitis B led to a ninefold greater likelihood of receiving special education:

> *This study found statistically significant evidence to suggest that boys in United States who were vaccinated with the triple series Hepatitis B vaccine . . . were more susceptible to developmental disability than were unvaccinated boys. . . . The odds of receiving EIS [special education] were approximately nine times as great for vaccinated boys (n = 46) as for unvaccinated boys (n = 7), after adjustment for confounders.*

The same researchers from SUNY Stony Brook published another study in 2010, this time looking at the relationship between receiving the hepatitis B series and autism. Published in the prestigious *Journal of Toxicology and Environmental Health*, "Hepatitis B Vaccination of Male Neonates and Autism Diagnosis" once again reached very clear conclusions: "Boys vaccinated as neonates had threefold greater odds for autism diagnosis compared to boys never vaccinated or vaccinated after the first month of life."[31] Journalist David Kirby appreciated the significance of the new findings, writing in the *Huffington Post*:

> [The study] *will be among the first university-based population studies to suggest an association between a vaccine and an increased risk for autism. And that would be in direct contradiction to all those MMR and thimerosal studies that purportedly found no such link.*

The two Goodman and Gallagher articles about hepatitis B raise many concerns. I've met pediatricians who feel that the hepatitis B vaccine specifically has triggered the epidemic of neurological disorders and autoimmunity we now see in our children. Hepatitis B was the first vaccine introduced after Congress indemnified vaccine makers from liability in 1986. The vaccine has a high dose of aluminum, which you will read in chapter 5 is likely a primary culprit of autism, and it's often given to babies on day one of life, which many immunologists feel is a huge mistake. These two studies raise major concerns, but I'm guessing you never knew either of these studies existed, which supports my point about scientists and PR firms.

In 2017, something amazing happened. Two separate studies comparing vaccinated and completely unvaccinated children actually got published. Unlike the Goodman and Gallagher studies above, which only explored a single vaccine (the rest of a child's vaccine status was simply not considered), these two new studies met the "gold standard"—they found children who had never received any vaccines and looked at their health outcomes in a variety of ways. The public health researchers from Jackson State University originally planned to publish a single study, until they looked at the data on children born prematurely, noting that the data on the difference in health outcomes for vaccinated versus unvaccinated premature infants was so dramatic it deserved its own study.

Published in the *Journal of Translational Science*, the first groundbreaking study was called, "Pilot Comparative Study on the Health of Vaccinated and Unvaccinated 6- to 12-Year-Old U.S. Children," and its results were so devastating to the US vaccine program that there wasn't a single media outlet in the country that covered its release.[32] The results of comparing vaccinated children to completely unvaccinated children were no surprise to me, my wife, or any of the autism parents I know, but perhaps would surprise others:

> *The vaccinated were less likely than the unvaccinated to have been diagnosed with chickenpox and pertussis, but more likely to have been diagnosed with pneumonia, otitis media, allergies and NDD* [neurodevelopmental disorders]. *After adjustment, vaccination, male gender, and preterm birth remained significantly associated with NDD.*

Specifically, vaccinated children were found to have a fourfold higher likelihood of having autism. I'm reminded of a quote by Dr. Daniel Neides of the Cleveland Clinic from chapter 2, who wondered if we were making trade-offs that aren't worth it. He said, "Some of the vaccines have helped reduce the incidence of childhood communicable diseases [like chickenpox and pertussis from the study above]. That's great news. But not at the expense of neurologic diseases like autism and ADHD increasing at alarming rates."[33]

Simultaneously, the Jackson State authors published a study in the same journal just looking at children born prematurely, titled "Preterm Birth, Vaccination and Neurodevelopmental Disorders: A Cross-Sectional Study of 6- to 12-Year-Old Vaccinated and Unvaccinated Children."[34] The results were disturbing, as the researchers found children born prematurely and vaccinated were fourteen times more likely to develop a neurodevelopmental disorder! The authors were appropriately concerned:

> *Preterm birth coupled with vaccination, however, was associated with a synergistic increase in the odds of NDD, suggesting the possibility that vaccination could precipitate adverse neurodevelopmental outcomes in preterm infants. These results provide clues to the epidemiology and causation of NDD but question the safety of current vaccination programs for preterm infants.*

Given what you've learned so far, are you surprised this study wasn't in the news? Five separate studies, all comparing a group of children vaccinated with a group of children unvaccinated, at least for a single vaccine. I'm guessing that for most readers this is the first time you've read about any of these studies. I think a fair question would be, "Why?" The answer is simple: Studies that might hurt the financial performance of pharmaceutical companies are not publicized by media outlets that derive advertising revenue from the pharmaceutical companies.

Are We Being Lied To?

Well, has it been asked and answered? Have scientists proven that vaccines do not cause autism? If you read this chapter with your mind even open a little, I know you know the answer to that question is, "not even close." When spokespeople for the vaccine industry (who often masquerade as concerned doctors or scientists) tell you the science has been done, and when they even get a bit exasperated that they are still answering this question, perhaps remember that this is all part of the Tobacco Playbook to distract, redirect, and delay. The science hasn't been done to "prove" vaccines don't cause autism. As you'll learn in chapter 5, in fact, the biological science is getting done, and it paints vaccines in a very different light.

CHAPTER 4

"The Reward Is Never Financial"

It is difficult to get a man to understand something when his salary
depends upon his not understanding it.

—Upton Sinclair

To go to such extreme—and desperate lengths—to annihilate Dr.
Wakefield (the person, note, not the science) some people must be
very afraid. Afraid, presumably, that parents might actually believe
something that is blatantly obvious: that is that all vaccines can cause
serious adverse reactions, including autism.[1]

—Dr. Richard Halvorsen, British doctor,
author of *The Truth about Vaccines*

D r. Stanley Plotkin is the godfather of the modern vaccine industry.
Now in his 80s, he literally wrote the book on vaccines; called
Plotkin's Vaccines, it's now in its seventh edition, and the textbook is recommended by Bill Gates as an "indispensable guide to the enhancement of
the well-being of our world."[2] In a 2013 poll of the Top 50 "most influential people in vaccines," Dr. Plotkin was voted number two, behind only
Bill Gates.[3]

Dr. Plotkin's intimate relationship with the vaccine industry knows no
boundaries. He's a vaccine inventor, company board member, peer reviewer,
professor, and mentor of all things vaccines. The number of awards Dr.
Plotkin has received for his service to vaccines would take up several pages
in this book, including the French Legion of Honor, the Sabin Gold Medal,
and the Maxwell Finland Award for Scientific Achievement.[4]

Dr. Plotkin's prize pupil, Dr. Paul Offit (ranked number six in the aforementioned poll), learned everything he knows about vaccines from Dr. Plotkin, and together they have shaped many of the talking points that govern the way vaccines are positioned to the public. They jointly shared in the riches of the development of the rotavirus vaccines, with each of them making a cool six million dollars when their invention was sold to Merck.[5] In early January of 2018, Dr. Plotkin almost added another superlative to his resume: expert witness.

A custody battle in Michigan between Lori Matheson and her ex-husband Michael Schmitt included a disagreement over vaccines for their shared child. The mother didn't want to vaccinate her daughter at all; the father did.[6] With the case making national headlines, Dr. Offit got involved with the case behind the scenes to support the father, along with the pharma-funded pro-vaccine nonprofit, Voices for Vaccines. Their big idea? Roll in Dr. Plotkin as the expert witness for the father. Who better to extoll the virtues of vaccination than the founder of the modern vaccine industry?

This would be a high-profile case, and Dr. Plotkin's testimony could set precedent for how these matters are adjudicated in the future. This was the first time Dr. Plotkin had agreed to serve as an expert witness on the subject of vaccines. It was also the first time Dr. Plotkin would have to testify under oath in a wide-ranging deposition conducted by the attorney for the mother in the case, Aaron Siri. Anytime an "expert witness" is offered up in a trial, the opposing counsel has the right to depose that witness in advance of the trial, and Mr. Siri exercised his rights, deposing Dr. Plotkin on January 11, 2018, at a location near Dr. Plotkin's megamansion in New Hope, Pennsylvania.

The deposition lasted eight hours. The next morning, January 12, Dr. Plotkin recused himself from being an expert witness in the case. In between, Mr. Siri exposed more truth about vaccines and the vaccine industry in one document than I've ever seen.

It's Never about the Money

Vaccine industry marketers have a unique ability to rationalize away any implication that there might be a profit motive behind their behavior. Dr. Offit in particular bemoans any hint that his motivations aren't pure:

But the part that hurts the most is the continued claim that we did this for the money. I don't know any scientist who does it for the money (you certainly don't make much in salary). You do it because it's fun and because you think you can contribute. And the reward for creating a vaccine was also never financial.[7]

Dr. Offit is discussing the six million dollars that he claims he received (other public estimates have been far higher) when a patent for the rotavirus vaccine for which he was a coinventor was sold to Merck. Unlike Dr. Offit, there are many people concerned that financial conflicts heavily impact vaccine policy making, so much so that the US Congress's Committee on Government Reform issued a blistering report on the very topic, titled "Conflicts of Interest in Vaccine Policy Making."[8] The conclusion was a stern rebuke:

The Committee's investigation has determined that conflict of interest rules employed by the FDA and the CDC have been weak, enforcement has been lax, and committee members with substantial ties to pharmaceutical companies have been given waivers to participate in committee proceedings.

Interestingly, the report was particularly critical of a doctor who served on a decision-making committee affiliated with CDC: Dr. Paul Offit. When a predecessor rotavirus vaccine was added to the recommended vaccine schedule in the United States, Dr. Offit voted in favor of adding it (while his own vaccine was still under development), but when that same vaccine was shown to be causing a high rate of a deadly bowel affliction, Dr. Offit abstained from supporting the vaccine's removal from the market (it was later removed). In an excellent investigation titled "Voting Himself Rich," Dan Olmsted and Mark Blaxill criticized Dr. Offit's "use of his former position on the CDC's Advisory Committee on Immunization Practices to help create the market for rotavirus vaccine—to effectively vote himself rich."[9]

As you're about to read, Dr. Plotkin equally considers himself to be above the fray, despite his gargantuan financial conflicts of interest. Sure, he takes millions of dollars from the vaccine industry, but that has nothing to do with the things he says about vaccines. Yeah, right!

The Plotkin Deposition

As a bespectacled Dr. Plotkin sat for his deposition wearing a dark suit and red tie, he had no idea his opposing counsel was one of the most informed people in the world on the topic of vaccines. A UC Berkeley School of Law honors graduate and former clerk for the Israeli Supreme Court, Mr. Siri is not your average lawyer. In 2015 Mr. Siri made headlines when he successfully defeated a flu shot mandate for children that had been imposed on citizens of New York City.[10] At the time Mr. Siri explained that "parents across the city who, in consultation with their doctors, made the decision that the risks outweighed the benefits for their particular child, had that right taken away from them by 11 unelected individuals sitting in the Board of Health right across the street."

Mr. Siri's cross-examination skills are formidable, and reading the deposition for the first time was one of the more satisfying moments in my time as an autism activist. The opposing lawyer representing Dr. Plotkin was severely outmatched, and I had to laugh that this was the brainchild of Dr. Offit. Did he not realize Dr. Plotkin would be deposed? Mr. Siri understood every trick, exaggeration, misstatement, and controversy, and he walked Dr. Plotkin into bear trap after bear trap the way Tom Cruise brought Jack Nicholson along in *A Few Good Men*, which is the movie I kept thinking of as I read the deposition. And watching the video of the deposition, I saw Dr. Plotkin grow more and more annoyed as the deposition progressed. I kept waiting for him to scream, "You can't handle the truth!"

Dr. Plotkin, along with Dr. Offit, has shaped many of the false narratives about vaccines that permeate our culture. From their perch at the Children's Hospital of Philadelphia, Drs. Plotkin and Offit are the go-to resource for any mainstream journalist writing about vaccines. Vaccines rarely harm, testing is thorough, they never cause autism, every child needs them, herd immunity must be maintained. All of these false narratives and exaggerations can trace their origins to Drs. Plotkin and Offit. But none of them has ever had to endure the scrutiny of being challenged under oath.

It's as close as we will ever get to deposing the vaccine industry itself, and it was a colossal blunder to allow Dr. Plotkin to be deposed, which he seemed to realize within the first hour of the deposition. It's hard to do a four-hundred-page document justice in a chapter, particularly because in many cases Mr. Siri would lead Dr. Plotkin down a lengthy path before exposing the lies or contradictions to his testimony, but I'll do my best. At the very least, I hope this will show you some of the ways the vaccine industry exaggerates, spins, and lies when the facts about vaccines don't suit their needs.

Conflicts of Interest

Mr. Siri opened by reminding Dr. Plotkin that he was testifying under "penalty of perjury" for any false statements, and Dr. Plotkin stated that his last deposition had been sometime in the 1960s but that he was "willing to help in this case." Mr. Siri then took Dr. Plotkin through his extensive travel schedule for 2017, at the end of which Dr. Plotkin confirmed that "probably about half" of the trips were sponsored by "companies developing vaccines."

Dr. Plotkin was asked if he knows the name, the age, and the vaccination status or has reviewed the medical records of the daughter of the parents involved in the court case. "I do not know" was the answer provided to every detail. Mr. Siri walked Dr. Plotkin through the name of every vaccine recommended by the CDC and asked Dr. Plotkin if the daughter in the case should receive the vaccine. Of course, Dr. Plotkin's answer was always yes. Mr. Siri established, with Dr. Plotkin's help, that "every vaccine that you [Dr. Plotkin] believe [daughter] should receive is produced by either Merck, Sanofi, GSK, or Pfizer, correct?"

Mr. Siri was then able to establish that Dr. Plotkin had received payments from these four vaccine manufacturers for at least the last thirty years, and that the dollar amounts are in the millions. Dr. Plotkin explained, "I'm sure it's a sizable amount of money." He further explained, "I've consulted for essentially all of the major manufacturers. I do not know how much I received. But I have certainly received payments from Merck, from Glaxo, from Pfizer, and many other entities."

Of course, it's no crime to consult to vaccine makers, or become a multimillionaire from doing so—it's Dr. Plotkin's job. It compromises your role as an expert witness, however. Mr. Siri quickly dug down into a pattern: nondisclosure and conflict. Mr. Siri first focused on a nonprofit organization that Dr. Plotkin was a "driving force" in creating, Voices for Vaccines. Dr. Plotkin asserted that the organization, a pro-vaccine advocacy organization, "receives no funding from any of the pharmaceutical companies, and that is on order to avoid any suggestion of a conflict of interest." It sounds like a line Dr. Plotkin has stated many times, and Mr. Siri then produced a tax return for Voices for Vaccines, showing support for the organization provided by the Task Force for Global Health, an industry-funded organization. Dr. Plotkin admitted that he "stands corrected."

Dr. Plotkin grew annoyed at all the questions about the money he has received from vaccine makers. The exchange is very telling:

> **Mr. Siri: You're here today opining that [daughter] should receive vaccines that are made by the big four pharmaceutical companies, correct?**
>
> Dr. Plotkin: I am, yes.
>
> **Mr. Siri: Okay. And you didn't anticipate that your financial dealings with those companies would be relevant in that issue?**
>
> Dr. Plotkin: I guess, no, I did not perceive that that was relevant to my opinion as to whether a child should receive vaccines. Vaccines have to be made by somebody. And, of course, in this world they're made by pharmaceutical companies who make profits on vaccines. And the fact that they make profits on vaccines has no bearing on whether those vaccines are good for a child or not.
>
> **Mr. Siri: So you think the fact that pharmaceutical companies make money on vaccines doesn't bias how they approach the promotion of their own products?**
>
> Dr. Plotkin: I imagine it biases them in favor of vaccines, but so does most of the scientific world.

Dr. Plotkin let Mr. Siri know that he "resent[s] very much the line of questioning that suggests that what I believe and what I've done have been done for financial reasons." He repeated the mantra from Dr. Offit above that "none of the things that I've done have been done for financial gain," even as Mr. Siri made it clear that Dr. Plotkin is a millionaire many times over because of his support of the vaccine industry.

In a crescendo to the conflict of interest questioning by Mr. Siri, we learned that Dr. Plotkin has a two-hundred-page resume, has been an author or coauthor of 794 published scientific studies, and is on the faculty of thirteen separate universities, his reach and influence perhaps unprecedented. But Dr. Plotkin's resume is also missing many critical details, including the names of all the vaccine makers who are currently paying him, as Mr. Siri pointed out:

*So in providing this CV to your, to defendant's counsel, you didn't
think disclosing your affiliations with the very companies whose
product you're saying [daughter] should receive, her pediatrician
purchase and provide to her, was necessary to disclose?*

Later Mr. Siri highlighted a 2011 report from the Institute of
Medicine in which Dr. Plotkin was listed as one of the reviewers of the
published study. Mr. Siri noted that Dr. Plotkin only has "University
of Pennsylvania" next to his name. "It doesn't disclose that at that time
you were working for all four of the major vaccine makers, correct?" Dr.
Plotkin responded: "No."

Mr. Siri then walked Dr. Plotkin through more than a dozen private
biotech companies—all developers of vaccines—where Dr. Plotkin served
as a compensated board member. None of his affiliations have been disclosed
anywhere. Finally, Mr. Siri quoted the *New England Journal of Medicine*,
which Dr. Plotkin had already affirmed is a highly credible journal:

Let me read you a different quote, again, by Dr. Angell [of the
NEJM] *in which she blames the issue with truths in medical
publishing, on individuals that use legitimacy of academia to push
pharmaceutical company agendas. Here's what she said about those
individuals. She says, "They serve as consultants to the same companies whose products they evaluate, join corporate advisory boards and
speakers bureaus, enter into patent and royalty arrangements, agree
to be the listed authors of articles ghostwritten by interested companies, promote drugs and devices at company-sponsored symposia, and
allow themselves be plied with expensive gifts and trips to luxurious
settings. Many also have equity interest in sponsoring companies."*

The whole time, Mr. Siri had been using this quote to establish Dr.
Plotkin's pattern of behavior. It was clear to everyone in the room that Dr.
Plotkin can check every box on the list of an editorial written by the editor
of the prestigious *New England Journal of Medicine* on why it is no longer
possible to believe clinical research, as pharmaceutical companies have so
thoroughly co-opted experts. It's clear that Dr. Plotkin is the poster child
for this phenomenon. Painstakingly, Mr. Siri asked Dr. Plotkin questions
about each of these ways that "experts" are co-opted:

"You consulted for the big four vaccine makers?"

"You're on the corporate advisory board of numerous vaccine developers, yes?"

"You have received royalties from the sale of one or more vaccines, correct?"

"You are listed as an author on at least one or more papers where individuals authoring papers receive compensation from vaccine makers, correct?"

"And you've taken numerous trips over the last 30 years to various parts of the world?"

Dr. Plotkin feebly answered "yes" to each question, the steam almost visibly rising from his head. And there we see, as clearly as you ever will, how thoroughly compromised people who purport to be disinterested parties really are when it comes to vaccines. How can people reaping millions from vaccine makers be the "expert witnesses" on the product?

Gardasil, Merck, and Data Manipulation

Earlier, Mr. Siri had established clearly that none of the vaccines for children were tested with a group of children who received an "inert placebo," making any conclusions drawn about side effects nearly impossible to corroborate. Dr. Plotkin was forced to agree. For Gardasil (the HPV vaccine), a different problem took place. There were actually three groups used during testing. One group received the vaccine. One group received a shot that only contained aluminum adjuvant, and one group received a true placebo, a shot of saline. The latter two groups (aluminum and saline), however, were combined when the data was reported, making it impossible to know if the true placebo group had a lower rate of adverse events than either Gardasil or the aluminum adjuvant.

Painstakingly, Mr. Siri took Dr. Plotkin through this extraordinary abuse of data. Overall, the Gardasil trial showed that 2.3 percent of the women who received either the vaccine or the combined aluminum/saline developed a systemic autoimmune condition within six months. Mr. Siri explained to Dr. Plotkin, and got him to confirm, that the saline group, had it been reported separately, actually had an adverse event rate of zero. "And then if we had a third column that was just the saline placebo, it would show 0 percent? . . . Wouldn't that have been a significant finding to report?"

Dr. Plotkin had no real answer: "I don't—you'd have to ask a statistician."

It's a remarkable exchange. Mr. Siri had just highlighted an extreme abuse of trust and data manipulation by Merck, Dr. Plotkin's primary benefactor.

Double Standards in Vaccine Testing

Mr. Siri then caught Dr. Plotkin in an extreme contradiction. He asked him about a recent study done by Dr. Peter Aaby in which Dr. Aaby looked at the impact of DTP vaccine in Africa and concluded the vaccine did more harm than good (discussed in chapter 2). Dr. Plotkin was familiar with the study, respected Dr. Aaby, but was dismissive of the findings, because Dr. Aaby "doesn't have randomly vaccinated or children who randomly receive pertussis vaccine or don't receive pertussis vaccine. . . . But in the absence of random administration, you don't know for sure whether it's the vaccine or other factors that are operating."

None of the licensed vaccines for children ever receive this sort of rigorous testing, and placebos are never used, as Mr. Siri quickly established. He also had Dr. Plotkin confirm how long the observation period is for vaccine trials and showed him a number of package inserts from the vaccines themselves.

Mr. Siri started with the hepatitis B vaccine. "How long does it say that safety was monitored after each dose?" Begrudgingly, Dr. Plotkin responded, "Five days." But, Mr. Siri wondered, is that "long enough to detect an autoimmune issue that arises after five days?" Dr. Plotkin stated the obvious: "No." Mr. Siri then asked, "Was there any control group in this trial?" Dr. Plotkin, who had just argued how important control groups are to cause and effect, was forced to answer truthfully, "It does not mention any control group, no."

Drilling down on the hepatitis B vaccine, Mr. Siri pulled out a different insert for a different hepatitis B vaccine that showed safety testing only took place for four days after administration. Dr. Plotkin confirmed the duration but stated, "I am willing to bet that they did collect reactions after four days." Mr. Siri pressed, since no documentation supported Dr. Plotkin's bet, and he was forced to admit it was "speculation." Apparently, rigorous testing is critical when finding fault with vaccines, but not when licensing them for use in millions of children.

This was such a revealing back and forth. Dr. Plotkin seemed genuinely surprised by how short the observation period was for vaccines; he was sure they must have done more monitoring later, but of course that would have been explained in the package insert, and it wasn't. Vaccine proponents lie about the "rigorous testing" vaccines have endured, but when you press them, they often point to how "safe" vaccines are that are already in use. In reality, we are dramatically underreporting vaccine injury, as Mr. Siri explained to Dr. Plotkin next:

Incomplete VAERS Data

> **Mr. Siri: Isn't it true that VAERS only receives a tiny fraction of the reportable adverse events after vaccination?**
>
> Dr. Plotkin: Well, I can't give you a percentage, but all physicians are asked to report putative reactions to the VAERS system. So I don't think the VAERS system covers a tiny portion of alleged reactions. I think, rather, probably most are reported.

> *Mr. Siri produced a study commissioned by HHS and run by Harvard Pilgrim. He showed Dr. Plotkin where the study says, "Fewer than 1 percent of vaccine adverse events are reported." He asked Dr. Plotkin to read it.*

> **Mr. Siri: Okay, so this study says that less than 1 percent of adverse events are reported to VAERS, right?**
>
> Dr. Plotkin: Well, I have to check that, but I think that's correct.

I probably let out my largest laugh during this exchange. Dr. Plotkin had the nerve to say that "probably most" vaccine reactions are reported. This is the mind-set of a vaccine developer who believes vaccines are always "safe and effective," no matter what the data says. It feels fanatical, really. He is one of the foremost experts on vaccines in the world, and he believes VAERS is capturing most vaccine injuries; simply unbelievable!

The Inadequate Pertussis Vaccine

As I mentioned in chapter 2, the reason there are guaranteed whooping cough (pertussis) outbreaks in the United States every year is that the vaccine for pertussis is pretty ineffective. Dr. Plotkin confirmed this:

> **Mr. Siri: How long does the current immunity last from the current acellular pertussis vaccine?**

Dr. Plotkin: Well, it lasts for probably on the order of five years, but the efficacy diminishes after two years or so. And the result is that there have been more pertussis in adolescents than we would like.

Mr. Siri was also able to establish that the vaccine for pertussis— DTaP—doesn't prevent people from being a carrier of whooping cough to others:

Mr. Siri: Does the cellular pertussis vaccine prevent the infection and transmission of pertussis in the person vaccinated with acellular pertussis vaccine?

Dr. Plotkin: It appears that the acellular vaccines don't protect the individual from carrying the organism as much as the so-called whole-cell pertussis vaccines did. . . . But there is a concern that the acellular vaccines may not protect an individual from passing the organism to another individual even if the vaccinated person doesn't get sick himself or herself.

I think very few people understand how inadequate this vaccine really is; it was nice for Dr. Plotkin to admit it. As I've said before, people often have this cartoonishly simple view of a vaccine: You get the shot; now you're immune—presto! It rarely works that way, and the explanation of DTaP's limitations makes that clear.

Experimenting on Marginalized and Vulnerable People

Mr. Siri brought up a topic that Dr. Plotkin did his best to avoid. He asked, "Have you ever used orphans to study an experimental vaccine?" Dr. Plotkin responded, "Yes." Mr. Siri then asked a horrifying question: "Have you ever used the mentally handicapped to study an experimental vaccine?" Dr. Plotkin does his best to evade the question:

Dr. Plotkin: I don't recollect ever doing studies in mentally handicapped individuals. At the time in the 1960s, it was not an uncommon practice.

Mr. Siri: So you're saying—I'm not clear on your answer. I'm sorry. Have you ever used mentally handicapped to study an experimental vaccine?

Dr. Plotkin: What I'm saying is I don't recall specifically having done that, but that in the 1960s, it was not unusual to do that. And I wouldn't deny that I may have done so.

Mr. Siri: Well, there's an article entitled "Attenuation of RA 27/3 Rubella Virus in WI-38 Human Diploid Cells." Are you familiar with that article?
Dr. Plotkin: Yes.

Mr. Siri: In that article, one of the things it says is 13 seronegative mentally retarded children were given RA 27/3 vaccine?
Dr. Plotkin: Okay. Well, then that's, in that case that's what I did.

Mr. Siri: Have you ever expressed that it's better to perform experiments on those less likely to be able to contribute to society, such as children with handicap, than with children without or adults without handicaps?
Dr. Plotkin: I don't remember specifically, but it's possible.

Mr. Siri: Do you remember ever writing to the editor of "Ethics on Human Experimentation"?
Dr. Plotkin: I don't remember specifically, but I may well have.

Mr. Siri: I'm going to hand you what's been marked as Exhibit 43. Do you recognize this letter you wrote to the editor?
Dr. Plotkin: Yes.

Mr. Siri: Did you write this letter?
Dr. Plotkin: Yes.

Mr. Siri: Is one of the things you wrote: "The question is whether we are to have experiments performed on fully functioning adults and on children who are potentially contributors to society or to perform initial studies in children and adults who are human in form but not in social potential?"
Dr. Plotkin: Yes.

Mr. Siri: Have you ever used babies of mothers in prison to study an experimental vaccine?
Dr. Plotkin: Yes.

Mr. Siri: Have you ever used individuals under colonial rule to study an experimental vaccine?
Dr. Plotkin: Yes.

I need to take a deep breath before I comment on this. My grandfather was adopted. My son is "mentally handicapped." I'm going to refrain from moralizing; feel free to draw your own conclusions. I'll just make two points: One, if you have "mentally handicapped" people as your test subjects, how will you know if the vaccine causes mental problems? Two, I think this shows you what the vaccine industry has always known: Vaccines are really dangerous. So when you test them on the populations that are the most hidden from society, and have the least power to complain, you can bury any disasters. It's profoundly depraved thinking. I'll just remind you that this doctor, and his medical ethics, built the modern vaccine industry.

Dismissal of Religious Objections

In the majority of US states, you can object to receiving a vaccine for religious reasons. Dr. Plotkin and his protégé, Dr. Paul Offit, have spearheaded talking points to combat these religious exemptions, arguing that biblical texts were written before the invention of vaccines, and that a parent denying a child vaccination on religious grounds is flying in the face of science and medicine that are "data-based systems, not beliefs."[11] Of course, they rely on their interpretation of vaccine injury data to make this argument. Mr. Siri pressed Dr. Plotkin on his thinking:

Mr. Siri: Do you believe that someone can have a valid religious objection to refusing a vaccine?
Dr. Plotkin: No.

Mr. Siri: Do you take issue with religious beliefs?
Dr. Plotkin: Yes.

Mr. Siri: You have said that, "Vaccination is always under attack by religious zealots who believe that the will of God includes death and disease"?
Dr. Plotkin: Yes.

Mr. Siri: You stand by that statement?

Dr. Plotkin: I absolutely do.

Mr. Siri: Are you an atheist?

Dr. Plotkin: Yes.

Mr. Siri: Do you accept that some people hold religious beliefs that are inherently unprovable?

Dr. Plotkin: Yes, I'm sure they do.

Dr. Offit, in consultation with Dr. Plotkin, has publicly been pushing this line of thinking quite a bit. Basically, they are saying, "There's no such thing as a religious objection to a vaccine." It's pretty crazy; the United States is founded on the idea that people cannot be compelled to do things that violate their beliefs. Dr. Plotkin doesn't think that way. Once again, it feels fanatical and intolerant, but that's just my opinion.

Doublespeak

Later, Mr. Siri discussed a 2011 Institute of Medicine report on vaccine safety. He read the report to Dr. Plotkin, summarizing, "so the IOM concluded of the 135 most commonly claimed injuries for vaccination, it didn't know whether or not the vaccines caused that." At this point, one of the more revealing exchanges takes place between Dr. Plotkin and Mr. Siri:

Mr. Siri: You know, you earlier stated that, you stated that hepatitis B is, doesn't cause encephalitis, right?

Dr. Plotkin: That's, that's my opinion, yes.

Mr. Siri: But the IOM, after doing its review, determined it couldn't find science to support a causal determination one way or another, correct?

Dr. Plotkin: Yes. But that means that they don't have evidence for the supposition.

Mr. Siri: That it either causes or doesn't cause?

Dr. Plotkin: Right.

Mr. Siri: They don't know?
Dr. Plotkin: They don't know because there aren't enough data.

Mr. Siri: Okay. But you have—
Dr. Plotkin: In the absence of data, my conclusion is that there are no, there's no proof that causation exists.

Mr. Siri: So if there's no data to show that it causes or doesn't cause—
Dr. Plotkin: Yes.

Mr. Siri: —your supposition is that—am I understanding that correctly?
Dr. Plotkin: Yes.

Mr. Siri: Is that it doesn't cause it?
Dr. Plotkin: That there's no proof that it does.

Mr. Siri: Okay. That's different than saying it doesn't cause it, correct?
Dr. Plotkin: Correct.

Mr. Siri: So when you were saying earlier when I asked you at the beginning of this whether certain vaccines caused certain conditions and you said, no, they don't, did you just mean that, no, there's not enough evidence to make a decision one way or another?
Dr. Plotkin: I mean that there's no knowledge known to me that they do certain things that are, that some may have alleged happen after vaccination.

Mr. Siri: Like, for example, you know, the IOM reviewed whether hepatitis B can cause lupus because of lots of reports of influenza can cause lupus. They concluded that there's insufficient evidence one way or another to make a determination. You indicated—
Dr. Plotkin: Right.

Mr. Siri: But you indicated earlier that those vaccines don't cause lupus. Your testimony, you're saying that you said no because you weren't aware of a mechanism by which it could cause it; is that right?
Dr. Plotkin: Yes. That's correct.

Mr. Siri: Okay. But the science really isn't available to make a determination on causation yet, right?

Dr. Plotkin: The science doesn't show that there is a relationship.

This hairsplitting by vaccine proponents drives me nuts. The Institute of Medicine report Mr. Siri is referring to makes three conclusions: Vaccines do cause certain side effects, they don't cause certain other side effects, and for certain side effects, we don't know whether they do because the work hasn't been done yet to find out, despite the fact that these side effects have been reported to the VAERS database. In Dr. Plotkin's world if the work hasn't been done, that means the vaccine doesn't cause it. It's crazy thinking, and not the kind of thinking any other prescription drug could survive, but in Dr. Plotkin's world, vaccines are innocent until proven guilty, so much so that an absence of data means the vaccines doesn't cause it—vaccines always get the benefit of the doubt.

DTaP, Autism, and the Burden of Proof

In reviewing the 2011 study from the Institute of Medicine, Mr. Siri asked Dr. Plotkin if he recollects what the IOM's conclusion was about whether DTaP vaccine can cause autism. Dr. Plotkin replied, "I'd have to look that up, but I feel confident that they do not cause autism."

Mr. Siri found the IOM's actual conclusion and had Dr. Plotkin read it: "The evidence is inadequate to accept or reject a causal relationship between diphtheria toxoid-, tetanus toxoid-, or the acellular pertussis-containing vaccine in autism."

Mr. Siri: So the IOM reviewed the available evidence with regard to whether Tdap or DTaP can cause autism, and their conclusion was the evidence doesn't exist to show whether DTaP or Tdap do or do not cause autism, correct?

At this point Mr. Siri made mincemeat of the oft-repeated claim by so many that "vaccines do not cause autism":

Mr. Siri: But since, Dr. Plotkin, we don't know whether DTaP or Tdap cause autism, right, it would be a bit premature to make the unequivocal, sweeping statement that vaccines do not cause autism, correct?

Dr. Plotkin: In the absence of evidence, one should not draw any conclusions except that there's no evidence. And so I don't infer from the absence of evidence about a million different things that they're necessarily true. One has to do studies to determine whether or not a phenomenon exists, and usually those studies are done because there's some suspicion that, of a relationship. But in, we have no suspicions, at least I don't, that autism is caused by DTaP.

Mr. Siri: Well, you may not have that suspicion, but it is one of the most commonly reported conditions, adverse events, which is why it was reviewed in this IOM report from DTaP/Tdap, which we discussed earlier. So I just, I'm not saying, I'm not asking you to say that vaccines do cause autism. I'm not asking that at all. I'm asking you, as a scientist, can you make the statement that vaccines do not cause autism if you don't know whether DTaP or Tdap cause autism?

Dr. Plotkin: As a scientist, I would say that I do not have evidence one way or the other.

Mr. Siri: And so for that reason, you're okay with telling the parent that DTaP/Tdap does not cause autism even though the science isn't there yet to support that claim?

Dr. Plotkin: Absolutely.

This exchange was so revealing for me. In fact, I only gave you the heart of it; it actually went on for many pages. Dr. Plotkin thinks it's okay to say, "Vaccines don't cause autism," even as the IOM has clearly said that with DTaP they don't have evidence either way. Why is it okay? Because in Dr. Plotkin's world, vaccines will never cause autism, because if they did his world as he knows it would basically end. The last exchange pushed me over the edge. Dr. Plotkin was more than happy to tell a parent DTaP doesn't cause autism, even though the IOM said evidence was "inadequate" to make any conclusion at all.

Immune Activation Is the Objective of Vaccines

One of the many extraordinary admissions that Dr. Plotkin provided concerns the relationship between vaccines and "immune activation," a topic you will soon understand intimately in chapter 5, as new science is demonstrating that immune activation events are the primary cause of autism.

> **Mr. Siri:** This is from California Institute [of Technology], CalTech. **That institution did a number of studies regarding—that group did a number of studies relating to immune activation and neurological disorder, correct?**
> Dr. Plotkin: Yes.

> **Mr. Siri: And they found a connection between immune activation and neurological historical disorders, correct?**
> Dr. Plotkin: Yes.

> **Mr. Siri: Okay. And one of the study's findings they had was that immune activation alters fetal brain development through interleukin-6, correct?**
> Dr. Plotkin: As I said before, IL-6 is an important cytokine. I would point out in relation to immune activation, that immune activation occurs as a result of disease and exposure to a variety of stimuli, not just vaccines.

> **Mr. Siri: But it can be caused by vaccines, correct?**
> Dr. Plotkin: Immune activation is the objective of vaccines.

When I first read Dr. Plotkin's testimony above, I gasped out loud. I know, if you're relatively new to this topic, you may be scratching your head: "What's the big deal?" The big deal is that science has converged, and it's converged on autism's causation: autism is caused by immune activation events, something vaccines are designed to trigger. Read on—chapter 5 will make the importance of his statement clear to you.

After reading a transcript of the deposition, I was struck with the following thoughts:

Dr. Plotkin appears sociopathic. The definition of the word is "lacks a sense of moral responsibility or social conscience." I'm not sure what else to call someone who runs vaccine trials on orphans, the mentally disabled, and babies of moms in prison and then pens an op-ed justifying using the mentally ill for medical trials. It's deeply disturbing thinking, and this is the man who has guided the vaccine industry's ideology for fifty years. He's also intolerant of anyone who may have a genuine religious objection to vaccines.

Dr. Plotkin employs scientific standards only when convenient. The DTP study in Africa doesn't meet his standards of science for having placebo controls, but vaccine safety trials do, despite having no controls and only monitoring adverse reactions for a few days. The Gardasil trial that hid its placebo numbers? You'll have to ask the statistician. I've seen this from so many pro-vaccine spokespeople—they will criticize any studies that question vaccine safety but never acknowledge the paucity of safety studies.

Dr. Plotkin is blind to the scale of vaccine injury. The exchange in which Dr. Plotkin figured the deeply flawed VAERS system captures most vaccine injury was revealing. He doesn't care about vaccine injury—the ends always justify the means. He's wrong about vaccine injury by at least a factor of one hundred times (because only 1 percent of vaccine injury is captured by VAERS). How could he not know that? Because knowing that is inconsistent with his worldview: Vaccines are safe, no matter what the data says.

Dr. Plotkin will never cross the autism line. In part two of this book, I will show you depositions from two of the leading autism scientists in the world, both of whom acknowledge that vaccines can and do cause autism. It's clear from how long Dr. Plotkin spends fighting Mr. Siri about the fact that the IOM stated that the data can neither prove nor deny a relationship between DTaP vaccine and autism that there is no world where Dr. Plotkin will acknowledge something that has become obvious to many. The mainstream has been denying the vaccine-autism link for so long—spearheaded by Drs. Plotkin and Offit—that admitting the connection at this point would probably be too much to bear.

Dr. Plotkin's flawed thinking is the vaccine industry's flawed thinking: Don't acknowledge vaccine injury. Don't acknowledge the weakness of safety studies. Employ scientific standards only when convenient. Never admit autism is connected to vaccines. Vaccines are always "safe and effective," no matter what the data says.

The Tobacco Playbook

In November 1998 a Master Settlement Agreement was reached between tobacco companies and attorneys general from forty-six states. Tobacco companies were finally accountable for at least some of the damage cigarettes had caused. But the first science implicating tobacco was a mouse study published in 1953 in which scientists demonstrated, clearly and unequivocally, that cigarette tar caused cancer.[12] The penalty of the settlement was $206 billion.[13] What did US District Judge Gladys E. Kessler find the tobacco companies guilty of? "Conspiracy."[14] There's that word again.

It took forty-five years for a reckoning because right after the mice study, to actively muddy the waters, tobacco companies formed the "Tobacco Industry Research Committee" so they could challenge all scientific evidence implicating tobacco. The organization provided hundreds of millions of dollars of funding for research at many of the leading institutions in the country that could sow doubt about the tobacco-cancer link. Producing "distracting research" that would sow endless doubt about a fast-emerging certainty became their primary goal. Committee members met with the leadership of every major newspaper, magazine, and television network, explaining their intent to fund a "research program devoted primarily to the public interest," which was really a euphemism for research that would exonerate tobacco, or at least muddy the scientific waters and generate as much doubt as possible about the link between smoking and lung cancer.[15]

Naomi Oreskes and Erik Conway, in their best-selling book *Merchants of Doubt*, explained how Big Tobacco exploited the vulnerabilities of science to their advantage, creating doubt at every turn in the road and effectively extending the industry's reckoning by four decades:

> By the late 1950s, mounting experimental and epidemiological data linked tobacco with cancer—which is why the industry took action to oppose it. In private, executives acknowledged this evidence. In hindsight it is fair to say—and science historians have said—that the link was already established beyond a reasonable doubt. Certainly no one could honestly say that science showed that smoking was safe. But science involves many details, many of which remained unclear, such as why some smokers get lung cancer and others do not.[16]

What if I told you that the only "Big" bigger than Big Tobacco was back in their heyday is today's Big Pharma, the very industry that makes all these vaccines? Big Pharma, one of the largest purchasers of advertisements in mainstream media,[17] and Big Pharma, the industry that spends the most on lobbying,[18] is the reason this fight about autism is taking so long. Don't believe me? From 1998 to 2009 the CDC was run by Dr. Julie Gerberding, where she presided over a massive expansion in the number of vaccines given to children and a massive explosion in the number of autism cases in the United States. Where did Dr. Gerberding go after resigning from the CDC? To serve as president of the vaccine division of Merck, the largest "Big Pharma" company in the world and the market leader in vaccines.[19] This is not an easy battle.

Let me remind you that the market for vaccines is expected to be worth $60 billion in 2020,[20] up from $170 million in the early 1980s.[21] Let me say that again. In the 1980s, with no childhood epidemics to speak of, the market for vaccinations was worth $170 million. Fast forward, and the market for vaccines has grown 350 times larger! In the 1960s the vaccine schedule in the United States called for three vaccines for childhood; today, as I said in chapter 2, it's thirty-eight (that's not a typo)—a more than twelvefold increase in the number of vaccines given to children.[22]

Autism is Tobacco 2.0, with manufactured doubt cast on every new discovery from determined parents, doctors, and scientists. Just like tobacco, we even have mice studies that show precisely how a vaccine can cause autism in the brain of a newborn. This evidence of "biological plausibility," now appearing in multiple scientific studies published since 2010, represents a tipping point for truth. History may not repeat, but it certainly rhymes.

People are fond of characterizing autism as "complex," but that obscures the simple explanation for what has happened to so many children, and why. In the 1970s the rate of autism was documented to be just under one in ten thousand children. Today one in thirty-six kids has autism—that's roughly 1.8 million school-age (four to seventeen) American children.[23] This also means there are 277 times more kids with autism today than there were thirty years ago. That's a gain of almost 30,000 percent! An epidemic this severe has to have a simple explanation, just as the lung cancer epidemic had a simple explanation, too.

The Tobacco Playbook is being expertly utilized by Big Pharma and their paid supporters—it almost seems like the very same PR firms and law firms that helped Big Tobacco are now helping Big Pharma . . . because they are. Literally. At the same time, it's astonishing how many people already know the truth about the autism epidemic and what's happening to our kids. Hundreds of scientists, thousands of doctors, and tens of thousands of parents, all saying the same thing. Heck, there's the camera man on *Larry King Live*, the makeup person on the set of *The Doctors*, the wife of the famous radio host, the *Time* magazine reporter who just can't tell the truth for fear of reprisal, or the board member at Autism Speaks, so many people know the truth. In fact, surveys show fully one-third of Americans today feel vaccines and autism are linked.[24] Attempts to dismiss people who "believe" vaccines cause autism as some sort of minuscule movement are not supported by the facts; hundreds of millions share my view and that of my wife and the many scientists, doctors, and parents you're about to meet in this book.

In retrospect, it seems unbelievable that it took people more than forty years to convincingly prove that inhaling hot tar multiple times a day would trigger lung cancer, but that's exactly what happened. The CEOs of all seven Big Tobacco companies stood before Congress, swearing to tell the truth, and then said (with a straight face, no less) that cigarettes were not addictive, nor was it clear that they were causing lung cancer. I remember the TV broadcast. It's an image I have never been able to shake. That congressional hearing took place in 1994, a full four years before the Master Settlement Agreement.

Perhaps not surprisingly, the very same strategies used to keep the tobacco debate alive have been employed in the debates about links between DDT and the loss of ecosystems, lead paint and children's IQs, coal and acid rain, asbestos and mesothelioma, CFCs and the ozone hole, Vioxx and heart attacks, and fossil fuels and global warming (to name just a tiny fraction of examples). This movie has been shown so many times before that I suppose it's harder to see it clearly in the moment. But the patterns are clearly established. Here's what we know about how corporations will behave in the face of mounting scientific evidence proving their product is causing harm:

1. Science will be utilized to manufacture doubt and manipulate the media and the public. This includes funding new science and paying experts to support the safety of a product causing harm.

This strategy was created and mastered by Big Tobacco and now, as I've mentioned, even has a name: The Tobacco Playbook.

2. Public relations firms will make a fortune from these deep-pocketed clients, and their job will be to meet with and alert members of the media on their client's sponsored science while refuting any science from the opposing side. This job is always easier if the industry causing harm is a large buyer of television, print, and other paid media. (The Tobacco Industry Research Committee was actually run by a PR firm, Hill & Knowlton.[25])

3. Aggressive lobbying will happen at the state and federal level and donations to politicians supporting industry views will rise. Where possible, lobbyists will write and promote laws supportive of the product, dismissive of health concerns, and protective of future liability. Their paid politicians will present and pass these laws.

4. Finally, real science will prevail. The truth will come out. And consumers will learn that the product in question causes harm, like the aforementioned mice study. This science will usually be hard to fund, condemned, and ruthlessly attacked, until enough courageous scientists publish the same information over and over again. Regulatory agencies will grudgingly respond. Few will see jail time, if any.

When the profits are big enough, corporations will do what they were formed to do: protect profits. This ruthless strategy continues today. Autism is arguably the most vicious, cruel, and dismissive battle yet. With so much at stake—money, careers, reputations—what happens when an inconvenient truth emerges? What happens when someone, somewhere speaks up and challenges the house of cards? Well, they need to be made an example of. Read on.

Getting Wakefielded

I've heard many researchers say, when considering whether or not to embark on studies or publish scientific results that may reflect poorly on vaccines, that they fear getting "Wakefielded." British doctor Dr. Andrew Wakefield's name has actually become a verb, and getting Wakefielded is something you most certainly want to avoid, as it spells a high probability of your career going up in flames.

Who do these researchers fear retribution from? It shouldn't be that hard to guess: the pharmaceutical industry, arguably the most financially powerful and ruthless commercial opponent the world has ever seen. I know that sounds dramatic, but consider the recent news that pharmaceutical executives knowingly conspired to create an opioid addiction epidemic. In their compelling critique, "The Opioid Epidemic: Fixing a Broken Pharmaceutical Market," Harvard medical scholars Ameet Sarpatwari, Michael S. Sinha, and Aaron S. Kesselheim put the behavior of pharmaceutical companies in painful relief:

> *Finally, to boost profits, pharmaceutical companies have often engaged in false or misleading marketing. Over the past twenty-five years, the industry has paid $35.7 billion to settle claims of illegal marketing, including making false or misleading claims or failing to disclose known risks. In 2012, for example, GlaxoSmithKline paid three billion dollars to settle civil claims and criminal charges that it downplayed the risk of the antidepressant paroxetine (Paxil) in adolescents, promoted the antidepressant bupropion (Wellbutrin) for unapproved uses, and hid data showing the increased risk of heart attacks from the diabetes drug rosiglitazone (Avandia). Although the then–largest healthcare fraud settlement in US history, the total penalty was "only a portion of the drug maker's profits from the drugs involved." Almost every major pharmaceutical company has been caught in similar marketing scandals. However, the industry remains highly profitable, supporting criticism that monetary penalties generally represent "a quite small percentage of . . . global revenue and often a manageable percentage of the revenue received from the product under scrutiny."* [26]

Vioxx, the pain reliever manufactured by Merck, caused five hundred thousand heart attacks. [27] This is the same Merck that is the largest vaccine maker in the world. During a class action lawsuit about Vioxx injury in Australia, internal Merck documents made the light of day, and they weren't pretty. Apparently, Merck had a "doctor hit list" of any doctors who were speaking poorly of Vioxx to their patients, and an internal email offered up that "we may need to seek them out and destroy them where they live." [28]

In the Federal Court in Melbourne, documents were produced showing that Merck would also "stop funding to institutions" and "interfere with academic appointments" if any academic institutions produced research questioning Vioxx's safety.[29] And this is for a product that Merck already knew, based on their own research, was causing heart attacks.

If all parents believed they had a one in thirty-six chance of their child developing autism from vaccines, the vaccination rates would plummet. And if the pharmaceutical industry were proven to have created an epidemic of autism of several million children worldwide, the economic liability would be astronomical. Just doing some basic math, the average cost of lifetime care for a person with autism is estimated to be $2.4 million dollars.[30] If every parent received that amount of money to care for just the 1.8 million American children with autism today (which is a low estimate of the total), the cost would be $4.32 trillion dollars. It would bankrupt the entire industry.

This is not a fight the pharmaceutical industry wants to lose, and in the press—where Dr. Wakefield's reputation has been annihilated—they take no prisoners.

Stonewalled

In the last four years, according to *STAT News*, advertising dollar spending by pharmaceutical companies in the United States has gone up 60 percent, to $5.2 billion, making the drug industry the second largest buyer of advertising, behind only the automotive industry.[31] CBS News recently reported that "nine out of 10 of the biggest pharmaceutical companies actually spend more on advertising than on R&D" and that "the U.S. spends more of its GDP on health care than 12 other developed countries."[32] Only two countries in the world allow drug advertising on TV—the United States and New Zealand—and the United States spends the most money per capita on prescription drugs in the world. In fact, a 2017 study noted, "Prescription drug spending per capita is far higher in the United States than in the nine other high-income countries considered."[33]

Sharyl Attkisson is a former investigative journalist with CBS News, and she's well known for hard-hitting, brave journalism that often challenges people and institutions in positions of power. In 2008 Ms. Attkisson produced a story about vaccine spokespeople, with a special focus on the aforementioned Dr. Paul Offit. The story opened ominously:

They're some of the most trusted voices in the defense of vaccine safety: the American Academy of Pediatrics, Every Child By Two, and pediatrician Dr. Paul Offit. But CBS News has found these three have something more in common—strong financial ties to the industry whose products they promote and defend.

Ms. Attkisson's story exposed Dr. Offit's "$1.5 million-dollar research chair at Children's Hospital, funded by Merck," and his "patent on an anti-diarrhea vaccine he developed with Merck," and that he was a "vaccine industry insider."[34]

Today her story on vaccine spokespeople corruption would never be able to run in a mainstream news outlet, as the corporate interests have perfected the art of the pushback. The general decline in advertising revenues available to mainstream print and electronic media has made media outlets extremely sensitive to alienating major advertisers. Pharmaceutical companies, and therefore vaccine makers, must be handled with kid gloves, at the expense of real reporting.

Ms. Attkisson has won five Emmy awards and the Edward R. Murrow Award for investigative reporting. She resigned from CBS in 2014, citing "an outsize influence by the network's corporate partners and a lack of dedication to investigative reporting."[35] After she left CBS, Ms. Attkisson penned a best-selling book, *Stonewalled*, which provided insights into how exactly pharmaceutical companies keep the media from reporting on the vaccine-autism issue. Here she is, discussing the first time she reported for CBS on the vaccine-autism conflict:

Minutes before one of my stories about childhood vaccinations and autism is to air, a spokesman for a nonprofit group called "Every Child By Two" calls the network in New York. The spokesperson evokes the name of former first lady Rosalynn Carter, who co-founded the group. . . . Resisting the pushback, we air the story as planned. . . . When we do, hired guns for pharmaceutical interests flood me and CBS News with emails, phone calls, and requests for meetings. They write letters to CBS attorneys. The spokesman for Secretary of Health and Human Services Tommy Thompson calls the CBS News Washington bureau chief to exert pressure to discredit our stories. Pharmaceutical company lawyers set up secretive meetings with

CBS officials in New York. Pharmaceutical interests contact CBS executives to complain.[36]

Later Ms. Attkisson reported on the Hannah Poling case where a child with autism had won a large award from the National Vaccine Injury Compensation Program's vaccine court (discussed in chapter 6). She explained that the pharmaceutical industry PR machine went into overdrive because of how damaging the story was, and their strategy "included a full-forced attack on me and my ongoing reporting."

After she ran her story, Ms. Attkisson learned that "PR Officials and a top attorney for vaccine maker Wyeth have managed to get a private meeting to spin two Evening News senior producers in New York about my reports." Ms. Attkisson's opinion was that meetings like this violate the code of investigative journalism, noting it's "unethical to offer the powerful corporate interest—who are also advertisers—special access, while those on the other side aren't given an audience to be heard."[37]

In the 1950s tobacco companies were doing the same thing to the press that pharmaceutical companies did to Ms. Attkisson. One of the primary PR firms working closely today with pharmaceutical companies is Hill & Knowlton, the same firm that helped Big Tobacco delay their day of reckoning by several decades.[38] Early on, Hill & Knowlton spearheaded a position that "there was 'no proof' that tobacco was bad" and they took their findings and concerns on a road show, meeting "men and women at the top of the American media industry."

They made it clear that they expected the "debate" about tobacco to be covered fairly, and their ad dollars bought them influence, balanced coverage, and several decades without accountability for all the death and disability their products were causing. Tobacco companies didn't leave it to the media to find all the facts; "they made sure they got them." This "balance campaign" included "aggressive dissemination and promotion to editors and publishers of 'information' that supported the industry's position."[39]

The *Lancet* Study

Which brings us back to Dr. Andrew Wakefield. Perhaps no lies are easier to disprove or easier for any reader to independently verify than the ones that have been manufactured about British gastroenterologist Dr. Andrew Wakefield, a doctor stripped of his medical license in Britain for a paper he copublished with twelve other doctors linking the MMR vaccine to autism. If you've only followed the vaccine-autism debate casually, you may have read in the media that Dr. Wakefield is a disgraced scientist who published fraudulent data linking the MMR vaccine to autism. And since Dr. Wakefield made everything up, you have nothing to worry about. Vaccines are perfectly safe and effective.

Dr. Andrew Wakefield was a highly respected gastroenterologist working at the Royal Free Hospital in London. In the mid-1990s he and his colleagues were surprised by a novel bowel condition they were finding in children with autism. It was unlike anything they had ever seen before. In 1998 Dr. Wakefield and twelve other colleagues published a single paper, only five pages in length, in the highly respected medical journal *The Lancet* announcing the discovery of this new bowel condition: Ileal-lymphoid-nodular hyperplasia.[40]

The paper explored the gastrointestinal health issues of twelve children with autism, as the authors made clear: "We investigated a consecutive series of children with chronic enterocolitis and regressive developmental disorder." The thirteen-member team of doctors who wrote the paper felt they had discovered a condition that may be unique to autism and that the condition merited further study, concluding: "We have identified a chronic enterocolitis in children that may be related to neuropsychiatric dysfunction."

The paper was a seminal work, the first time that gastrointestinal symptoms and autism had been tied together, something that today is treated as medical fact. This paper is viewed as the pioneer of the gut-brain connection in autism and has been cited in more than two hundred other studies. The conclusions of the paper, from the standpoint of gastroenterology, have been replicated on dozens of occasions.

The paper's other conclusion, which was really more commentary than science, was what created all the controversy, and ultimately the witch hunt against Dr. Wakefield. Of the twelve children in the study, the parents of eight of the children had noted that the regression into autism happened after their child had received the MMR vaccine. The study authors debated these parental reports and decided to include that information in the study. That's all. As the thirteen coauthors stated in the conclusion of the paper:

In most cases, onset of symptoms was after measles, mumps, and rubella immunisation. Further investigations are needed to examine this syndrome and its possible relation to this vaccine.

Most people don't believe me when I explain to them how minor the mention of vaccines was in the infamous, five-page-long "*Lancet* study." Moreover, they have no idea that Dr. Wakefield had twelve other coauthors or that there never was any data about vaccines and autism in the paper itself. One of the many false narratives is that Dr. Wakefield "faked the data" about vaccines and autism, but that would be impossible. There was no data! The scientists reported parental reports of a relationship between vaccines and autism, nothing more, and were very clear that they felt more study was needed. You'll likely be shocked that they also said this in the paper: "We did not prove an association between measles, mumps, and rubella vaccine and the syndrome described."

How can a paper that dutifully reported the feedback of the parents of eight children, that clearly stated they had not found an association between the MMR vaccine and autism, and that encouraged more study of this issue cause such a scandal? Moreover, Dr. Wakefield's recommendations concerning vaccines at a press conference to discuss the paper seemed very reasonable, if not downright conservative. As Dr. Wakefield recounts:

The important thing to say is that back in 1996–1997 I was made aware of children developing autism, regressive autism, following exposure in many cases to the measles mumps rubella vaccine. Such was my concern about the safety of that vaccine that I went back and reviewed every safety study, every pre-licensing study of the MMR vaccine and other measles containing vaccines before they were put into children and after. And I was appalled with the quality of that science. It really was totally below par and that has been reiterated by other authoritative sources since. I compiled my observations into a 200-page report which I am seeking to put online once I get permission from my lawyers. And that report was the basis of my impression that the MMR vaccine was inadequately tested for safety certainly compared with the single vaccines and therefore that was the basis of my recommendation in 1998 at the press conference that parents should have the option of the single vaccines.[41]

Dr. Wakefield recommended that parents in England, rather than getting the combination MMR vaccine, consider getting three separate vaccines for measles, mumps, and rubella. That's it.

I just want to pause for a moment. If you really don't think that the pharmaceutical industry will mobilize forces to seek and destroy a doctor who says unflattering things about one of their products, I hope Dr. Wakefield's experience will give you pause. How can reporting the parental feedback of eight children constitute the "elaborate fraud" that Dr. Wakefield was later accused of?

In 2004, facing extreme pressure and the threat of losing their careers, ten of the original coauthors of *The Lancet* paper issued a statement, published in *The Lancet*, titled "Retraction of an Interpretation." The coauthors wrote:

> *We wish to make it clear that in this paper no causal link was established between MMR vaccine and autism as the data were insufficient.*[42]

Of course, to anyone who actually read the original paper, this is a statement of the obvious since no one, including Dr. Wakefield, ever represented that the "data" in the paper was sufficient to draw a vaccine-autism link, since there wasn't any data. This short statement by the coauthors was used to further isolate Dr. Wakefield and one of his coauthors, Dr. John Walker-Smith, who were both unwilling to sign their names to what they viewed as a retraction they were being coerced to do, and that violated their professional ethics. Accordingly, Drs. Wakefield and Walker-Smith were put on "trial."

Dr. Wakefield's "trial" in the United Kingdom was not in front of a court but rather in front of the General Medical Council, the governing body in the UK for the licensing of doctors. It's here that Drs. Wakefield and Walker-Smith were stripped of their medical licenses. What's never reported is that soon after the GMC's ruling, Dr. Walker-Smith chose to take his case to a real court, the UK's High Court, and had all charges reversed:

> *The judge quashed a GMC finding of professional misconduct. Mr Justice Mitting called for changes in the way General Medical Council fitness to practise panel hearings are conducted in the future saying: "It would be a misfortune if this were to happen again." Prof*

Walker–Smith, who retired in 2001, said: "I am extremely pleased with the outcome of my appeal."[43]

A final aspect of Dr. Wakefield's study that's never addressed in the press is the feedback from the parents of the twelve children in *The Lancet* study itself. I've personally talked with several of these parents, and they remain convinced that vaccines caused their children's autism and that Dr. Wakefield has been vilified. Isabelle Thomas, the mother of twins in the study, has been one of the more outspoken parents, writing:

> *Dr. Andrew Wakefield listened to the concerns of many parents about their sick children suffering with bowel conditions and a form of Autism, a bowel condition and brain damage that was ignored by other professionals. These parents were demonstrably "black listed" for saying their children became ill after the MMR vaccine. Parents were speaking about this situation years before Dr. Wakefield came on the scene and our government also knew about these concerns years before the Lancet study yet they did nothing to investigate, leaving hundreds of other children at risk of side effects. Our government did not listen to parents but accused them of making the symptoms up and threatening to take their children away if they did not stop making a connection with MMR vaccine. As a result, these children and young adults live in a great deal of pain to this day (one doctor saying to my son "we believe you believe you are in pain"). . . . How long does it take the UK government to learn that cover-up is invariably a more serious matter than the original crime or mistake?[44]*

It's hard to make sense of the Dr. Wakefield witch hunt when you understand the details of his paper, the actual conclusions drawn, the fact that he had twelve coauthors, the recommendations he publicly made about vaccinating, the reversal of Dr. Walker-Smith's GMC sentencing, and the feedback from parents within the study itself. Moreover, to say that Dr. Wakefield's paper was fraudulent and therefore vaccines are safe would fail any logic test, since Dr. Wakefield's paper did no analysis or study whatsoever about the relationship between a single vaccine (MMR) and autism but rather simply reported parental feedback. And on every other vaccine children receive, the paper was silent. Anyone who claims that because Dr. Wakefield's data was fraudulent and therefore the DTP, hep B, polio, Hib, flu, and varicella vaccines are all safe is hoping you never do your own research.

What's more amazing to me is how much more incriminating science we now have, directly implicating vaccines in the epidemic of autism. We actually have very real data! In most cases it's biological science that demonstrates exactly how a vaccine can trigger autism. And the dozens of study authors of these new studies are making declarations about vaccines far bolder than anything Dr. Wakefield ever said, and yet somehow the demonic mythology around Dr. Wakefield persists.

The Truth Can't Be Hidden Forever

Despite the fact that tobacco took four decades to come to its day of reckoning, it happened, and I take great solace in that. In fact, it has fueled me time and again when really all I wanted to do was beat my head against the wall as the pharma-funded PR juggernaut crushed the vaccine injury story at every turn. And it happened because truth has a way of bubbling to the surface against the odds. In the case of vaccines and autism, there's so much truth, so many affected children, so many loud and active parents, and new people brought into this fight every day.

The drumbeat will continue, the truth will get louder, and the next section will explain how much truth we already have through published scientific research—in the courtroom and through the stories of tens of thousands of parents. I think the real shame of Dr. Wakefield getting "Wakefielded" was best captured in a statement he made about the impact of *The Lancet* study, and who is really paying the price:

> *The damage done to my reputation and to that of my colleagues as well as the personal price for pursuing a valid scientific question while putting the patients' interests above all others is trivial compared with the impact of these falsehoods on the children's access to appropriate and necessary care. My experience is intended as a cynical example to discourage others. As a consequence, many physicians in the United Kingdom and United States will not risk providing the care that is due to these children. There is a pervasive and openly*

stated bias against funding and publication of this work, and I have
been excluded from presenting at meetings on the instructions of the
sponsoring pharmaceutical company. It has been an effective exercise
in public relations and selling newspapers. But it will fail—it will
fail because nature cannot be deceived. It has always been a privilege
working with these children and their families. It is my hope that
before too long the tide will turn.[45]

The Line We Will Not Cross

As we slowly built up our forces in the late 1960s in Vietnam, a prevailing ideology in the US government was that if Vietnam fell to the Communists, there would be a domino effect throughout Asia, and we'd see more countries fall to Communism, including Japan and South Korea. This fear of a far greater problem was used to justify the time, expense, and loss of life that followed. And it turned out to be untrue.

The public health system in the United States is consumed by a similar ideology. Admitting any problem with the present vaccine schedule or, God forbid, removing a vaccine is something that must not be done, the thinking goes, because it could cause the entire vaccine program to collapse if there's any loss of confidence on the part of the public. At the end of the day, the vaccine program does rely on a complicit public. If most parents believed there was a nearly 3 percent chance of their child developing autism if they were vaccinated, you can imagine the impact on the vaccine program. In 2001, during deliberations for an IOM study that would be released in 2004, the study's leader, Dr. Kathleen Stratton, made an admission during deliberations that only came to light through a Freedom of Information Act (FOIA) request:

> *The point of no return, the line we will not cross in public policy is to*
> *pull the vaccine, change the schedule.*[46]

Dr. Stratton is articulating a widely held view in public health, which I believe to be completely contrived. And she made her comment before any of the data had been reviewed—the fix was in! Trying to convince the public that vaccines are always "safe and effective" forces officials to lie, exaggerate, and cajole the public. A backlash is inevitable as more and more people discover the truth for themselves. It's part of what has created the dynamic we have today where so many scientists and doctors know the truth, and they're choosing to say so publicly.

On a more sickening level, I've heard public health officials who basically say, "Even if vaccines do cause autism, it's a justifiable outcome for a robust vaccine program." Really, that thinking does exist in public health. So what if we destroy the lives of 3 percent of the kids? It's worth it to protect the other 97 percent. It's insane. It never works, over the long term, to lie to the public, especially with medical procedures. Parents just want accurate information. They want to understand the true risk versus reward of getting their child vaccinated. Like any cover-up, the choice public health officials are making right now is just postponing the day of reckoning.

Truth always comes out in the end. Can we just get on with it?

PART TWO

The Truth about Vaccines and Autism

CHAPTER 5

Emerging Science and Vaccine-Induced Autism

A scientific discovery is not an event; it's a process, and often it takes
time for the full picture to come into clear focus.
—Naomi Oreskes and Erik Conway,
Merchants of Doubt

S ince 2004 there have been eleven groundbreaking discoveries in separate
but related scientific fields that, taken together, reveal the cause of autism.
Because of this science, we now know that autism is created by immune
activation events in the brain during critical phases of brain development,
typically by the time a child is thirty-six months old, and that these immune
activation events in the brain can be triggered by the aluminum adjuvant in
vaccines. While the first of these discoveries occurred in 2004, the critical
missing pieces have only fallen into place since 2010. What you're about to
read is arguably the most important chapter in this book; in it I will walk you
through each of these eleven discoveries and its significance.

These discoveries have been made and then published in peer-reviewed
journals by scientists from all over the world in many different disci-
plines. Dr. Carlos Pardo-Villamizar of Johns Hopkins is a neurologist.
Dr. Christopher Exley of Keele University in England is a professor of
bioinorganic chemistry. Dr. Paul Patterson of Caltech was a professor
of biological sciences (he passed in 2014). Dr. Romain Gherardi of the
Université Paris-Est specializes in neuromuscular diseases. I could go on,

but my point is that this is how science works: Scientific understanding rarely comes into focus from a single breakthrough study; more often it comes from a collective and cumulative picture—in this case, of how autism is created and triggered—that emerges over time.

A 2017 article in *University Affairs* explained how slowly science and medicine can move:

> *Not many patients would be happy to hear that there's a lag of about 17 years between when health scientists learn something significant from rigorous research and when health practitioners change their patient care as a result.*[1]

This time lag between when rigorous research is published and when patient care changes in a clinical setting is really significant—and unbearably frustrating. This is true of all medicine but especially when it comes to autism because there are kids everywhere who urgently need us to understand this science yesterday, not fifteen years from now or whenever the lumbering, bureaucratic (and frankly corrupt) public health establishment gets with the program.

When my son was diagnosed with autism in 2004, nothing I'm about to share with you had yet been discovered. I didn't even know that the brain had its own, distinct immune system (it does). Even now, most of what I'm about to walk you through is not widely known or recognized, except among the scientists doing the work, many of whom have recently chosen to become publicly vocal (at great risk to their careers). But here's what I hope everyone will take away from this chapter: Actually, the science now *exists*—in abundance. It's up to the adults in the room to read it, understand it, and change these devastating policies as soon as possible in order to end the autism epidemic.

So what are the eleven key discoveries? Read on:

Discovery #1: In 2004 Dr. Carlos Pardo-Villamizar at Johns Hopkins University discovers that autism brains are permanently inflamed.

In late 2004 the press release from Johns Hopkins proclaimed, "Brain's Immune System Triggered in Autism."[2] Titled "Neuroglial Activation and Neuroinflammation in the Brain of Patients with Autism,"[3] Dr. Pardo-Villamizar's research demonstrated "an active neuroinflammatory process" in the brains of people with autism, in what was the first time scientists looked at the actual brains of people with autism.

Dr. Paul Patterson of Caltech, the scientist behind Discovery #2, provided one of the best explanations for the importance of Dr. Pardo-Villamizar's work:

> *There is also very striking evidence of immune dysregulation in the brain itself. . . . A group led by Carlos Pardo at Johns Hopkins found what they're calling a "neural inflammation" in postmortem examination of brains of patients with autism who died between the ages of eight and 44 years. But these people weren't infected—they died of such things as drowning or heart attacks. The study found that the microglial cells, which act as the brain's own immune system, were activated. The study also found amazing increases of certain cytokines in the brain, and of others in the cerebro-spinal fluid. This is a landmark paper, in my opinion. It presents the first evidence that there's an ongoing, permanent immune–system activation in the brains of autistic people. It's a subclinical state, because there's no overt infection. But it's there.*[4]

This passage is so important, I want to walk you through it in a bit more detail. We learn, for the first time, that these autism brains have an immune system in a permanent, active state. It also mentions, for the first time, the discovery that certain "cytokines" are highly elevated. Cytokines are small proteins released by the immune system to tell other cells how to behave. They are also biomarkers for inflammation. Dr. Pardo-Villamizar didn't know it yet, but scientists would soon identify certain cytokines that are clear markers for immune activation that all brains with autism seem to share.

I've been haunted by Dr. Patterson's quote ever since I first read it, because of this one line: "There's an ongoing, permanent immune-system activation in the brains of autistic people."

I can't help but think, "Is this what my son is experiencing?" His head always seems to hurt. Sometimes he slaps himself in the head, he often seeks head pressure, seemingly to alleviate discomfort. Is his brain permanently swollen and in a state of subclinical infection? And if it is, how in the world did it get that way? What created this condition? What triggered it? And of course, how do I reduce the inflammation and help him feel better?

Dr. Pardo-Villamizar and colleagues were the first to find this "microglial activation" in the brains of children with autism, and this finding has now been replicated many times. As just one example, a study from Japan in 2013—"Microglial Activation in Young Adults with Autism Spectrum Disorder"—found the same thing:

> *In conclusion, the present PET measurements revealed marked activation of microglia in multiple brain regions of young adults with ASD. The results strongly support the contention that immune abnormalities contribute to the etiology of ASD.*[5]

At the time Dr. Pardo-Villamizar and his colleagues weren't sure why the brains were inflamed; they just knew they were:

> *These findings reinforce the theory that immune response in the brain is involved in autism, although it is not yet clear whether the inflammation is a consequence of disease or a cause of it, or both.*[6]

Soon enough, through ten additional discoveries, that answer has become clear.

Discovery #2: In 2005 Dr. Paul Patterson at the California Institute of Technology discovers that immune activation events lead to autism.

Dr. Patterson credits Dr. Pardo-Villamizar's 2005 paper with forcing him to research what, exactly, causes a brain to develop autism. Over the next nine years, until his passing in 2014, Dr. Patterson would develop a robust body of work that today has created scientific certainty: Immune activation events in the brain at critical times of brain development lead to autism. As his obituary explained:

> *[His] research focused on interactions between the nervous and immune systems—a connection that was not universally acknowledged in the early days of neuroscience. . . . He became intrigued by epidemiological studies that had linked a severe viral or bacterial infection during pregnancy with the increased risk of a woman's giving birth to a child with a neurodevelopmental disorder such as schizophrenia or autism. Patterson and his coworkers reproduced this human effect in mice using a viral mimic that triggers an infection-like immune response in the mother, producing in the*

offspring the core behavioral symptoms associated with autism and schizophrenia.[7]

In 2006 Dr. Patterson introduced the complex interaction between the immune system and neurodevelopment through an article in the journal *Engineering & Science*, titled "Pregnancy, Immunity, Schizophrenia, and Autism."[8] This is the foundational work for the modern understanding of how autism is triggered, and it's widely accepted today by leading scientists. Dr. Patterson explained his discovery in lay terms:

> *As we learn more about the connections between the brain and the immune system, we find that these seemingly independent networks of cells are, in fact, continually talking to each other. As an adult, the activation of your immune system causes many striking changes in your behavior—increased sleep, loss of appetite, less social inter- action—and, of course, headaches. Conversely, stress in your life (as perceived by your brain) can influence immune function—the brain regulates immune organs, such as the spleen, via the autonomic nervous system. Recent evidence shows that this brain-immune conversation actually starts during the development of the embryo, where the state of the mother's immune system can alter the growth of cells in the fetal brain. As we shall see, such alterations can lead to an increased risk of schizophrenia or autism in the offspring.*

If a pregnant mother becomes sick (virus, bacteria) while pregnant—an event that "activates" her immune system—that activation can impact the neurodevelopment of the fetus, potentially leading to neurological problems after birth. This is where the term "immune activation event" comes from, and it's an immune activation event that can lead to autism. Dr. Patterson's work was largely focused on pregnant mothers, and what he termed "Maternal Immune Activation." In his 2006 seminal paper, Dr. Patterson asked a foreboding question; he was well aware of where the science might lead in the next few years:

> *Should we really be promoting universal maternal vaccination? . . . Remember that double-stranded RNA experiment—we activated the immune system, and it caused all these downstream effects on*

the fetus. And what does a vaccination do? It activates the immune system. That's the point of vaccination. In practice, not all pregnant women receive flu shots, and I think that universal vaccination of pregnant women could get us into a whole new set of problems.

Dr. Patterson tied the immune system and brain together in ways previously not recognized. Even better? His theories have since been replicated many times. In 2012 Dr. Patterson and his colleagues produced a paper—"Maternal Immune Activation Yields Offspring Displaying Mouse Versions of the Three Core Symptoms of Autism"—which was more autism specific and reached a similar conclusion:

These results indicate that MIA yields male offspring with deficient social and communicative behavior, as well as high levels of repetitive behaviors, all of which are hallmarks of autism.[9]

In 2014 the MIND Institute at UC Davis published "Activation of the Maternal Immune System during Pregnancy Alters Behavioral Development of Rhesus Monkey Offspring."[10] This study took Dr. Patterson's work in mice and replicated it in monkeys. Why do monkeys matter? The study authors explained:

Maternal infection during pregnancy is associated with an increased risk of schizophrenia and autism in the offspring. Supporting this correlation, experimentally activating the maternal immune system during pregnancy in rodents produces offspring with abnormal brain and behavioral development. We have developed a nonhuman primate model to bridge the gap between clinical populations and rodent models of maternal immune activation (MIA).

The MIND Institute scientists saw results similar to what had been found in mice:

In this rhesus monkey model, MIA yields offspring with abnormal repetitive behaviors, communication, and social interactions. These results extended the findings in rodent MIA models to more human-like behaviors resembling those in both autism and schizophrenia.

Discovery #3: The cytokine interleukin-6 is the key biomarker for immune activation.

If you're an autism parent, you may have heard the expression "cytokine storm." In 2006 Dr. Patterson and his colleagues were speculating that the immune system's cytokines, which are cell modulators released during times of infection, might be responsible for altering the brain development of the fetus during gestation:

> *Cytokines are produced by the white blood cells, and their levels in the blood increase when we get an infection.... We think that maternal immune activation alters brain circuits.... There's that permanent, subclinical, altered immune state in the autistic brain—those increased cytokine levels.... Are they [cytokines] actually interacting with the brain in an ongoing fashion, with consequences visible in the patients' behavior? I favor [the cytokine] hypothesis.*

Just a year after Dr. Patterson published his article about maternal immune activation (MIA) in 2006, he and his colleagues produced the first study that presented their understanding of cytokines at a more detailed level. Knowing that MIA was producing offspring with neurological disorders (in their mouse model), they wanted to find out what—exactly WHAT—was causing the altered brain development. They hypothesized it was a cytokine (there are many), but which one? As Patterson and his colleagues noted, "however, the mechanism by which MIA causes long-term behavioral deficits in the offspring is unknown"—that is, until they discovered it:

> *Here we show that the cytokine interleukin-6 (IL-6) is critical for mediating the behavioral and transcriptional changes in the offspring. A single maternal injection of IL-6 on day 12.5 of mouse pregnancy causes prepulse inhibition (PPI) and latent inhibition (LI) deficits in the adult offspring.*[11]

Patterson and his colleagues injected pregnant mice with a specific cytokine—interleukin-6 (IL-6)— and saw changes in the neurology of their offspring.

Other studies support Dr. Patterson's findings. For example, "Brain IL-6 Elevation Causes Neuronal Circuitry Imbalances and Mediates

Autism-Like Behaviors" was published in the journal *Biochimica et Biophysica Acta* in 2012:

> *In summary, our study supports a critical role of IL-6 elevation in modulating autism-like behaviors through impairments on synapse formation, dendritic spine development, as well as on neuronal circuit balance. These findings suggest that manipulation of IL-6 may be a promising avenue for therapeutic interventions.*[12]

What's the takeaway of these first three discoveries? We now know with certainty that immune activation events in the brain, at critical moments of brain development, can create autism. We also know that IL-6, a cytokine of the brain's immune system, is a biomarker for immune activation, meaning that when the IL-6 level is elevated, we know immune activation is present.

Discovery #4: Immune activation can take place after birth.
Dr. Patterson's important work remained focused on immune activation events that happened during gestation, but a recent study published in the journal *Neuropsychopharmacology* in January 2018 from Harvard affiliate McLean Hospital showed that immune activation events after birth can trigger conditions of autism, too:

> *While previous research in laboratory animals has established that immune activation during critical prenatal (before birth) developmental periods can later produce the core features of ASD, including decreased social interaction, aberrant communication, and increased repetitive behavior, we wanted to evaluate whether postnatal (during infancy) immune activation could also produce other symptom clusters that are often seen in ASD and related conditions.*
>
> *Our findings demonstrate that early-life immune activation can lead to long-lasting physiologic perturbations that resemble medical comorbidities often seen in ASD and other neuropsychiatric conditions.*[13]

The primary limitation of Dr. Patterson's pioneering work on immune activation is that he never did any studies like this one to bridge the divide between a child in gestation and a child during infancy. If immune activation events after birth could also trigger the development of autism, then something besides the mother would have to trigger the immune activation.

Vaccine Papers, a website written and maintained by scientists who think vaccines should be held to the same scientific standards as other drugs, addresses this topic of postnatal immune activation:

> *Diverse evidence indicates that the brain can be adversely affected by postnatal immune activation. Postnatal immune activation experiments, human case reports, and consideration of brain development timelines suggest that the human brain is vulnerable to immune activation injury for years after birth.*

So far, the science has shown us how autism can be created by an immune activation event at a critical phase of brain development. But what can cause, or trigger that immune activation event? We know that a maternal infection can cause an immune activation event; Dr. Patterson proved this. But what about an illness or infection after a child is born? Could, for example, a bout of the flu trigger autism? And if so, how would that explain the permanent, ongoing immune system activation of the brains of people with autism that Dr. Pardo-Villamizar discovered? Are vaccines actually important to prevent autism if, in fact, a childhood infection would be enough to trigger an immune activation event and create autism? To answer these questions, we turn to the work of a researcher in Canada named Christopher Shaw who, almost by accident, opened the door in 2009, after which a cascade of subsequent research followed.

Discovery #5: Aluminum adjuvant in vaccines produces behavior and motor function deficits.

Dr. Christopher Shaw of the University of British Columbia in Canada found himself faced with a simple question that science could help answer: Were vaccines causing Gulf War syndrome in Canadian soldiers? His laboratory became the first one to ever test the aluminum used in vaccines in a biological setting, in a study published in 2009.[14] Dr. Shaw and his colleagues "examined the potential toxicity of aluminum hydroxide in male, outbred CD-1 mice injected subcutaneously in two equivalent-to-human doses." As he recounts:

We did the really simple experiment of taking the same stuff out of the vaccines, the aluminum hydroxide, and injecting it into mice, into the muscles, to see what would happen if we tried to mimic the vaccine schedule.[15]

Dr. Shaw's findings were troubling, and they demonstrated neurological problems in mice who received the aluminum injections after they were born:

We were quite surprised to see how rapidly the behavioral symptoms emerged. They showed not only behavioral deficits of motor function but they ultimately showed cognitive deficits as well. Once we sacrificed the animals and started looking inside their brains and spinal cords, we found massive damage to motor neurons.

Once Dr. Shaw realized how toxic aluminum adjuvant appeared to be to the neurological system of the mice, an obvious question emerged: What about the aluminum adjuvant in all of the pediatric vaccines?

Aluminum compounds (both Al hydroxide and Al phosphate) are currently used as adjuvants in the hepatitis A, hepatitis B, diphtheria-tetanus-pertussis (DTaP, Tdap), *Haemophilus influenzae* type b (Hib), human papillomavirus (HPV), and pneumococcus (PCV) vaccines, which are all part of the childhood schedule for vaccines.

The amount of aluminum being injected into children's bodies skyrocketed beginning in the early 1990s for two reasons: (1) more vaccines were added to the schedule and (2) the number of kids receiving all vaccines rose (from 50 to 60 percent in the mid-1980s to over 90 percent today). A fully vaccinated child in the mid-1980s would have been injected with 1,250 micrograms of aluminum by his eighteen-month birthday. A fully vaccinated child today is injected with 4,925 micrograms of aluminum, a near quadrupling.

Aluminum makes most vaccines "work." It's not the weakened strain of the hepatitis B virus (called the antigen), for example, that provokes an immune response when a child receives the hepatitis B vaccine. It's the aluminum adjuvant that provokes the immune response. When you understand aluminum's role and what a vaccine adjuvant is intended to do, the next question becomes obvious: Could an ingredient in vaccines whose

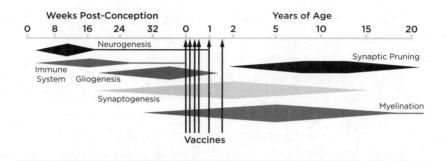

Figure 5.1. How Vaccination Corresponds to Brain Development. Arrows indicate vaccines given at 0, 2, 4, 6, 12, and 15–18 months. Data from Centers for Disease Control and Prevention. Chart adapted from Semple et al., "Brain Development in Rodents and Humans: Identifying Benchmarks of Maturation and Vulnerability to Injury Across Species," *Progress in Neurobiology*, 106/107 (July–August 2013): 1–16.

purpose is to hyperstimulate the immune system trigger immune activation events in the brain at critical points during brain development?"

One of the charts that woke me up to how risky vaccinating infants can be is shown in figure 5.1 and illustrates how the timing of the infant vaccination schedule matches up to critical phases of brain development. As you can see, an infant's brain continues to develop long after a child is born, and vaccines are injected during many of the most critical phases. Remember how worried Dr. Patterson was about vaccinating pregnant women with the flu shot? Well, as of today, the vaccination rate for pregnant women with the flu shot is only 35 percent.[16] And most pregnant women who do receive vaccines while pregnant only get two vaccines: flu and DTaP. Infants, on the other hand, receive twenty different vaccines by their first birthday, and vaccination rates in the United States are above 90 percent. If vaccinating pregnant women might produce some unintended immune activation, vaccinating infants still undergoing brain development might in fact be catastrophic.

It's important to understand that aluminum was grandfathered into pediatric vaccines without safety testing. You might want to read that again. Injecting aluminum has never been tested in the pediatric population. Dr. Shaw and his colleague, Dr. Lucija Tomljenovic, addressed this omission in a 2011 study they published in *Current Medicinal Chemistry* titled, "Aluminum Vaccine Adjuvants: Are They Safe?"[17] They wrote:

Aluminum is an experimentally demonstrated neurotoxin and the most commonly used vaccine adjuvant. Despite almost 90 years of widespread use of aluminum adjuvants, medical science's understanding about their mechanisms of action is still remarkably poor. There is also a concerning scarcity of data on toxicology and pharmacokinetics of these compounds. In spite of this, the notion that aluminum in vaccines is safe appears to be widely accepted. Experimental research, however, clearly shows that aluminum adjuvants have a potential to induce serious immunological disorders in humans. In particular, aluminum in adjuvant form carries a risk for autoimmunity, long-term brain inflammation and associated neurological complications and may thus have profound and widespread adverse health consequences.

In 2012 Drs. Shaw and Tomljenovic published another paper, "Mechanisms of Aluminum Adjuvant Toxicity and Autoimmunity in Pediatric Populations," in which they expressed grave concerns about the limited understanding of aluminum adjuvants' toxicity:

It is somewhat surprising to find that in spite of over 80 years of use, the safety of Al adjuvants continues to rest on assumptions rather than scientific evidence. For example, nothing is known about the toxicology and pharmacokinetics of Al adjuvants in infants and children. . . . Yet, in spite of these observations children continue regularly to be exposed to much higher levels of Al adjuvants than adults, via routine childhood vaccination programmes.[18]

The two scientists called for an urgent reevaluation of the safety profile of aluminum adjuvant–containing vaccines:

However, the existing data (or lack thereof) raise questions on whether the current vaccines aimed at pediatric populations can be accepted as having adequate safety profiles. Because infants and children represent those who may be most at risk for complications following vaccination, a more rigorous evaluation of potential vaccine-related adverse health impacts in pediatric populations than what has been provided to date is urgently needed.

Discovery #6: Aluminum adjuvant in vaccines, injected into the body, can be carried to the brain by macrophages.

In 2013 French scientists Drs. Romain Gherardi and Josette Cadusseau from the Université Paris-Est demonstrated that aluminum adjuvant, when injected into the body of a mouse, ended up in the brain one year later, in a study titled, "Slow CCL2-Dependent Translocation of Biopersistent Particles from Muscle to Brain." The study authors expressed serious concerns about this very new discovery:

> *However, continuously escalating doses of this poorly biodegradable adjuvant in the population may become insidiously unsafe, especially in the case of overimmunization or immature/altered blood brain barrier.*[19]

"Insidiously unsafe" should cause any parent worry. Unfortunately, the very thing they express real concern about—escalating doses—is exactly what has been happening to children since the early 1990s, when the immunization schedule in the United States and all over the world more than tripled, largely due to new vaccines being introduced that contain aluminum adjuvant.

There was another nuance to this French discovery that's very important to understand. CCL-2 is a cytokine that "recruits monocytes, memory T cells, and dendritic cells to the sites of inflammation produced by either tissue injury or infection."[20] In lay terms CCL-2 sounds an alarm to the immune system, and "macrophages" come running. Macrophages are the immune system's garbagemen, and they travel the body eating up debris, infections, and so on. When aluminum adjuvant enters the body, it's not recognized by the body because it's a foreign, man-made substance. The macrophages grab it, but they don't have the means to eliminate it, so they carry it, and bring it to soft tissue places in the body, like the brain. And guess what the brain's immune system does when it encounters the aluminum, a foreign substance it doesn't recognize? It reacts. Said differently, it activates.

Discovery #7: Aluminum adjuvant stays in the brain for much longer than anyone realized.

In 2015 another study from the same group of scientists at the Université Paris-Est, "Biopersistence and Brain Translocation of Aluminum Adjuvants of Vaccines," showed that aluminum adjuvant slowly makes its way to the brain, where it then stays, possibly forever. [21]

The French scientists explained that aluminum adjuvant can generate a long-term immune response because of its "biopersistence," which basically means our body has no ability to rid itself of aluminum adjuvant, because it's a man-made substance we have no natural designs to eliminate:

> *Thus alum and other poorly biodegradable materials taken up at the periphery by phagocytes circulate in the lymphatic and blood circulation and can enter the brain using a Trojan horse mechanism similar to that used by infectious particles. Previous experiments have shown that alum administration can cause CNS dysfunction and damage, casting doubts on the exact level of alum safety.*

I think this is a moment worth tying something together that we learned a while back. Remember Dr. Paul Patterson? He said, "There's an ongoing, permanent immune-system activation in the brains of autistic people." What if the brain's immune system is just sitting there, in a constant battle with the aluminum, that it doesn't know how to get out of the body? What if that's what's causing the inflammation Dr. Pardo-Villamizar talked about back in 2005?

Discovery #8: Small Doses of Aluminum Adjuvant Are Actually More Dangerous.

In the fall of 2016, an important and revealing study done on aluminum adjuvant, "Non-linear Dose-Response of Aluminium Hydroxide Adjuvant Particles: Selective Low Dose Neurotoxicity," provided more bad news, and insight. [22] This study's conclusions revolutionized our understanding of aluminum adjuvant. From the journal *Toxicology* the French study authors were very concerned about the widespread use of aluminum adjuvant:

> *Concerns about its [aluminum adjuvant's] safety emerged following recognition of its unexpectedly long-lasting biopersistence within immune cells in some individuals, and reports of chronic fatigue syndrome, cognitive dysfunction, myalgia, dysautonomia and autoimmune/inflammatory features temporally linked to multiple Al-containing vaccine administrations.*

They also discovered, through mouse models, an alarming and unique characteristic of aluminum adjuvant: Low, consistent doses were *more* neurotoxic than a single bolus (large) dose:

> *We conclude that Alhydrogel [aluminum adjuvant] injected at low dose in mouse muscle may selectively induce long-term Al cerebral accumulation and neurotoxic effects. To explain this unexpected result, an avenue that could be explored in the future relates to the adjuvant size since the injected suspensions corresponding to the lowest dose, but not to the highest doses, exclusively contained small agglomerates in the bacteria-size range known to favour capture and, presumably, transportation by monocyte-lineage cells. In any event, the view that Alhydrogel neurotoxicity obeys "the dose makes the poison" rule of classical chemical toxicity appears overly simplistic.*

Vaccine Papers provides more insight:

> *Remarkably, the study found that the lowest dosage (200 mcg/Kg) was the most toxic! For many outcomes, the 400 and 800 mcg/Kg dosages had no observable adverse effects, but the 200 mcg/Kg dosage did. The low toxicity of the higher dosages appears to be a consequence of dosage-dependent inflammation at the injection site. The high dosages caused intense inflammation at the injection site, forming "granulomas." The 200 mcg/Kg dosage did not produce granulomas. . . . This suggests that it is more dangerous and harmful to administer numerous small injections of Al adjuvant, compared to a large single injection capable of inducing a granuloma.*

The French scientists also disputed the way the FDA and CDC currently think about aluminum adjuvant toxicity, basically saying that the current approach is wrong: "As a possible consequence, comparing vaccine adjuvant exposure to other non-relevant aluminium exposures, e.g. soluble aluminium and other routes of exposure, may not represent valid approaches."

The French scientists finished with a conclusion that all parents should find troubling: "In the context of massive development of vaccine-based strategies worldwide, the present study may suggest that aluminium adjuvant toxicokinetics and safety require reevaluation."

This conclusion raises an obvious question: How is the safety of aluminum calibrated by the FDA and CDC for use in pediatric vaccines? It's hard to believe, but the entire basis for declaring that aluminum adjuvant can be safely injected into the bodies of newborns is based on a single study published by a single FDA scientist, Dr. Robert J. Mitkus, in 2011.[23] "Updated Aluminum Pharmacokinetics Following Infant Exposures through Diet and Vaccination" appears to be a reassuring response to any concerns parents might have, which Dr. Mitkus directly addresses in the study's abstract:

> Because concerns have been expressed by the public that aluminum in vaccines may pose a risk to infants, we developed an up-to-date analysis of the safety of aluminum adjuvants.

What would be lost on the average layperson is that the only biological science Dr. Mitkus considered in making his safety assessment was a single study that infused (rather than injected) aluminum citrate (rather than aluminum hydroxide) into adults (rather than babies). It's hard to put this seemingly minor detail in proper context. In no other drug on the planet (except for vaccines) would safety standards ever be determined without using the actual product (aluminum hydroxide) administered in the proper way (intramuscular injection), into the proper patient population (infants).

Vaccine Papers provides additional perspective on Dr. Mitkus's study:

> Mitkus 2011 is the best scientific evidence vaccine promoters have for defending Al adjuvant safety. It is fatally flawed and incredibly bad. It is not based on any toxicity experiments with actual Al adjuvant. It ignores key studies that contradict the assumptions it is based on. . . . Aluminum adjuvant nanoparticles are very different from dissolved aluminum ions. Consequently, the only scientifically-valid way to establish the safety of injected aluminum adjuvant, is by experiments with injected aluminum adjuvant. Studies of ingested, soluble aluminum salts cannot establish the safety of Al adjuvant. Models of only dissolved aluminum cannot be used to determine the toxicity of the particles. Ignoring the toxicity of Al adjuvant particles is scientifically indefensible. Why do the vaccine promoters rely on

oral ingestion studies to defend Al adjuvant safety? It is because they have no experimental research showing that injecting Al adjuvant is safe! They are empty-handed.

In early 2018 a paper published in the prestigious *Journal of Inorganic Biochemistry* took dead aim at the safety standards used for vaccine aluminum adjuvant. Titled, "Critical Analysis of Reference Studies on the Toxicokinetics of Aluminum-Based Adjuvants," the paper addressed the limitations of studies, in particular Dr. Mitkus's, that both the FDA and the CDC have relied on to declare vaccine aluminum "safe" to be injected into children.[24] The study authors, from France and the U.K., included most of the leading experts in the world on the neurotoxicity of aluminum, including Dr. Romain Gherardi, Dr. Guillemette Crepeaux, and Dr. Christopher Exley. Their criticism was incisive:

To date, aluminum adjuvants per se have, perhaps surprisingly, not been the subject of any official experimental investigation, and this being in spite of the well-established neurotoxicity of aluminum.

The study authors also mention a laundry list of countries that have produced studies implicating aluminum-containing vaccines in chronic illness:

The occurrence of myalgia and arthralgia, chronic fatigue and neurological disorders following multiple injections of aluminum-containing vaccines against hepatitis B, tetanus and human papilloma virus (HPV) has been reported in many countries: Australia, Canada, Denmark, France, United Kingdom, Italy, Israel, Japan, Mexico, Portugal, and USA.

The gist of their paper? None of the studies done to date on aluminum safety actually tell us if aluminum is, in fact, safe. All the study authors of this paper have done their own biological studies of aluminum adjuvant and found it to be highly neurotoxic. Their conclusion:

Both paucity and serious weaknesses of reference studies strongly suggest that novel experimental studies of Al adjuvants toxicokinetics should be performed on the long-term, including both neonatal and adult exposures, to ensure their safety and restore population confidence in Al-containing vaccines.

Words like "paucity" and "serious weaknesses" are not words you want to hear when you are the CDC or the FDA and your job is to certify that something is safe when it appears that's not remotely true. Then again, "paucity" and "serious weakness" are not words you want to hear when you are a parent and your job is to protect the life of your child.

Discovery #9: Aluminum causes immune activation in the brain.

A study from the Middle East published in 2015 provides a critical bridge between aluminum adjuvant and IL-6, which is the cytokine released during an immune activation event. In this case, scientists were using aluminum to induce Alzheimer's in rats, which they appear to have done successfully, showing that aluminum caused a fourfold increase in IL-6:

The results also showed that aluminum administration increased the hippocampus pro-inflammatory cytokines TNF-α by 3.8-fold, IL-6 by 4-fold, and iNOS by 3.8-fold compared to the normal control group.[25]

This study is critical in connecting several discoveries together. We know immune activation events in the brain can trigger autism. We know aluminum is highly neurotoxic and poorly studied, but we need clear evidence that aluminum can—by itself—trigger an immune activation event. As you already learned, one of the key biomarkers of an immune activation event is the cytokine IL-6, which this study showed was triggered by aluminum. Moreover, this injected aluminum triggered IL-6 in the brains of the rats, which means the aluminum found its way through the body and into the brain, which we already knew it would do.

Discovery #10: Hepatitis B vaccine induces IL-6 in postnatal rats.

When this paper was published in China, it didn't make national news or create a reaction from the CDC, even though it should have. Some of it was probably the name, quite a mouthful: "Neonatal Vaccination with Bacillus Calmette–Guérin and Hepatitis B Vaccines Modulates Hippocampal

Synaptic Plasticity in Rats." And the scientists weren't looking to prove vaccines can trigger autism, even though they did. You had to appreciate all of Patterson's work. You had to understand the IL-6 connection to immune activation and to autism. You had to appreciate the new insights about aluminum adjuvant toxicity, the low dose implications, and that aluminum adjuvant was ending up in the brain. And you had to read a paper from China that covered a lot of other ground.[26]

Vaccine Papers has written extensively about this study:

> *This is the first study to test the effects of immune activation by vaccination on brain development. All other studies of immune activation have used essentially pathological conditions that mimic infection and induce a strong fever. . . . This 2016 study demonstrates that vaccines can affect brain development via immune activation. Hence, the immune activation experiments are relevant to vaccines. . . . The hep B vaccine increased IL-6 in the hippocampus (the only brain region analyzed for cytokines).*

And the Vaccine Papers scientists continue, explaining the timing of the injury to the rats vaccinated with the Hep B vaccine:

> *An important finding in the rat BCG/Hep B study is that many of the effects of hep B vaccine did not appear until age 8 weeks. This finding undermines claims of vaccine safety, which are almost always based on short-term outcomes of a few days or weeks. Furthermore, 8 weeks is a long time in rats. 8-week old rats are almost fully mature adults. This suggests that adverse effects of vaccines may take years or decades to appear in humans. This is consistent with what is known about immune activation and schizophrenia. Immune activation in the fetus can cause schizophrenia 20–30 years later.*

This study is extraordinary. There were three different groups of rats: rats receiving a BCG vaccine (not given in the United States), rats receiving the hepatitis B vaccine (given on day one of life in the United States), and a control group with no vaccine. The BCG vaccine does *not* contain aluminum adjuvant, and the impact on the rats' brains from BCG was actually positive! The hep B vaccine rats, however, showed the kind of immune activation event we are seeing in autism (high IL-6). This is biological proof of the link between a vaccine given to a postnatal animal inducing an immune activation event, including the cytokine marker for autism, IL-6. A scientific first.

In late 2016 the same Chinese scientists replicated their own work, this time focusing exclusively on the biological impact of the hepatitis B vaccine in a paper titled, "Neonatal Hepatitis B Vaccination Impaired the Behavior and Neurogenesis of Mice Transiently in Early Adulthood." Their results were confirmatory and very disturbing, including bringing up the risk of autism explicitly: "This work reveals for the first time that early HBV vaccination induces impairments in behavior and hippocampal neurogenesis. This work provides innovative data supporting the long suspected potential association of HBV with certain neuropsychiatric disorders such as autism and multiple sclerosis."[27]

Discovery #11: High Levels of Aluminum Are Uniquely Located in Brain Tissue of People with Autism.

In early December 2017 Dr. Christopher Exley of Keele University in England and his colleagues published a paper that for the first time looked at the brain tissue of subjects with autism to determine the level of aluminum found within it.[28] With the most complete database of aluminum levels in human brains in the world (over one hundred), Professor Exley and his colleagues were in a great position to put the results of their new study in proper context, as Professor Exley said in explaining the groundbreaking results:

> *While the aluminium content of each of the 5 brains* [of people with autism] *was shockingly high it was the location of the aluminium in the brain tissue which served as the standout observation. . . . The new evidence strongly suggests that aluminium is entering the brain in ASD via pro-inflammatory cells which have become loaded up with aluminium in the blood and/or lymph, much as has been demonstrated for monocytes at injection sites for vaccines including aluminium adjuvants.*[29]

Dr. Exley's quote includes a reference to "monocytes at injection sites" and an interaction between monocytes and aluminum that is critical to appreciate. A "monocyte" is a type of white blood cell. One form of mono-cyte is a "macrophage," which we already discussed. Dr. Exley is saying that macrophages are escorting aluminum injected from a vaccine directly into the brain. The location of the aluminum within the autism brains is the most important finding of Exley's study, because it serves as a marker for the route the aluminum took to get to the brain. In a private email to the director of the National Institute of Mental Health, Dr. Exley explained that the location of aluminum in the brain proved to him "that aluminium adjuvant could be transported to the brain from a vaccine injection site." In a blog post, Dr. Exley expanded on that same point:

> I have seen the same cells that we will see at an injection site [from vaccination] carrying a cargo of aluminum into the brain tissue of individuals who died with autism.

Eleven Discoveries Light a Clear Path to Autism

Figure 5.2 shows in simple terms how aluminum adjuvant can trig-ger autism, as demonstrated by the published science. Science shows that autism is caused by an immune activation event. The adjuvant in vaccines—aluminum adjuvant—can activate the brain's immune system and is more neurotoxic than previously realized. Aluminum can trigger IL-6, the key cytokine implicated in autism. Chinese scientists—for the first time anywhere in the world—used a vaccine to trigger an immune activation event and recorded elevated levels of IL-6 in rats. And British scientists discovered extraordinarily high levels of alumi-num in the brains of people with autism, particularly inside cells, the

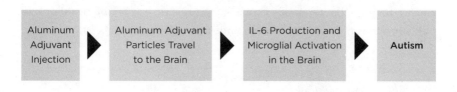

Figure 5.2. How Aluminum Adjuvant Can Trigger Autism. Courtesy of the Vaccine Papers.

macrophages, that served to transport the aluminum into the brain from the injection site.

I can't help but tie everything I read and see here to my own son's experience. Born in 2002, my son seemed to get sicker with every vaccine appointment, and his head always seemed to be hurting. And with each vaccine appointment, unusual behaviors and odd movements began to appear. A really sad reminder of this reality appeared in a study published in 2017 in *Nature* that described how children with autism developed enlarged foreheads:

> *Brain enlargement has been observed in children with autism spectrum disorder (ASD), but the timing of this phenomenon, and the relationship between ASD and the appearance of behavioural symptoms, are unknown. Retrospective head circumference and longitudinal brain volume studies of two-year olds followed up at four years of age have provided evidence that increased brain volume may emerge early in development.*[30]

Wouldn't the above theory about how autism is triggered do a pretty good job of explaining why these children have large (swollen) heads? As you know, the immune activation event leads to what Dr. Patterson called "an ongoing, permanent immune-system activation in the brains of autistic people." And guess what: Permanent immune system activation means inflammation . . . which would lead to a "large brain" and a "swollen forehead." Is that why children with autism are known to head bang? Perhaps you would, too, if your brain was in a state of permanent inflammation.

Aluminum's newly discovered role in triggering immune activation events in the brain changes everything about the science of vaccines and autism, because it establishes a clear biological basis for how a vaccine can cause autism. In late 2017 Dr. Exley expressed the risk he was taking by talking so publicly about the vaccine-autism connection with some dark humor:

> *I am very prudent. I only put my neck on the guillotine when it is absolutely necessary. And that time is now.*[31]

What will it take for our health authorities to stand up and face the truth? We have new, credible biological science showing us that we are deliberately damaging our babies, and likely creating the autism epidemic. As Dr. Christopher Exley said:

> *We need to think carefully, is this vaccine a life-saving vaccine or not? If it isn't, don't have it with an aluminum adjuvant.*[32]

Why a Biological Basis Matters

In 1953 Adele B. Croninger, working out of her research laboratory located on the campus of Washington University in St. Louis, painted the fated white mice three times a week with a liquid solution of cigarette tar. In her recollection of the experiment she recalled that "after about eight months, these animals first lost the hair on the painted area and then little warts, or papilloma as we call them, appeared . . . and in the 11th month of painting, we had our first cancer."[33] Ms. Croninger's meticulous laboratory work represented a landmark moment in science. From this experiment with mice, the first domino fell, and the result was the ultimate legal, marketing, and moral censure of the most powerful industry on earth at the time, Big Tobacco.

Ms. Croninger's 1953 study was published in the journal *Cancer Research*.[34] The title of the paper foreshadowed its catastrophic conclusions, "Experimental Production of Carcinoma with Cigarette Tar." In the study, eighty-one mice were painted with the cigarette tar and 59 percent developed papillomas [tumors], while 44 percent developed skin cancer. Ms. Croninger and her study authors noted that "it is not known which fraction or fractions in tobacco tars are carcinogenic," but they felt further study in this area was "urgent" in the hopes that it might promote "some practical aspects of cancer prevention."

Ms. Croninger's work is an excellent example of biological science, a scientific approach, whereby a clear cause-and-effect relationship can be established between a potentially toxic substance (tobacco tar) and a laboratory animal. Her 1953 study generated panic within the tobacco industry because the results were unassailable: Tobacco tar and cancer were linked.

In autism science we now have our own mice studies, most published since 2010, and they are demonstrating exactly how vaccines can trigger autism. Unlike bogus epidemiological studies you read about in part 1 where very narrow components of the vaccine schedule (MMR, thimerosal) are analyzed with population data that can be manipulated, biological science has a much harder time hiding from the truth.

Critically, I want to address the MMR vaccine for a moment, for two reasons. First, many parents I know blame the MMR vaccine appointment as the one where their child slipped into autism. Second, the MMR vaccine, because it's a live virus vaccine, does not contain aluminum adjuvant. How could this be? In many ways, MMR actually makes the aluminum adjuvant story more airtight. MMR, using live viruses, provokes a very strong response from the immune system and triggers the release of a macrophage transport mechanism known as MCP-1. As Vaccine Papers explains:

> When MCP-1 is produced by microglia, macrophages from around the body travel into the brain. . . . "MCP" stands for "macrophage chemoattractant protein," which of course describes its primary function of summoning macrophages. . . . MCP-1 production is stimulated by some types of immune activation. Hence, a vaccine that stimulates MCP-1 may cause AANs [aluminum adjuvant nanoparticles] (e.g. from prior vaccines) to move into the brain. Some infections or toxins induce MCP-1. Interestingly, Al adjuvant induces MCP-1, suggesting that it may stimulate its own transport. . . . We can speculate that AANs from vaccines may remain "dormant" for years, until MCP-1 production is stimulated. The MCP-1 will cause macrophages containing AANs to mobilize and transport AANs into the brain and other sensitive tissues. This may explain some of the damage from the MMR vaccine. MMR is given at 15–18 months of age, which is after Al-containing vaccines are given (at 0, 2, 4, and 6 months). The measles vaccine can stimulate MCP-1 production. Therefore, the MMR vaccine may stimulate the movement of AANs (received from prior vaccines) into the brain. This may explain how MMR could cause Al toxicity, even though it does not contain aluminum adjuvant.

In lay terms, the MMR vaccine, which isn't typically given until a child is thirteen months old (and has already received twenty other vaccines), serves to round up all the aluminum already in the body and bring it right to the brain, by summoning macrophages to accelerate the transport of aluminum. This would certainly help explain the many children I know who experienced seizures and regression immediately following the MMR vaccine.

In 1999, in response to a new law (the FDA Modernization Act), the FDA publicly announced that mercury levels in pediatric vaccines—through a preservative called thimerosal, which I discussed in chapter 3—exceeded safety standards. With autism rates beginning to skyrocket and many parents seeing changes in their children after vaccine appointments, the mercury hypothesis was valid. Unlike with aluminum, vaccines don't "need" thimerosal to be effective; the only role it plays is as an antibacterial in multidose vaccine vials. When the switch was made to single-dose vials, the need for thimerosal disappeared, and it was largely removed from vaccines by 2003. Since that time a "natural experiment" has reduced the likelihood that thimerosal has played a primary role in autism, although injecting infants with mercury remains a profoundly dangerous thing to do and no doubt has caused harm. In fact, even the CDC published a study showing thimerosal increased tics, a neurological disorder, in children. Unlike aluminum adjuvant, thimerosal does not hyperstimulate the immune system, which, with the benefit of all the newly published science, explains why aluminum, rather than mercury, appears to be the likely trigger for immune activation in the brains of infants, causing autism. As Vaccine Papers explains:

> *There is evidence that thimerosal in vaccines causes harm. It is idiotic to inject thimerosal in any amount into infants or pregnant women.*

Three Extraordinary Letters

In mid-2017 three of the leading scientists in the world who have spearheaded many of these important discoveries did something extraordinary: They wrote private letters to the directors of the three agencies that make up the US public health service: the CDC, the Food and Drug Administration (FDA), and the National Institutes of Health. Their letters were a warning about the newly discovered dangers of aluminum adjuvant and its relationship to autism. I was heartened, and a little astonished, when I read each of their letters, each one drafted on the letterhead of their respective university. Here are three excerpts:

From Dr. Christopher Shaw of the University of British Columbia:

We have studied the impact of aluminum adjuvants in animal models of neurological disease, including autism spectrum disorder (ASD). . . . These studies and the broader existing literature regarding aluminum toxicity, lead almost invariably to the conclusion that aluminum in any chemical form is always neurotoxic when administered to humans. Further, I am convinced that aluminum adjuvants in vaccines may contribute to neurological disorders across the lifespan. In adults, such adjuvant may induce macrophagic myofasciitis, a disease with neuropathological aspects. In children, there is growing evidence that aluminum adjuvants may disrupt developmental processes in the central nervous system and therefore contribute to ASD in susceptible children. . . . In regard to the above, it is my belief that the CDC's claim on its website that "Vaccines Do Not Cause Autism" is wholly unsupported.

From Dr. Romain Gherardi of the Université Paris-Est:

I am an expert in the field of aluminum adjuvants toxicity in humans and animal models. I have been working in this field since the initial description of the Al vaccine-induced macrophagic myofasciitis in 1998. Since that time I have written 40 peer-reviewed scientific publications and one book on this subject. I strongly support the contention that aluminum adjuvants in vaccines may have a role in the etiology of autism spectrum disorder (ASD). My view is founded on a significant and burgeoning body of peer-reviewed scientific evidence which makes the link between ASD and exposure to aluminum through vaccinations and other sources.

From Dr. Christopher Exley of Keele University:

I am an expert in the field of aluminum adjuvants and aluminum toxicity. I have been working in this field for more than 30 years during which time I have written in excess of 150 peer-reviewed scientific publications on this subject. . . . As an expert in the field of aluminum adjuvants and aluminum toxicity I solemnly declare that more research on the role of aluminum adjuvant in vaccines and neurological disorders, including ASD, is essential and urgently required.

A French Nobel Laureate Speaks Up

In late 2017 a mandatory vaccination decree arose in France, spearheaded by French prime minister Édouard Philippe. Mr. Philippe's task was challenging, due to general sentiment in France about vaccinations, according to *The Independent*:

> *A recent survey found more than three out of 10 French people don't trust vaccines, with just 52 per cent of participants saying the benefits of vaccination outweigh the risks.*[35]

Compounding France's challenges of passing a mandatory vaccination law, Dr. Luc Montagnier, arguably the most famous scientist in France, decided to step into the debate about vaccines soon after Prime Minister Philippe announced his intentions. Dr. Montagnier, a French virologist, is, by every standard, a bona fide science rock star, having won the Nobel Prize in medicine in 2008 for his discovery of HIV and proving that it led to AIDS. Dr. Montagnier has won dozens of prestigious awards and is a member of both the Academy of Sciences and the Academy of Medicine.

In early November of 2017, Dr. Montagnier held a press conference against the "vaccine dictatorship" at the Theatre Michel in Paris to discuss the proposed mandatory vaccination law. Dr. Montagnier was joined on stage by another heavyweight of the scientific world, Dr. Henri Joyeux, a former professor of oncology and laureate of the prestigious Antoine Lacassagne Cancer Prize of the Ligue Nationale contre le Cancer. Their comments were startling in their honesty and clarity, loudly warning the French populace on the dangers of vaccines.

Dr. Montagnier opened his press conference by explaining that his motivation was to "launch an alert to all France and the world" and that he and Dr. Joyeux "urge members [of the French parliament] not to vote in favour of this law, which goes against the interests of children's health and imposes an industrial and administrative diktat on doctors and families."

The two doctors dropped their own bomb about aluminum, sounding very much like all the other aluminum scientists previously discussed:

> *The sum of the proposed vaccines gives the infant an excessive amount of aluminum, a bio-persistent adjuvant which has demonstrated its harmfulness locally at the injection site and also its penetration in*

the form of aggregates to the brain and other areas of the body (Bone, Kidneys) as has been demonstrated in the dust-breathing workers during the extraction of bauxite (Occupational Diseases). In addition, aluminum in veterinary vaccines has been found to be toxic to animals, directly or indirectly responsible for sarcoma (cancers) in the vaccination area within 3 years of vaccination and in other areas of the body. 5 years later: Ostéosarcomes, fibrosarcomes, chondrosarcomes, limbs, chest and abdomen. Would our cats be better treated than our children, since aluminum was removed from veterinary vaccines by a Sanofi subsidiary?

Blessed by Dr. Patterson's Colleagues

Paul Patterson, the scientist from Caltech who first helped us understand how an immune activation event can trigger autism, passed away in 2014. However, after a February 2017 blog post I wrote about all his pioneering work and the other discoveries, I heard directly from his widow Carolyn, who wrote me the following in an email:

> *I shared your article with several people who had worked with PHP [Dr. Paul Patterson], and they all were favorable about your conclusions. As scientists, none of them would go against the vaccination theory, per se, but they were also aware of the numerous anecdotes of changes in behavior, around 18 months, in a set of children—which corresponds to the time when vaccinations are given. They were inspired by your connections and appreciative of your ingenuity.*[36]

I want to make several points about Carolyn Patterson's email. First, the group of studies I just shared with you and how they all interrelate were viewed "favorably" by Dr. Patterson's protégés. Second, despite their favorable view, his widow felt compelled to tell me that none of these scientists would "go against" the vaccination theory, meaning they're scared to endorse the vaccine-autism connection (because they don't want to be "Wakefielded"). This is how taboo the vaccine-autism connection is in the mainstream world of science. Even protégés of Dr. Paul Patterson, the scientists in perhaps the best position to understand exactly how a vaccine could cause autism, are scared to touch the topic. In the same email Ms.

Patterson told me the story of her sister's baby boy: "My sister and her husband had a baby boy 18 months before we had our son. He turned out to be on the autism spectrum, and while he was a 'late talker,' my sister noticed a profound difference after he had his immunizations at 18 months," she said. "My sister had his blood levels tested, and he was always extremely heavy with metals in his blood," she continued.

Dr. Paul Patterson's nephew regressed after his vaccines—Paul Patterson, the man who discovered how immune activation events lead to autism.

I've often wondered about scientists who know the truth about the cause of autism but have yet to say anything publicly. How do they live with themselves? As one example, I feel that Caltech's Dr. Patterson, were he still alive, would be standing with scientists like Professor Exley and publicly telling the truth about immune activations events, vaccines, and his own nephew. But what about so many others?

In late 2016 two scientists, in legal depositions, affirmed everything I could have hoped for, and more. And not just any scientists, but Drs. Andrew Zimmerman and Richard Kelley, arguably the two leading mainstream autism scientists in the world. Their intimate relationship with the "vaccine court" almost ended the autism epidemic in 2009, and their ongoing willingness to tell the truth will likely contribute to the ending, I hope very soon.

CHAPTER 6

The Clear Legal Basis that Vaccines Cause Autism

I also find, with a high degree of medical certainty, that the set of immunizations administered to Yates at age 11 months while he was ill was the immediate cause of his autistic regression because of the effect of these immunizations to further impair the ability of his weakened mitochondria to supply adequate amounts of energy for the brain, the highest-energy consuming tissue in the body.

—Dr. Richard Kelley, Professor of Pediatrics,
Johns Hopkins University (Kennedy Krieger Institute)[1]

There are only a few people in the world I believe could end the autism epidemic single-handedly. The director of the CDC would be one, the president of the American Academy of Pediatrics probably another. Dr. Andrew Zimmerman, the former director of medical research at the prestigious Kennedy Krieger Institute at Johns Hopkins University, would be the third.

For years Dr. Zimmerman served as a go-to expert in "vaccine court" to dispute parental claims that vaccines caused their children's autism. And as the reigning national expert on the topic of autism in the scientific community, Dr. Zimmerman's opinions held tremendous weight: His written testimony helped deny the claims of the families of more than five thousand children with autism during an Omnibus Autism Proceeding in 2009 in vaccine court, as I will explain in a moment.

In the late 1990s a young doctor fresh out of medical school joined the Kennedy Krieger Institute in Baltimore as a resident and worked closely with Dr. Zimmerman. His name was Jon Poling. In 2000 Dr. Poling's nineteen-month-old daughter, Hannah, experienced a massive regression into autism after her vaccinations, much as happened to my son. Unlike my son, Hannah's parents had access to the most sophisticated autism research center in the world, and Dr. Zimmerman and several of his colleagues, including Dr. Richard Kelley, who was serving as director of Kennedy Krieger's laboratory, tried to figure out what had happened to her, and why.

Of course, everyone at Kennedy Krieger initially approached the idea that vaccines had played a role in Hannah's regression skeptically, including Dr. Poling himself. He was a decidedly mainstream neurologist, having attended Georgetown to get both his MD and PhD. He and his wife Teri had fully vaccinated Hannah, and he'd explain many times over the next few years that he wouldn't have believed it if he hadn't seen it himself.

Through an unexpected series of events, Dr. Poling and Dr. Zimmerman, colleagues at the most prestigious autism research facility in the world, nearly ended the autism epidemic in 2008. Because of Hannah Poling, Dr. Zimmerman became convinced that vaccines are indeed capable of causing autism under certain circumstances, representing a change in his previously held positions. Like any good scientist, Dr. Zimmerman appeared willing to go where the evidence took him, even toward something as inconvenient as a vaccine-autism connection.

Dr. Zimmerman's professional opinion about what caused Hannah's autism, given the tremendous weight he carried within the scientific community and his long-time role as an expert witness, triggered a panic at both the CDC and the Department of Justice. It led to a quick twenty-million-dollar settlement with the Polings in 2010, but not before Hannah's story became worldwide news.[2]

I've always had so many questions about the Hannah Poling case, Dr. Zimmerman, Dr. Kelley, and Dr. Poling. Soon after the news spectacle, the Polings disappeared from the public, never to be heard from again. Sources have told me that the Department of Justice made it clear to the Polings that if they wanted to receive their vaccine court compensation, they needed to keep quiet. They appear to have complied.

Very recently, however, Drs. Zimmerman and Kelley privately agreed to serve as expert witnesses in the first vaccine injury trial of any kind in a regular courtroom in more than thirty years. The trial is a medical negligence case in Tennessee, alleging that a pediatrician allowed a child to develop autism by vaccinating him when there was clearly excessive risk, based on previous reactions he'd had to vaccines. The boy's name is Yates Hazlehurst, and he was one of three "test cases" in the aforementioned Omnibus Autism Proceeding back in 2009—only a year prior to the DOJ's settlement with the Poling family—a case that was lost partially based on the written testimony of Dr. Zimmerman.[3]

Drs. Zimmerman and Kelley, under oath, provided depositions for the trial as expert witnesses. What's significant is that in the future they would be testifying on *behalf* of the Hazlehurst family, confirming that in Yates's case, vaccines caused his autism. Yes, you read that right. In 2009 the Omnibus Autism Proceeding concluded that Yates Hazlehurst's autism was not caused by vaccination, a decision based partially on Dr. Zimmerman's testimony—and a decision that, significantly, served as the basis for denying claims to more than five thousand other children.

Fast forward to 2017, and Drs. Kelley and Zimmerman are expert witnesses for the same child, and they are both saying, "with a reasonable degree of scientific certainty," that vaccines caused Yates's autism.

Confused yet? I know I was. Let's start at the beginning.

The "Vaccine Court"

If vaccines cause autism, you'd think "vaccine court" would be a great place to find the evidence for it. Compensated claims typically include extensive details about timelines, medical tests, and doctors' opinions. They read more like case reports in medical journals than legal settlements.

Established through the National Childhood Vaccine Injury Act of 1986, the original purpose of the vaccine court (officially called the United States Court of Federal Claims special masters) was to quickly and expeditiously pay any claims made by American citizens for vaccine injury. The vaccine court is buried within the Department of Health and Human Services (HHS), and when you petition the vaccine court because of a vaccine injury, you're actually suing the federal government, and the lawyer representing the government (and therefore opposing your claim) will be a Department of Justice lawyer. Due process in vaccine court is nonexistent. There's no jury, just a single court-appointed "special master" who hears your case and makes a decision.

Since 1989, when the vaccine court began to operate, these special masters have awarded more than $3.8 billion to vaccine-injured Americans (children and adults).[4] Of the total cases filed since the court came into existence in 1998, there have been twelve hundred claims filed for death and eighteen thousand filed for injury. The DTP vaccine is the most common vaccine for claims to be filed against, with MMR in second place. Of the people who file claims with the court, approximately 34 percent end up receiving compensation; 2017 was actually the single biggest year for claims paid, with just over $282 million.

Rolf Hazlehurst, an assistant attorney general from Tennessee, has been an outspoken critic of the vaccine court, particularly since he had to fight his way through it as a claimant on behalf of his son Yates, who he believes developed autism as a result of his vaccinations. In a memorandum to the US Congress in 2013, Rolf Hazlehurst described the court:

> *Vaccine court is not a court of law. It is an administrative proceeding in which the most basic rules of law do not apply. In vaccine court, the Rules of Discovery, Evidence and Civil Procedure do not apply. There is also no judge or jury. In vaccine court, the American legal system has been replaced by what is known as a special master. A special master is an appointed government attorney.[5]*

Why Does the Vaccine Court Exist?

This may seem like an elementary question, but it's not. The purpose of the vaccine court is to protect the vaccine program, not to monitor vaccine safety or mete out justice. The year the vaccine court began operating—1989—is important to this story, because that's also the birth year many point to as the beginning of a meteoric rise in the number of children with autism. Three other potentially monumental things happened in 1989: the hepatitis B vaccine was licensed, the Hib vaccine was licensed, and, for the first time, a second dose of the MMR vaccine was recommended for all American children.

When the vaccine court was established in 1986, there were only three vaccines given in the United States—DTP, polio, and MMR—and vaccination rates hovered between 50 and 60 percent nationally.[6] Today, there are eleven vaccines for children, given in multiple doses, with vaccination rates hovering around 90 percent nationally. There is an enormous difference between the market the vaccine court was created to "protect" and the market today. In raw numbers there are nearly four times as many vaccine doses given each year to children than there were in 1986, even though the US population has only grown by 0.3 in that same time period.

Beginning in 1989, the US vaccine schedule quickly morphed from the one the vaccine court was created to support to a far larger schedule with more complexity. This isn't a coincidence; the vaccine court removed all liability from vaccine makers, greatly altering the risk/reward calculation in their favor.

When the court was established, the word "autism" was never even discussed. By the late 2000s autism almost brought the entire court, and the vaccine program, to a screeching halt.

Changes Make It Nearly Impossible to Win Claims

Few people know that the vaccine court amended its rules in 1995 to make it harder to win a claim in vaccine court, largely due to the increasing number of claims made as the vaccine schedule became bloated. By revising its Vaccine Injury Table—a list of "accepted" injuries from various vaccines, the court quietly made the standard for proving a vaccine injury much higher. As one simple example, claims for DTP shots causing brain injury were paid on roughly 25 percent of filed cases before the 1995 changes and only 5.4 percent of cases after the changes were made, a decrease of more than 80 percent.[7] Testifying before Congress in 1999, Barbara Loe Fisher, the president of the National Vaccine Information Center, explained:

> *The principal reason why the Vaccine Injury Compensation Program has become highly adversarial and is turning away three out of four claimants is that the Department of Health and Human Services (DHHS), with the assistance of the Department of Justice (DOJ), has wielded its discretionary authority to all but eliminate a just list of compensable events in the Vaccine Injury Table, thereby destroying the guiding tenet of presumption.[8]*

Recognizing vaccine injury is no easy task; few doctors are able to recognize any of the signs. As I first mentioned in chapter 2, the United States has a vaccine injury reporting system called the Vaccine Adverse Event Reporting System (VAERS) database. Estimates are that VAERS captures roughly 1 percent of all vaccine injuries.[9] How many vaccine injuries actually make it into vaccine court? A fraction of a fraction of a fraction of 1 percent. (I can't find any accurate data, but the number is clearly tiny or the vaccine court would have exploded in size.)

The burden is on the parents to track "adverse events," despite the fact that pediatricians almost never explain all of the possible side effects. Parents might be told to expect redness at the injection site, swelling, maybe some fussiness or mild fever. Nothing some infant Tylenol can't fix.

Perusing the website of a vaccine court attorney today, you can see how strongly the decks are stacked against those injured by vaccines. Richard Gage & Associates, one of the top vaccine lawyers in the country, lets potential clients know that "obtaining compensation for a vaccine injury is a complex, sometimes extremely difficult process."[10] Parents of a child who received compensation shared their view about what the experience was like:

> DOJ [Department of Justice] attorneys were disrespectful and combative. . . . The Compensation Program should be about compensation and not about defense of the vaccine program.[11]

A critical report from November 2014 about the vaccine court produced by the Government Accountability Office (a federal agency) found the court wasn't accomplishing what it had been purportedly created to do: to make vaccine injury compensation quick and fair.[12] The report noted that most claims take "multiple years to adjudicate" with 51 percent taking more than five years.

Parents who have filed claims in the court report that the compensation program has an "adversarial environment" and a statute of limitations (three years from the date of injuries being exhibited) that reduces the likelihood that parents can even file claims. This is far worse when it comes to autism, a condition that wasn't even contemplated when the court was created.

As Mr. Hazlehurst's memo further explains:

> The procedural "catch 22" of vaccine court works as follows. Under the Vaccine Act, before the parents of a vaccine-injured child may

file a lawsuit in a court of law, they must first timely file a claim in vaccine court. However, the Vaccine Act has a 3-year statute of limitations, which begins to run upon the first symptom of injury. Under the CDC vaccine schedule children receive their first vaccinations either at birth or 2 months of age. However, in most cases, children are not diagnosed with autism until they are 3 or 4 years old. Therefore, by the time the child is diagnosed with autism, the statute of limitations has run in vaccine court and the parents are forever denied the right to proceed with a lawsuit in a court of law.[13]

In a 1998 article for the *Washington Post*, journalist Arthur Allen criticized the changing standards of the vaccine court and explained the excruciating (and ultimately losing) journey of a family whose son had become extremely disabled from the DTP vaccine.[14] With the changes to the Vaccine Injury Table, Mr. Allen noted, "the burden of proof in most cases now lies with the petitioners, and that is a tricky business, because proof is an elusive matter in ailments of the brain." Mr. Allen caught the former medical director of the Vaccine Injury Compensation Program, Dr. Geoffrey Evans, in a vulnerable moment, explaining the true purpose of the vaccine court:

There's a larger issue, too. They want parents to immunize their children, and for that they want the record to show that vaccines are safe. "I'm not going to say that awarding too many people will undermine vaccine safety, but I look on the Internet, and I see that our statistics are taken out of context," says [Dr. Geoffrey] Evans, the medical director of the compensation program.

I want to highlight something Mr. Allen wrote above: "They want the record to show that vaccines are safe." Dr. Evans viewed his job as protecting the vaccine program, and he made it clear that awarding "too many people" for vaccine injury could very much "undermine" vaccine safety.

Why does this matter? Because shortly after Dr. Evans made this comment, the court was flooded with claims—claims from way "too many people" for something that no one had even discussed when the vaccine court was created in 1986: autism.

Omnibus Autism Proceeding (OAP)

By 2002, four years after Mr. Allen's article in the *Washington Post*, the vaccine court was overwhelmed with hundreds of claims for autism, a previously rare disorder (at the time) that was experiencing an explosive rise. Lawyers were warning the court that thousands more claims were headed their way. Chief Special Master (the head judge of the vaccine court) Gary Golkiewicz, in response, issued an order in July of 2002 to address an "unusual situation" facing the court:[15]

> *This situation arises out of concern in recent years that certain childhood vaccinations might be causing or contributing to an apparent increase in the diagnosis of a type of serious neurodevelopmental disorder known as "autism spectrum disorder," or "autism" for short.*

The vaccine court's solution for handling so many claims was complex, painstaking, and ultimately catastrophic for the families involved. In simple terms, the vaccine court took more than 5,500 claims from parents alleging vaccines caused their child's autism and put them into a single group. Six "test cases," which were later narrowed to three, were singled out from these 5,500 claims, and the results of the test cases would impact the totality of claims made in the court. Parents were given the choice to opt in to the Omnibus Proceeding, putting them at the mercy of the outcome of the test cases, or opt out and file a separate claim in the court themselves. Most decided to opt in.

Unfortunately, seven years passed between the formation of the OAP and the final judgment by the special masters, and in that time many special interests found ways to intervene and corrupt the proceedings, as Wayne Rohde explained in his 2014 book, *The Vaccine Court*:

> *The OAP, for all the good intentions it was designed to achieve, quickly became a corrupt legal proceeding, all to accommodate the pharmaceutical industry, the medical community, and our government, instead of determining compensation for thousands of vaccine-injured children and the tens of thousands to come in the future.*[16]

As the attorneys representing the 5,500 claims began to organize themselves, the choice of test cases became incredibly important to the outcome of the proceedings, as well as the first opportunity to corrupt the legal proceedings.

Hannah Poling: The Unassailable Test Case

As the lawyers representing the families sifted through the claims to find the perfect test cases to represent the Omnibus Proceeding, one case stood out for its robustness and defensibility: Hannah Poling, the daughter of Dr. Jon Poling of the world-renowned Kennedy Krieger Institute.

The government, however, had an advantage that would allow it to tilt the proceedings in its favor: They could settle any claim from any family at any time, including the claims being put forth as possible "test cases." The Department of Justice attorneys learned that Dr. Zimmerman believed Hannah Poling's autism had indeed been caused by her vaccines. On November 30, 2007, Dr. Zimmerman penned a two-page letter to the Polings' attorney, Clifford Shoemaker, explaining that with a "reasonable degree of medical certainty," he believed:

> *The cause for regressive encephalopathy in Hannah at age 19 months was underlying mitochondrial dysfunction, exacerbated by vaccine-induced fever and immune stimulation that exceeded metabolic energy reserves. This acute expenditure of metabolic reserves led to permanent irreversible brain injury. Thus, if not for this event [her vaccinations], Hannah may have led a normal and productive life. Presently, I predict Hannah will have a normal lifespan but with significant lifelong disability.*[17]

Dr. Zimmerman's medical explanations, some of which made it into the public realm, have at times been twisted by vaccine proponents. Make no mistake: What Dr. Zimmerman is saying here is that vaccines caused Hannah's autism. His recent depositions make this clear.

Mitochondrial Disorders: Common or Not?

I want to take a quick departure to explain "mitochondrial disorder." It's an abnormality in metabolism, and if a child has a mitochondrial disorder, her cellular energy level is low, and she is more at risk of having a vaccine pushing her over the edge and causing a bad reaction, including developing autism. A child with a mitochondrial disorder is at higher risk for an immune activation event after vaccination. Vaccine proponents desperately want to portray mitochondrial disorders as rare, but that's not the case, with the data showing that anywhere from 20 to 50 percent of children with autism have some type of mitochondrial disorder.[18] Worse, mitochondrial disorders are sometimes genetic but can also be caused by the toxins in the environment. So a healthy child could receive one load of vaccines and develop a mitochondrial disorder and then receive a second load and develop autism.

Mitochondrial disorder as a preexisting risk to regressive autism is what Hannah Poling taught the Kennedy Krieger doctors. Based on her data, they realized there is a "vulnerable subset" of children who regress into autism after vaccines because they have mitochondrial issues that may not be detected. Hannah's mitochondrial disorder, which her dad repeatedly explained to the press was not rare at all, was what vaccine proponents would use to try to confuse the issue, to the annoyance of Dr. Poling.

In 2006 a paper titled, "Developmental Regression and Mitochondrial Dysfunction in a Child with Autism" was published in the *Journal of Child Neurology*.[19] It was a case report of a single child, Hannah Poling, and it told her entire story. The authors? Dr. Jon Poling and Dr. Andrew Zimmerman. Reading the study, you realize how Dr. Zimmerman and others at the Kennedy Krieger Institute were able to change their minds about the vaccine-autism connection: Hannah's experience caused them to go back and revisit their clinical data, as they explain:

> *The subtle laboratory abnormities identified in this case led us to retrospectively evaluate the laboratory records of other patients with autism. Records from the Kennedy Krieger Institute between January 1995 and September 2002 were selected.*

This study received almost no publicity back in 2006, but part of its discussion was foreboding:

> *Young children who have dysfunctional cellular energy metabolism therefore might be more prone to undergo autistic regression between 18 and 30 months of age if they also have infections or immunizations at the same time.*

What's important to recognize is that the Kennedy Krieger doctors came to their new point of view through careful research of their entire patient population of autistic children. Hannah Poling was the catalyst, not the basis, for their conclusions.

Twenty Million Dollars to Go Away

In late 2007, with the Omnibus Proceeding well underway (a final ruling would be delivered in 2009) and with Hannah Poling's case officially presented as one of the three tests cases for the OAP, the Justice Department lawyers did something that likely saved the vaccine court and the industry it exists to protect: They settled the Hannah Poling case and removed it from the OAP. As Dr. Jon Poling explained:

> We are obviously pleased with the HHS decision to concede our case, but we had NOTHING to do with the concession. This was a unilateral decision from HHS (recall that HHS is the respondent, rather than the vaccine maker, as manufacturers have blanket liability protection afforded by the Vaccine Injury Program established in 1986). I will not speculate on the obvious question—why concede? Hannah's case was positioned to set precedent as a test case in the Omnibus Autism Proceedings for potentially thousands of other cases.[20]

HHS conceded the Poling case to save the vaccine industry and keep Dr. Zimmerman's opinion from becoming public. Imagine the national backlash that would have ensued if Americans had heard the truth on TV and in the media: Vaccines caused autism, and the US government paid to silence the family whose case proves it beyond doubt. Think back to the purpose of the vaccine court: to show that vaccines are safe. Hannah's case put that purpose at risk. Like most settled cases in vaccine court, Hannah's was settled confidentially (with a gag order on the family) in late 2007. Most of us would have never heard of Hannah Poling, if one of the attorneys representing the families hadn't leaked the settlement document to journalist David Kirby in early 2008.

It's absolutely mystifying to read the entirety of the Poling family's winning judgment. It's a step-by-step explanation for how a child regresses into autism through multiple vaccine appointments, replete with ongoing doctor visits, emergency room trips, and recurring loss of previously attained developmental milestones.[21] For an autism dad like me, it triggers a bad case of PTSD, with so many parallels to our experience with Jamison.

Like many children, Hannah "consistently met her developmental milestones during the first eighteen months of her life."[22] On July 19, 2000, Hannah received five vaccinations at one appointment (DTaP, Hib, MMR, Varivax, and IPV), and her mother, a trial attorney, reported that Hannah "developed a fever of 102.3 degrees two days after her immunizations and was lethargic, irritable, and cried for long periods of time." Twelve days after her vaccine appointment, Hannah "presented to the Pediatric Center with a 101–102 degree temperature, a diminished appetite, and small red dots on her chest." She was diagnosed by the emergency room staff with "a post-varicella vaccination rash."

The judgment continues with a seemingly endless list of trips to doctors and emergency rooms for ear infections, inconsolable crying, painful urination, bowel distress, and many other physical problems. Finally, in February of 2001, roughly seven months after Hannah's fateful vaccine appointment, she received an autism diagnosis from Kennedy Krieger by Dr. Andrew Zimmerman himself, and he noted that Hannah had regressive brain damage after her vaccine appointment. And with tortured language reminiscent of President Clinton defending his infidelities, the vaccine court admitted that vaccines caused Hannah's autism:

> In sum, DVIC [Division of Vaccine Injury Compensation] has concluded that the facts of this case meet the statutory criteria for demonstrating that the vaccinations CHILD [Hannah Poling] received on July 19, 2000, significantly aggravated an underlying mitochondrial disorder, which predisposed her to deficits in cellular energy metabolism, and manifested as a regressive encephalopathy with features of autism spectrum disorder. Therefore, respondent recommends that compensation be awarded to petitioners.[23]

Dr. Zimmerman's opinion had triggered the settlement in Hannah's case. Earlier, Dr. Zimmerman had provided a separate opinion about one of the other test cases, that of Michelle Cedillo. He felt that Michelle's autism had not been caused by vaccines, and a written memo he provided would be a primary reason that all three remaining test cases would lose in the

Omnibus, impacting 5,500 families. No one knew that Dr. Zimmerman held a different opinion about Hannah Poling. Rolf Hazlehurst, in his memo to the US Congress, spelled out this hypocrisy:

> *The government never intended for the American people to know about the Poling case and has fought hard to keep it under seal. By conceding the Poling case, the government prevented Dr. Andrew Zimmerman from taking the witness stand, in which case it could be shown that one expert witness provided two very different reports. The first report was very publicly used against the petitioners [in the other test cases]. The second was used to compensate one child and in the process the government kept the evidence in her case under seal. The evidence placed under seal is strong evidence of how vaccines can cause autism.*

Mr. Hazlehurst was able to get the sealed details of the Hannah Poling case, which included the complete opinion of Dr. Zimmerman. He writes:

> *The written opinion of the government's own expert witness in the field of neurology clearly reflects that he is of the opinion that the vaccines in question were a direct cause in the development of autism by Hannah Poling. Again, Poling v HHS would have been the fourth test case in the Omnibus Autism Proceeding if the government had not conceded the Poling case. The sealed evidence includes the expert opinion of the government's own expert witness, which explains how vaccines can cause autism.*

After Dr. Zimmerman gave his private opinion about Hannah Poling's case, he was effectively uninvited from being part of the vaccine court. He was never part of the actual Omnibus Autism Proceeding (beyond a memo he had written earlier), and he never had a chance to form an opinion about Yates Hazlehurst. He became a liability to the vaccine court.

Hannah Makes National News

Hannah Poling's leaked case spurred the vaccine industry into damage-control mode, as Hannah's story led most mainstream news coverage for several nights, especially on CNN, right in the CDC's Atlanta backyard. Julie Gerberding, at the time the CDC's director, appeared live, arguing, "The government has made absolutely no statement indicating that vaccines are a cause of autism. This does not represent anything other than a very specific situation and a very sad situation as far as the family of the affected child."[24] The "spin," of course, was that Hannah's case was exceptionally rare.

That would be the spin time and again: Hannah's case was unique, she had a "mitochondrial dysfunction," it had no bearing on the larger debate about vaccines and autism. Dr. Jon Poling deemed it a complete mischaracterization of the facts, writing, "The only thing unique about my little girl's case is the level of medical documentation—5 to 20% of patients with ASDs have mitochondrial dysfunction [a number today we know is higher]."[25] In an interview on CNN with Dr. Sanjay Gupta, Dr. Poling would make his case even more emphatically:

Dr. Gupta: We've talked to a lot of experts about this, and they say that vaccines in no way cause autism. You're a neurologist, you're also the father of Hannah; what do you say?

Dr. Poling: The Department of Health and Human Services conceded that my daughter's medical problems, which are autism, encephalopathy, seizures, were brought on by vaccination.

Dr. Gupta: But that's startling for a lot of people to hear, because we've been taught for so long there's so many good things about vaccines, but in your daughter's case it turned out to be a problem?

Dr. Poling: I wouldn't have believed it until it happened to me. As a doctor, until it happened to me, until I saw the regression, until I saw a normal 18-month-old toddler descend into autism, I wouldn't have believed it was possible.

Dr. Gupta: The experts I've talked to, including the director of the CDC, Dr. Julie Gerberding, say, "That was a rare case, that is not likely to be the norm, that's likely to be an exception." What do you say to that?

Dr. Poling: Well, I think a lot of media outlets have put out a statement that says, "rare underlying genetic mitochondrial disease." Now that's five words. Four of those are not accurate in the sense that we know now—we didn't know back in 2001—that mitochondrial dysfunction is not rare. Two, we don't know if it was underlying or if something that developed later. The only correct word is mitochondrial.

Dr. Gupta: So what you believe is that Hannah did have some sort of predisposition and then vaccines tipped her over the edge into developing autism. What is your belief now?

Dr. Poling: Well, I don't think vaccines are the only way that you can tip over a child like Hannah to regress and have an encephalopathy and regress into autism. There are probably multiple triggers. In my daughter clearly it was vaccinations; that was our experience.[26]

Writing for the *Huffington Post*, investigative journalist David Kirby echoed Dr. Poling, noting that "some reports estimate the rate of mito-chondrial dysfunction in autism to be 20% or more. And the rate among children with the regressive sub-type of autism is likely higher still."[27] What if mitochondrial dysfunction was the predisposition that made kids with autism particularly vulnerable to vaccines? As Mr. Kirby continued, "What's needed most urgently, if possible, is a quick, affordable and effi-cient method of testing children for low cellular energy, perhaps before vaccination even begins."

Mr. Kirby continued to press the case with HHS, trying to understand how many other Hannah Poling–like cases there might be hiding under seal. The doublespeak he received in a letter from David Bowman in the HHS's office of communications played word games:

> *The government has never compensated, nor has it ever been ordered to compensate, any case based on a determination that autism was actually caused by vaccines. We have compensated cases in which children exhibited an encephalopathy, or general brain disease. Encephalopathy may be accompanied by a medical progression of an array of symptoms including autistic behavior, autism, or seizures. Some children who have been compensated for vaccine injuries may have shown signs of autism before the decision to compensate, or may ultimately end up with autism or autistic symptoms, but we do not track cases on this basis.[28]*

Mr. Bowman is trying to be artful with semantics. Autism is not a diagnosis you receive based on a medical test, a gene test, or with any sort of lab report. It's a behavioral diagnosis that has been relegated to the psychiatric back forty for decades. It is listed in the *DSM*, the *Diagnostic and Statistical Manual of Mental Disorders*.[29] There is no medical test for autism. Autism is a documented observation that a child has enough exhibited speech, language, and social impairment symptoms to qualify for a diagnosis. Therefore, someone with "regressive autistic symptoms" has autism. A child with an encephalopathy and "autistic behavior" has autism. When Hannah Poling suffered "regressive encephalopathy with features of autism disorder," she had autism, which is her official diagnosis. What Mr. Bowman is really saying is that they have compensated vaccine injury cases of children who have autism as a result of their vaccine injury, but they will never say so directly, because that will scare the public. Soon after Mr. Bowman's statement, this became even more evident.

Mary Holland and Lou Conte

Soon after conceding Hannah's case, the Omnibus court ruled against the roughly 5,500 families and exonerated vaccines as the cause of autism. For many parents the Omnibus ruling in February 2009 represented the final insult for their children: no government compensation for their child's suffering.

Hannah Poling's case also caught the eye of two parents of children with autism: Mary Holland and Lou Conte. Ms. Holland is an NYU law professor, and Mr. Conte is the father of triplet boys, two of whom have autism; author of *Vaccine Injuries*; and (now) retired assistant commissioner in the Westchester County, New York, Department of Probations. They were intrigued by the Hannah Poling case and began to wonder if there was any truth to one of the vaccine court's "dirty secrets" exposed by Mr. Bowman's response to David Kirby. Some parents of children with autism who had chosen to sidestep the Omnibus proceedings knew the secret of the court: If you mention the word *autism* in your injury claim, you'll lose. Brain damage? Fine. Encephalopathy? No problem. Autism? No, vaccines don't cause autism; you lose.

Ms. Holland and Mr. Conte wondered, was the vaccine court compensating the families of autistic children, so long as they played along? What they learned was that maybe Hannah Poling's case was not so unique.

Bailey Banks

Just one month after the Omnibus ruling against the 5,500 families, a leaked case in March of 2009 should have destroyed the CDC's position that Hannah Poling was an isolated case. In a clear ruling on the 2007 case of a ten-year-old autistic child named Bailey Banks, the vaccine court noted, "The MMR vaccine at issue actually caused the conditions from which Bailey suffered and continues to suffer."[30] The court found that Bailey's family proved that the MMR vaccine had caused a brain inflammation illness known as ADEM, which lead to his autism:

> The Court found that Bailey's ADEM was both caused-in-fact and proximately caused by his vaccination. It is well-understood that the vaccination at issue can cause ADEM, and the Court found, based upon a full reading and hearing of the pertinent facts in this case, that it did actually cause the ADEM. Furthermore, Bailey's ADEM was severe enough to cause lasting, residual damage, and retarded his developmental progress, which fits under the generalized heading of Pervasive Developmental Delay, or PDD [an autism spectrum disorder]. The Court found that Bailey would not have suffered this delay but for the administration of the MMR vaccine, and that this chain of causation was . . . a proximate sequence of cause and effect leading inexorably from vaccination to Pervasive Developmental Delay.

So the vaccine court doesn't acknowledge that vaccines can cause autism—except when the vaccine court acknowledges that vaccines can cause autism. In the case of Bailey Banks, they were willing to recognize that his PDD (part of the autism spectrum) was caused by the MMR, perhaps because the case took place before the final Omnibus judgment. In the case of the Banks family, they had chosen not to join the OAP and to pursue their claim individually. This turned out to be a prudent move, as the awarded money would help provide for Bailey's lifelong needs. Writing about the Banks decision in 2009, David Kirby and Robert F. Kennedy Jr. took to the mainstream press in an op-ed for the *Huffington Post*:

> In many other successful cases, attorneys elected to steer clear of the hot button autism issue altogether and seek recovery instead for the underlying brain damage that caused their client's autism. . . . The

vaccine court, in other words, seems quite willing to award millions of dollars in taxpayer funded compensation to vaccine-injured autistic children, so long as they don't have to call the injury by the loaded term "autism."[31]

Unanswered Questions

Joined by attorneys Robert Krakow and Lisa Colin, Ms. Holland and Mr. Conte went to work, asking a simple question, "Is the Vaccine Injury Compensation Program ('VICP') of the U.S. Court of Federal Claims a fair forum?"[32] They decided to conduct an investigation, and possibly publish a study, depending on what they found. They took direct aim at the Omnibus Proceeding:

> *Are the cases of "autism" that the VICP [Vaccine Injury Compensation Program] rejected in the Omnibus Autism Proceeding really different from the cases of "encephalopathy" and "residual seizure disorder" that the VICP has compensated before and since? Is it possible the VICP rejected cases of "autism" because of the hot-button label and not because of real differences in injuries or evidence?*

Of course, they soon discovered what you probably have already deduced: that the court has in fact been compensating cases of autism called other things since the inception of the program. After digging through thousands of claims, many with sealed and confidential decisions that kept firm conclusions from being drawn, they were still able to find eighty-three cases of children with an autism diagnosis who had been compensated for "vaccine induced brain damage."

Holland and Conte began to compile their results in earnest. For a court that had recently reassured the world that vaccines don't cause autism, this was a devastating finding. Worse for the vaccine court, the study authors decided to include interview responses they received from some of the families who had received compensation from the court in their study. The study authors asked, "How is your child's life today?" Some of the responses follow:

- "[She] is profoundly autistic. [She] is non-verbal, has major behavioral issues, is self-injurious . . . classic and very severe autism."

- "[He] has no speech, no functional use of his hands. . . . He is not potty trained. He is very sensory defensive, flaps his hands, and makes moaning noises."
- "[She] is a 'giant baby.' . . . She functions at the level of a 2-year old. . . . [She] has frequent periods of frustration, extreme rage, and self-injurious behavior."

Those are parental responses from just three of the eighty-three compensated children. The study authors also asked, "Was your child's claim resolved fairly?" One family responded, "No, it was a war." Another noted, "The attorney for the government was absolutely horrible. She was cold, insulting, and did whatever she could to keep us from getting compensated."

Keep in mind that these eighty-three cases were a fraction of compensated cases, the majority of which remain sealed and confidential to this day. There could be hundreds more; we just don't know. Discussing this report in their book *Vaccine Injuries*, the aforementioned Lou Conte and Tony Lyons explained that "despite requests filed under the Freedom of Information Act, the government blocked investigative access to the vast majority of cases."[33] Conte and Lyons also reached out to former vaccine court employees and reported on those findings:

> One retired employee stated emphatically that the development of autism in the presence of severe encephalopathy was understood by those in the program on both sides of the bar. . . . Another retired employee also confirmed that autism was seen as an indication of brain damage in vaccine injury.

A Bombshell Report

The study spearheaded by Ms. Holland and Mr. Conte was front-page news. Published in the spring of 2011 in the *Pace Environmental Law Review*, "Unanswered Questions from the Vaccine Injury Compensation Program: A Review of Compensated Cases of Vaccine-Induced Brain Injury" challenged the legitimacy of the vaccine court and showed that the courts had found, at least eighty-three times, that the medical standard for vaccines causing autism had been met. One report excerpt explained:

It is notable that over a twenty-year period the VICP did not publicly acknowledge an apparent vaccine-encephalopathy-autism link. While in the early years of the program there might have been no particular attention to this association, certainly by the late 1990's, the question of vaccine injury and autism was one of general public interest. The findings of so many cases of autism among compensated cases calls into question HHS's assertions on the topic.

Fox News broke the "bombshell report" on their May 16, 2011, nightly news broadcast. Lead reporter Alisyn Camerota noted that "the Feds have been quietly compensating children injured by vaccines; these are children who have autism. All of this despite the public denials."[34] Ms. Camerota explained she had interviewed one of the compensated parents, who told Fox News she had been told to stay quiet and that she feared losing the annuity she received from the government for her child's vaccine injury by publicly commenting. Ms. Camerota explained that the federal government had issued a statement in response to the study, affirming that vaccines don't cause autism. Finally, Ms. Holland appeared on screen and issued an eloquent rebuke of the federal government's public position:

Remember that these case decisions that were compensated by the federal government were based on science. They had ample scientific and medical evidence before them. We rely on the fact that the government used the best science available to decide that these were cases of vaccine injury. What we've added to this debate, Alisyn, is that these kids have autism. In addition, there are an awful lot of kids whose families allege that they have autism and when they use that word, they didn't get compensation.

Many of the families of the eighty-three children joined Ms. Holland and her coauthors in a public press conference on the steps of the vaccine court. They demanded a congressional investigation. They said the vaccine court isn't working. They explained the vaccine court's "dirty secret," that children with vaccine-induced autism are routinely compensated, meeting the vaccine court's high hurdle for proof, so long as they avoid the word *autism.* It was a bombshell, the kind of study published in a peer-reviewed law journal that on perhaps any other topic would produce an immediate congressional investigation, like the Flint drinking water crisis in 2016. Except it didn't.

The Congressional Hearing That Almost Happened

In November 2013 the House of Representatives Oversight and Government Reform Committee's chairman, Representative Darrell Issa (R-CA) announced his committee's plans to hold a hearing about the National Vaccine Injury Compensation Program.[35] The pharmaceutical industry attacked the hearing with all its resources. Every Child By Two, a vaccine industry-funded advocacy group, circulated a letter to all members of Congress deriding the need for hearings.[36] Amy Pisani, director of Every Child By Two, asserted that the activists pushing for a hearing "have a long history of claiming that vaccines cause autism" and that "to dismantle the National Vaccine Injury Compensation Program in order to appease fringe groups that have had their day in court would be a great disservice to public health."

Had parents ever gotten their day in court? Mr. Hazlehurst, in his memo to the Government Reform committee, didn't think so. "In 1986, the United States Congress took away the American citizens' right to legitimately question vaccine safety in a court of law. Two of the most fundamental rights of an American, the right to a trial by jury and a trial under the rules of law were taken away," he wrote in his memo. "The Vaccine Act created a vaccine program which is an invitation for abuse of power. The Zimmerman issue [Dr. Zimmerman, his testimony sealed in the Hannah Poling case] is but one of many deeply disturbing actions which have occurred in the vaccine program. The actions of the United States Department of Health and Human Services and the United States Department of Justice during the Omnibus Autism Proceeding warrant an investigation by the Congress of the United States."

Despite the alarming and compelling evidence that the vaccine court was burying cases of vaccine-induced autism, Representative Issa blinked and "postponed" the 2013 scheduled hearing. Mr. Conte assessed the delay for the *Age of Autism* blog:

> *The staffers [in the US Congress] that said that the hearing was postponed because this issue is so divisive were right. The hearing*

on the NVICP would have re-ignited the vaccine injury–autism controversy right smack in the middle of a Congress already beset with conflicts. Taking on the powerful pharmaceutical industry AND the federal public health establishment would be a daunting task. But the autism problem won't go away. It is certainly reasonable to believe that the passage of the 1986 Vaccine Act that started the NVICP also triggered the autism epidemic. Autism and the NVICP are intertwined and the program will never be viable until it opens the books and finally discloses the truth of vaccine injury.[37]

As of the writing of this book, the hearings have never happened. But that's not where the story ends.

After the Omnibus loss, Rolf Hazlehurst reached out to Dr. Zimmerman. Remember that after the Polings's settlement, Dr. Zimmerman was effectively uninvited from serving as an expert witness in vaccine court. He was never part of the actual Omnibus Autism Proceeding (beyond a memo he had written earlier), and he never had a chance to form an opinion about Yates Hazlehurst.

Long before the Omnibus proceedings, in the early 2000s, however, Yates had been a patient at Kennedy Krieger. Dr. Zimmerman's team had learned many things in the ensuing years, and he was more than happy to look at Yates's medical records again with this new knowledge. What Dr. Zimmerman and his team found was a child who looked very much like Hannah Poling. The doctors found that Yates's test results showed that he, too, had a mitochondrial disorder that led to his regressive autism, and Dr. Zimmerman said he would share that opinion with anyone who asked. Dr. Richard Kelley reached the same conclusions independently and also told the Hazlehurst family he'd be happy to support Yates.

As of the writing of this chapter (in mid-2018), Drs. Andrew Zimmerman and Richard Kelley are scheduled to testify in September in a civil suit brought on by the Hazlehurst family against the doctor who vaccinated Yates. Because they will be in a normal, open courtroom, we will all have the opportunity to hear from these experts when they take the witness stand.

For now, I'm one of a handful of people in the world who has copies of the depositions of Drs. Zimmerman[38] and Kelley[39]. So I know—and soon you will, too—that these depositions confirm their opinions that Yates Hazlehurst—remember, one of the original test case children in the OAP—had the same mitochondrial deficit that Hannah Poling had, and that vaccines caused his autism.

Had this information been in play back in 2009, the outcome of the OAP, and the current state of the autism epidemic, would be very different. The professional opinions of two of the most respected autism scientists (and, according to them, many of their colleagues) in the world affirm the whole point of this book: Vaccines can, and do, cause autism.

My biggest fear is that Yates's case will be settled before it goes to trial. I won't begrudge the Hazlehurst family, of course; they need money to care for Yates, who is nearly an adult now, and a settlement would mean money for Yates. But I'm hoping to see the vaccine-autism connection on trial, in a real courtroom, with Drs. Zimmerman and Kelley on the stand, telling the truth, in front of a real jury, with the same legal standard every drug is held to, except for vaccines. It could—it *should*—change this entire debate forever.

In a way, though, the trial itself doesn't really matter. The two doctors have already been deposed. They've said what they've said. The trial doesn't change any of that. We have their words, under oath, forever now. For that I'm grateful.

A Landmark Case: Yates Hazlehurst

Yates Hazlehurst had a horrible reaction to his vaccines when he was six months old. His pediatrician should have identified Yates as a child who should never be vaccinated again. Instead, he was given a full load of vaccinations at twelve months of age, while sick and taking antibiotics, and he regressed into autism. Furthermore, Yates's pediatricians never informed the Hazlehurst family of the possible risks of vaccines, which is their responsibility. Without "informed consent" you have medical malpractice.

Those are the allegations from his father, Rolf, an assistant district attorney in the state of Tennessee. He's suing Yates's former pediatricians at the Jackson Clinic in Jackson, Tennessee, for medical malpractice. Because of the convoluted rules of the vaccine court, this is the first time in thirty years a vaccine injury case will be presented in a normal courtroom, and it's also the first time the question of whether vaccines cause autism will be litigated in front of a jury. Mr. Hazlehurst, a skilled prosecutor, has been navigating his son's case now for seventeen years and had to meet every complex hurdle of vaccine court before he could file a lawsuit in "open court." It's literally the only case in the world.

Yates's case already made national news in late 2016 when the Hazlehursts' attorney, Bryan Smith, in preparing for the trial, subpoenaed Dr. William Thompson, the CDC scientist-turned-whistle-blower who confessed to the falsification of a 2004 study he coauthored denying a link between MMR vaccine and autism (discussed in chapter 3).[40] Dr. Thomas Friedan, at the time head of the CDC, successfully blocked Dr. Thompson from testifying, claiming in a letter to Mr. Smith, "Dr. William Thompson's deposition testimony would not substantially promote the objectives of CDC or HHS [Health and Human Services]."[41]

I can only imagine how alarmed the Jackson Clinic's defense team must have felt when they learned that Zimmerman and Kelley had agreed to testify as expert witnesses. As standard practice, the opposing counsel (along with Mr. Hazlehurst's attorney) were given the opportunity to depose both Dr. Zimmerman and Dr. Kelley, which they did in late 2016. What follows are some of the more astonishing highlights from those two depositions.[42]

As an autism activist for more than a dozen years, reading these comments from two of the most respected autism scientists in the world gave me a huge boost of hope that the autism epidemic may actually be closer to ending than most people think. Read on: I'll do my best to put all of their comments in proper context along the way.

Dr. Zimmerman on What Happened to Yates Hazlehurst

Lawyer: As succinctly as you can tell me, describe the opinions that you hold in this case.

Dr. Zimmerman: My opinion is that—that the Yates child—Yates Hazlehurst had a regressive onset of autism following administration of vaccines and at the same time he had an ear infection, both of which—both factors created inflammation and within 12 to 14 days after the immunization he began regressing. I saw Yates some years later in Baltimore County Krieger Institute and did some testing to look for signs of mitochondrial dysfunction. And these were later evaluated by Dr. Richard Kelley. And subsequently I did not see Yates for follow-up but learned that he was found to have a mitochondrial disorder. And it is my opinion that it is the underlying mitochondrial disorder that created the susceptibility factor in Yates that led to his autistic regression and change in brain function.

One of the three test cases from the OAP, Yates Hazlehurst, has the same diagnosis as Hannah Poling. Again, if this had been known at the time, we might have seen much faster progress in ending the autism epidemic.

Dr. Kelley on the Percentage of Kids Who Have Autism Based on Mitochondrial Dysfunction

Lawyer: Would you say that you are an expert in mitochondrial dysfunction but not in autism? Would that be a fair way to describe it?

Dr. Kelley: I am an expert in mitochondrial disease. And I am an expert in the aspect of autism that pertains to the roughly 25, 30, 40 percent of children who have autism based on mitochondrial dysfunction.

The leading expert in the country just said that between 25 and 40 percent of children with autism have mitochondrial dysfunction. So now we know that Hannah Poling and Yates Hazlehurst's cases are not rare. Writing in the *Atlanta Journal-Constitution* back in 2008, Dr. Jon Poling made this point:

> *Emerging evidence suggests that mitochondrial dysfunction may not be rare at all among children with autism. . . . In fact, mitochondrial dysfunction may be the most common medical condition associated with autism. . . . National public health leaders, including those at CDC, must now recognize the paradigm shift caused by this biological marker with regard to their current position of dispelling a vaccine-autism link. In light of the Hannah Poling concession, science must determine more precisely how large the mitochondrial autism subpopulation is.*[43]

Dr. Zimmerman on His Colleagues and the Poling Case

Lawyer: Do other people in your field, reputable physicians in your field, hold the opinion that vaccines can cause the type of inflammatory response that can lead to a regressive autism?

Dr. Zimmerman: Yes.

Lawyer: And you have been involved and testified in cases in the vaccine court?

Dr. Zimmerman: Yes.

Lawyer: And that theory has been accepted by the vaccine court in certain cases that have led to compensation of children who were injured as a result of a vaccine?

Dr. Zimmerman: The only one I'm aware of who was compensated was Poling, and I don't believe that actually went to court.

Lawyer: But actually the same theory that you have in this case was the same theory generally that you had in Poling?

Dr. Zimmerman: Correct.

Lawyer: And it's your understanding that Poling did receive compensation from the vaccine compensation program for a vaccine-related injury that led to autism?

Dr. Zimmerman: Yes.

Can we just pause right here? Dr. Andrew Zimmerman, scientific titan in the field of autism and at the time a neurologist at Harvard Medical School, confirmed that his colleagues—reputable physicians in his field—share the opinion that vaccines can cause autism.

As it relates to Hannah Poling's case, Dr. Zimmerman confirms that she was awarded compensation because vaccines caused her autism without any of the CDC's qualifications about her case being "exceptionally rare."

Dr. Zimmerman on Vaccines, Inflammation, and Regression

Lawyer: There can be some type of triggering inflammatory response that can cause or lead to regressive autism?

Dr. Zimmerman: Correct.

Lawyer: And that science is accepted by the people in your field?

Dr. Zimmerman: Yes.

Lawyer: Other reputable physicians in your field?

Dr. Zimmerman: Right. People who work in the field of autism see, commonly see a relationship between infection, inflammation, and onset of regression.

Lawyer: And vaccines can cause the type of inflammatory response, in fact they're designed to—to cause the type of inflammatory response that can lead to or trigger a regressive autism?

Dr. Zimmerman: They're designed to lead to an immune response, and that may compound the immune response from an infection.

Lawyer: So in other words, kids who have this underlying mitochondrial disorder who are—have an ongoing infection are at an even higher risk of an injury from the vaccine?

Dr. Zimmerman: When combined, yes.

Lawyer: And as I understand it, sort of the key period or where a child's brain is more at risk for these types of, or is more susceptible to these types of risk is somewhere around a year to 18 months?

Dr. Zimmerman: Or 24 months, in that area.

I need to make an important point. Dr. Zimmerman is a clinician. He sees children with autism every day. He diagnoses them, and he tries to help them get better. The "inflammatory response" he's talking about is the "immune activation event" Dr. Patterson from Caltech discovered. Dr. Patterson was a neuroscientist and a developmental biologist. They are using slightly different words, and looking through a slightly different lens, to describe the exact same phenomenon. Neurotoxicologists, another kind of scientist, study things like aluminum and macrophages to explain why immune activation events happen. The lenses are slightly different for these different kinds of scientists, but the stories all line up.

What Dr. Zimmerman confirms is that the leading scientists understand that immune activation events lead to autism. The only question left is how often those immune activation events are triggered by vaccines. Some of the time, most of the time, or all the time?

Dr. Zimmerman on Epidemiology at CDC and Prevention

Lawyer: How about the Centers for Disease Control? Its position is vaccines do not cause autism?

Dr. Zimmerman: Correct.

Lawyer: And [the CDC] is well respected?

Dr. Zimmerman: Of course.

Lawyer: And they do sound research and reach conclusions that are scientifically valid and sound in your judgment?

Dr. Zimmerman: Based on epidemiological studies in the past, but I think we are in a new era when a lot of research is being done now that helps us to understand the underlying metabolic basis of autism, and I think this is going to change our approach to the problem.

Lawyer: But that hasn't happened yet, has it?

Dr. Zimmerman: It hasn't reached the epidemiological level at this point. We are in the midst of active research in this area and this is—I don't expect that it's going to change the overall picture of immunizations, but I expect that it is going to change the way we approach the problem.

Lawyer: Meaning what?

Dr. Zimmerman: Once we have the biomarkers for the patients who have susceptibility of regression following immunizations, it will change our approach to—to treatment of the children, to identify the children who are at risk.

Lawyer: So in your opinion, looking forward is, what you contemplate will happen, the change you see is the treatment of autistic children?

Dr. Zimmerman: I think it will change the treatment, but more importantly I think it will prevent the development of autism in quite a few children. Currently about 30 percent of children with autism undergo regression, and we would like very much to understand the metabolic basis for that and how we can prevent it.

This is slightly confusing, and so important. What Dr. Zimmerman is saying is that the CDC's epidemiological studies lack the statistical power to find the vaccine-autism connection. I wish Dr. Zimmerman was better versed in the extreme inadequacy of these studies. He doesn't point out that only one vaccine (MMR) and one ingredient (thimerosal) have ever even been studied (see chapter 3), but what he does do is basically explain that no, the CDC isn't "lying" when they say vaccines don't cause autism; they're just basing their conclusions on studies that aren't designed to find a connection. Moreover, Dr. Zimmerman explains that the science continues to evolve and that the CDC's positions are outdated by the new science that he's seeing.

Dr. Zimmerman also makes one heartening comment and one explosive comment. He says the science is moving to identify children who may be at risk of regressing into autism if they are vaccinated, so that these children can be protected ahead of time. Also, he implies that perhaps 30 percent of children with autism have the same profile as Hannah Poling and Yates Hazlehurst—not exactly rare.

Dr. Kelley Exposes the AAP and CDC Doublespeak

Lawyer: Do you agree with the statement that vaccines do not cause autism?
Dr. Kelley: No.

Lawyer: Is it generally accepted in the medical community that vaccines do not cause autism?
Dr. Kelley: It is a common opinion.

Lawyer: It is generally accepted in the medical field that vaccines do not cause autism?
Dr. Kelley: I have no basis to judge that. It is most often when physicians are commenting on that they say there is no proven association.

Lawyer: Do you know the position of the American Academy of Pediatrics about any link between vaccines and autism?
Dr. Kelley: Yes. They also say there is no proven association.

Lawyer: Do you agree with the position of the American Academy of Pediatrics?

Dr. Kelley: I agree with their position as a public health measure. I don't agree with it scientifically.

Lawyer: You are actually arguing for a link between vaccines and autism in this case, aren't you?

Dr. Kelley: I am.

Lawyer: And that is contrary to the medical literature, isn't it?

Dr. Kelley: It's not contrary to the medical literature that I read. It is contrary to certain published articles by very authoritative groups who say there is no proven association in large cohort studies.

Lawyer: Your opinion is contrary to, say, the opinion of the CDC, correct?

Dr. Kelley: It is contrary to their conclusion. It is not contrary to their data.

My favorite quote here is, "It is contrary to their conclusion. It is not contrary to their data." He's making the point that the CDC does its best to frame its studies' conclusions in a certain way—which is always that vaccines are safe and effective—even if the data doesn't actually support it. Dr. Kelley, unfortunately, seems to think this dishonesty is justified as a "public health measure." I couldn't disagree more and will discuss this below.

Dr. Zimmerman on the AAP's Position on Vaccines and Autism

Lawyer: Tell me if you can identify this page, Doctor.

Dr. Zimmerman: This is from the American Academy of Pediatrics on vaccine safety.

Lawyer: And then down in the next paragraph it says, "Research has been conducted on all these topics, and the studies continue to find vaccines to be a safe and effective way to prevent serious diseases." Did I read [this] correctly?

Dr. Zimmerman: Yes.

Lawyer: And then it says here, "These studies do not show any link between autism and MMR, thimerosal, multiple vaccines given at once, fevers, or seizures. Did I read that correctly?

Dr. Zimmerman: Yes.

Lawyer: And you agree with that, right?

Dr. Zimmerman: Yes, with the exception that these are epidemiological studies and do not incorporate our new knowledge at this point.

This is the same point Dr. Kelley just made about the position the CDC has on vaccines and autism. He's not saying the CDC or AAP (of which he is a member) are lying when they say, "Vaccines do not cause autism." He's saying they are relying on flawed and outdated science.

Dr. Kelley on the CDC and Dr. William Thompson

Lawyer: Is it your position that the Centers for Disease Control is somehow engaged in some kind of fraud with regard to its position on vaccines and autism?

Dr. Kelley: That has been reported. Dr. Thompson, a whistleblower, has said that.

Lawyer: I'm interested in whether you are going to take that position and express that view that the Centers for Disease Control is somehow guilty of fraud?

Dr. Kelley: I don't have an opinion to say. They are clever in how they publish data to avoid public attention that there is an association. But I can understand why they did that. That is a bit of a cover-up. But it was done for a good reason, so to speak.

Okay, this drives me crazy. One of the things you see in the depositions of both Dr. Kelley and Dr. Zimmerman is that they really try to toe the line that vaccines are generally "safe and effective" and most children should get them. Dr. Kelley appears to be giving CDC a hall pass for playing with data, since it was "done for a good reason." The implication is that there is no reason good enough to risk the vaccine program. Ever. Even when autism is nearing 3 percent of our children. This is madness.

I appreciate that Dr. Kelley acknowledges that Dr. William Thompson, a CDC scientist-turned-whistle-blower, did allege fraud at CDC, but trust will keep eroding until public health officials tell the truth about the vaccine-autism connection.

Dr. Zimmerman on Children He Sees at Harvard

Lawyer: You actually see children in your clinic daily, weekly, with autism that has resulted from an underlying mitochondrial disorder?

Dr. Zimmerman: Yes.

Lawyer: And when you see those children, you go about trying to figure out what may have been the triggering event or the causative event of the regressive autism?

Dr. Zimmerman: Yes.

Lawyer: And in your practice you look at vaccines as one potential cause for a regressive autism in a child—for children like Yates?

Dr. Zimmerman: Potential, yes. And then we—we're trying very hard to treat them.

Dr. Zimmerman confirms that vaccines are on the table as a possible cause of autism for all the children whom he sees. I also want to point out that in reading Dr. Zimmerman's entire deposition, I really saw his humanity, and his honesty. He sees these children every day. Unlike *NeuroTribes'* Steven Silberman, Dr. Zimmerman isn't romanticizing autism; he knows how devastating a disability it is, for the affected kids and their families. It's clear he wants to help these children recover, and to prevent children from developing regressive autism in the first place.

Dr. Zimmerman on Epidemiological Studies versus Clinical Observations

Lawyer: There is a difference between determining a causative link between, say, vaccines and regressive autism and epidemiological studies versus making a connection for a particular patient in a clinical setting?

Dr. Zimmerman: Very different approach.

Lawyer: Can you explain that a little bit?

Dr. Zimmerman: Well, an epidemiological study looks at a large group, but it may not be able to detect a small subgroup. And what we're really looking at is a different approach where we go—we start not from the large group but from the individual.

I'm reminded here of a quote from the late Dr. Bernadine Healy, who used to run the prestigious National Institutes of Health. During the Hannah Poling media frenzy, Dr. Healy stood up and told the truth, and she was roundly criticized for it (of course) and labeled an "anti-vaxxer." What she said back in 2008 sounds just like what Dr. Zimmerman said:

> *This is the time when we do have the opportunity to understand whether or not there are susceptible children, perhaps genetically, perhaps they have a metabolic issue, mitochondrial disorder, immunulogical issue, that makes them more susceptible to vaccines plural, or to one particular vaccine, or to a component of vaccine, like mercury. So we now, in these times, have to, I think, take another look at that hypothesis; not deny it. And I think we have the tools today that we didn't have ten years ago, that we didn't have twenty years ago, to try and tease that out and find out if indeed there is that susceptible group. Why is this important? A susceptible group does not mean that vaccines are not good. What a susceptible group will tell us is that maybe there is a group of individuals, or a group of children, that shouldn't have a particular vaccine or shouldn't have vaccine on the same schedule. I do not believe that if we identified a susceptibility group, if we identified a particular risk factor for vaccines, or if we found out that maybe they should be spread out a little longer, I do not believe the public would lose faith in vaccines.*[44]

Dr. Healy offered up so much common sense, and Dr. Zimmerman just said the same thing—there may be children who are more vulnerable to vaccines. Let's figure out who they are before they get vaccinated.

Dr. Kelley on the Risks of Multiple Vaccines at Once

Lawyer: You said you can't identify the specific vaccine that triggered, that led to the regressive autism, but the set of vaccines were the trigger?

Dr. Kelley: That is correct. In the sense that each vaccine creates some degree of inflammation. And one would interpret the events that there was a sufficient inflammatory event from the vaccinations all together that caused the deterioration. If one gave those vaccines individually over a period of a couple weeks, then it might not have been any event. It's the summation of the inflammatory response.

I couldn't believe this exchange. The CDC and AAP have statements on their websites reassuring parents that multiple vaccines in one visit are perfectly safe, and here's a leading autism doctor saying the opposite. Here's a quote provided by the AAP:

> Current studies do not support the hypothesis that multiple vaccines overwhelm, weaken, or "use up" the immune system. On the contrary, young infants have an enormous capacity to respond to multiple vaccines, as well as to the many other challenges present in the environment.[45]

Dr. Zimmerman on the Omnibus Autism Proceeding

Lawyer: It's my understanding that you had written a report in that case [test case for Michelle Cedillo] and were set to testify but then were pulled by the US government after you told them that you believe that there were exceptions to the general rule?

Dr. Zimmerman: I don't know if there was a connection between the two events, but that's the way it happened temporally.

Lawyer: In other words, you told them that you felt that there were exceptions like Yates Hazlehurst and Hannah Poling, and other people that actually did have an injury due to vaccines and then after that you were pulled out of the case. Is that true?

Dr. Zimmerman: That's the way it happened, yes. . . . And the reason I believe that I was not called to testify in the Cedillo case was that I told them that I think there are rare exceptions, like Poling, and therefore I was not asked to testify.

It's pretty clear what happened. Rather than face the implications of Dr. Zimmerman's evolved understanding of the vaccine-autism link, they sent him packing but were more than happy to use his written testimony for their purposes. I'm not a lawyer, but if some or all of that isn't fraud, then I don't know what is. It's a firm reminder that the vaccine court's purpose is to protect the vaccine program, not end the autism epidemic.

My Thoughts about These Two Depositions

The two depositions total more than 250 pages, and I've now read them several times. These are such important historical documents that I believe they will contribute to the end of the autism epidemic, and I have so many comments to make. First, I just want to say that I'm grateful to Drs. Zimmerman and Kelley for being honest, and for their willingness to let their comments be recorded for posterity. They both confirm that vaccines can trigger autism in certain vulnerable children. It's really now just a matter of how many. Here's what really struck me:

My book could just be this one chapter. If you still think all the hundreds of thousands of parents screaming that vaccines caused their kid's autism are just flat-earthers, or tinfoil hat wearers, or just looking for someone to blame, I can no longer help you. I just showed you the words—provided under oath—of two of the leading autism scientists in the world who were both key expert witnesses for the vaccine court's lawyers, and they've just told you the truth and also said that many of their colleagues feel the same way. Vaccines cause autism in some kids. Period. Full stop. We're just left to figure out how many kids.

They treat regressive autism like a binary event. Their view seems to be that vaccines tip some children into regressive autism, while other kids are spared. It's sort of like they view it as a dodged bullet—it either lodges in your body or misses you completely, creating two stark outcomes. But that's not actually what happens. We know vaccines also cause autoimmunity and many other issues in the body. And, what about all the other neurological disorders that are epidemic in kids? Perhaps a mild reaction to all these vaccines manifests as ADHD, anxiety, or a learning disability? They don't see those kids in their clinics. They see autism. What if it's not black and white? What if there's severe injury or mild injury, but never no injury at all? Something that can trigger a disability as devastating as autism could well be responsible for smaller conditions, too, like a tornado that uproots some trees but can also pick up and move a house if the circumstances are right. In my estimation, a kid with eczema, a learning disability, and a deadly peanut allergy is also vaccine injured, just in a different way. If vaccines can push some kids into autism, as Drs. Zimmerman and Kelley clearly believe they can, doesn't that open the door for everything else?

They're unwilling to consider that the original "mitochondrial dysfunction" might also be caused by vaccines. Before Dr. Jon Poling disappeared from the public, I had the chance to talk with him a few times, back in 2008. He made it clear that he'd never know if Hannah's mitochondrial issues predated her first vaccines. Said differently, mitochondrial disorders may in fact be *caused* by the first vaccines a child receives, and then later rounds push them into autism. This is never discussed by Drs. Zimmerman and Kelley; perhaps it's just too big to consider.

Maybe some of the kids who don't have an obvious regression got tipped into autism much earlier in their lives, like after their two-month appointment rather than their twelve-month appointment. We really have no idea. They also never discuss maternal vaccines during gestation, even though that was Dr. Paul Patterson's original concern. What if a child "born with autism" is simply the victim of a vaccine the mother received?

Drs. Zimmerman and Kelley are not toxicologists. They don't understand things like the "biopersistence" of aluminum and the way it hangs out in the brain. They don't discuss the fact that it's the aluminum actually generating the inflammation, which is the whole purpose for aluminum, or that once it's done doing that it just sits there in the brain. That's not how they look at the world. They don't ever mention Dr. Pardo-Villamizar's work that found autism brains in a simmering, permanent state of inflammation. Aluminum has so many downstream consequences for the body.

This is one of the limitations of dealing with the scientific community that I find frustrating. People like Dr. Christopher Exley and Dr. Christopher Shaw don't spend time with people like Dr. Zimmerman to create a more holistic view of how autism is being created. We now know that the tiny injections of aluminum, given time and again, can be devastating to the developing brain. Dr. Kelley, in particular, is really focused on what happens during the twelve-month vaccine appointments, but for most American children, that's actually their fifth vaccine appointment (birth, two-month, four-month, six-month are the first four). What if a child is already suffering from previous toxicity? It's just not something they are looking at.

Drs. Zimmerman and Kelley really try to remain steadfastly pro-vaccine. I'm frustrated by this. Dr. Kelley even gives his patients an anti-inflammatory (montelukast) before he vaccinates them, if he thinks they are "at risk." He believes this reduces the likelihood the at-risk child will tip into autism. He's basically using a pharmaceutical drug to suppress an immune activation event for a medical procedure whose purpose is immune activation. Doesn't that seem a little crazy?

They never mention delaying vaccines, spacing them out, or not giving some of the less important vaccines, like hep B, influenza, varicella, or rotavirus. They are trying very hard to tow the party line; all of their ideas are for how to identify vulnerable kids prior to vaccination. This is a noble pursuit, for sure, and I applaud it, but I think you need to come at this problem from both sides: Identify the vulnerable children, and make the vaccine schedule way, way safer, and smaller. This is a topic they clearly will not touch.

Dr. Kelley makes a revealing comment when he mentions a special master (of the vaccine court) who was very concerned about any inference at all that vaccines could cause autism, because of the effect the message could have on parental behavior. Who needs truth when you have a vaccine program to implement? I'm even more disturbed by Dr. Kelley's comments about how the CDC misrepresents the data for "public health reasons" so that makes it okay. No, it doesn't. Lying is lying, and when the truth finally seeps out, as it's doing, the destroyed trust will be far more difficult to repair.

They never criticize the narrowness of the studies CDC, AAP, and IOM rely on to declare "vaccines don't cause autism." Both doctors clarify that the conclusions of CDC, AAP, and IOM are based on large-scale epidemiology that wouldn't find a vulnerable subset of children, because large-scale studies typically miss these kids. But they never mention that these studies also only looked at a single vaccine (MMR) and a single ingredient (thimerosal). They perpetuate the myth that vaccines and autism have been studied, when they really haven't been. Given their training, expertise, experience, authority, and power, I hold them—I think quite reasonably—to a higher standard to understand the science. **Finally, we really have no idea how many of the children with autism got that way due to their vaccines.** I've heard that 50 percent or more of autism parents blame vaccines. My son's story is almost exactly like the stories of Yates Hazlehurst and Hannah Poling. Ear infections, illness, antibiotics, and obvious vaccine reactions kept happening to him until he finally disappeared. My pediatricians were every bit as careless as the ones at the Jackson Clinic. The thing is, most of the autism parents I know, and I know a lot, have the same story. Not all, but certainly most—thousands of parents I've heard from directly.

The thing I do is, I turn back the clock to the old autism numbers. I look at the one in ten thousand number from Wisconsin in the 1970s that was so accurately and thoroughly derived. Where the hell have all these kids come from, and why do so many parents blame vaccines? One in thirty-six kids is insanity. "Vaccines" is far and away the most biologically plausible explanation for what has happened. There is no such thing as a genetic epidemic, and the few studies of 100 percent unvaccinated kids show dramatically lower numbers of neurological disorders. It adds up. It's not *if* vaccines cause autism, it's *how many* of the cases? And therefore, how many cases do we know we can prevent? Dr. Kelley actually helps us here. He at least estimates that 25 to 50 percent of kids with autism have mitochondrial dysfunction, which means all those kids are at risk for vaccine-induced regression. As I said earlier, the way these two doctors look at the world misses many kids who are injured by vaccine in year one of their lives, so I think the number is far higher than 50 percent of kids with autism who got it because of vaccines, but no one knows for sure.

Even with my criticisms, I consider these two doctors to be heroes who have taken extraordinary risk by telling the truth. I've asked Rolf Hazlehurst this question, "How the hell can these guys be helping you? Don't they realize how serious this is? How much they could destroy their careers? A 'Wakefielding' is surely headed their way soon, no?" Rolf thinks they are high-integrity scientists and that when asked, they tell the truth. They go where the facts take them. And they have empathy. They see kids with autism every day. Autism is not a mild disability. They want to prevent kids from regressing into autism. The only way they can do that is by telling the truth about what is causing at least some of the cases. Rolf also thinks age is an issue, with both scientists in their 70s. Regarding Dr. Zimmerman, Rolf tells me, "I think he wants to set the record straight before he dies."

CHAPTER 7

The Critical Mass of Parents All Saying the Same Thing

Here's the key lesson that I learned, which applies to all pediatricians: Listen to parents. It is a basic tenet of being a pediatrician. Little children and those with significant developmental delays cannot speak for themselves. They cannot report what ails them. We must rely on those who know them well to offer their observations and interpretations of their children's behavior.

—Dr. Lisa Shulman, associate professor of pediatrics, Albert Einstein College of Medicine[1]

It's June 2017. The "Vaxxed Bus" rounds the bend and comes into view. I'm sitting in the outdoor patio of Kyra's Bakeshop, a popular gluten-free bakery in the heart of Lake Oswego, Oregon, an idyllic town just south of Portland. The giant black RV with the word "VAXXED" painted along the length of both sides in massive red and white letters looks like some kind of rebel assault vehicle, out of place in this well-to-do town where nothing bad ever seems to happen. The customers sitting near me suddenly look uneasy. And I transform before their eyes from a random, middle-aged dude to a member of the Rebel Alliance as I stand up and head out to the parking lot to greet the bus.

The Vaxxed Bus was the brainchild of an irrepressible British model turned autism mom named Polly Tommey. Polly and I, like many autism parents, are connected by our deep grief and passion for answers. She watched her son Billy descend into autism after a vaccine appointment, and she's endowed with the same reservoir of anger that propels me, too.

Polly's waving through the window as the bus pulls up. She's been on a multimonth tour, making her way across the country. The bus stops are often met by local press accounts of the "anti-vaccine" bus arriving to scare the populace, along with dozens of parents eager to tell their stories about how vaccines harmed their children and damaged their families.

I had first met Polly a year earlier in Seattle, when the documentary film *Vaxxed* was premiering across the country. *Vaxxed* details the confessions of a single CDC scientist, Dr. William Thompson, who became a federal whistle-blower when he admitted that a study he'd coauthored in 2004 assessing the relationship between the MMR and autism—diminishing the connection—had been falsified. He tells of scientists meeting in a private office at CDC headquarters to combine their data sources and destroy them. It's an ugly story, and it distills the autism fight down to its essence: corruption and lies hiding in plain sight, and public health authorities and doctors who continue marching, pretending as though nothing is wrong.

I traveled from my home in Oregon to Seattle at Polly's request, unprepared for the emotional upheaval I was about to experience. She knew of my activism and had invited me to sit on a Q&A panel following each screening over the course of a couple of days. I wasn't concerned about it. I've been immersed in this subject for years, I'm confident I know what I'm talking about, and I could anticipate the questions that would be asked by concerned parents (and maybe a few trolls). Maybe one of my answers, I thought, could save a child from the fate that befell my boy.

What unmoored me, however, was a tradition initiated by the *Vaxxed* team following each screening. As the lights came up after the first screening I attended and we panelists walked down the aisles for the Q&A, Polly made a request on her portable mic. "If you or a family member has been injured by a vaccine, please stand up." Easily half the audience rose, in quiet solidarity. Emotion flooded my head, throat, and heart. It was the same— the sheer number of people, the overwhelming emotion—following every screening. Polly, I realized, had already experienced this a few hundred times.

The Vaxxed Bus is now parked. It takes up a good portion of Kyra's parking lot, and I'm guessing this bus will be the talk of Lake Oswego for a few days. I've brought my son, Jamison, with me. He's fourteen. His autism prevents him from understanding the reasons for the bus that's just pulled up, or its relationship to him—his interest is much more focused on the kombucha and paleo muffin I just bought him. Polly hops off the bus, and we hug, happy to know the other is still fighting. The depth of our loyalty to the mission we share is an unspoken, and permanent, bond.

In another stroke of awareness-building brilliance, Polly has turned the Vaxxed Bus into a mobile shrine. The parent of every vaccine-injured child who has visited the bus has been given the opportunity to write his or her child's name, with a white paint pen, on the black bus. The collection of names is reminiscent of the Vietnam memorial in Washington, DC. Each name is numbered, and by the time it's my turn, there are more than four thousand. More than four thousand kids, each one memorialized. Each life altered. Each family devastated. I grab the pen. I write Jamison's name. It's emotional. It sucks. It's everywhere.

Dr. Bernard Rimland and DAN!

More than a decade earlier, I was part of another audience of parents who "stood up" at the request of autism pioneer Dr. Bernard Rimland. It was September 2004, and I was in San Diego for a "Defeat Autism Now!" conference, a semiannual event that started in 2001. DAN! was an organization of doctors who were treating autistic children biomedically through diet, nutrition, heavy metal removal, and immune system support, a topic I will discuss in more detail in chapter 10. Sadly, DAN! fizzled after Dr. Rimland's passing in 2006, but many of the former DAN! doctors continue to practice.

Bernie, as most autism parents affectionately called Dr. Rimland, stood at the front of the massive conference space, where more than a thousand parents listened intently, hoping for answers. This was a special DAN! conference, however: A news crew for the CBS show *60 Minutes* was following Dr. Rimland for a special about him, and the large conference space included several CBS cameras. Dr. Rimland addressed the packed house.

"Please, if you are the parent of an autistic child, please stand up."

At once, most of the people in the room rose. I stood and felt the waves of emotion as the scale of our shared pain hit me. At that point, I was very new to the autism community. My son had been diagnosed only a few months earlier.

"If your child is one of those who became autistic after receiving a vaccination and you believe it was the vaccine that caused your child's autism," Dr. Rimland continued, "please raise your hand."[2]

Practically every hand in the room went up.

"If you can document with videotapes or photographs or whatever that your child was normal and became autistic after the vaccine, wave your arms."

The whole room moved with waving arms, looking more like a rock concert than an autism conference.

Dr. Rimland chuckled, looking to the film crew, "Okay. Did you get that? Let's hope it gets on CBS."

The film of that moment can still be found on YouTube, frozen in time, perhaps to remind future generations how long the truth has been known. As you probably can guess, that scene didn't make it on to *60 Minutes*.

Hear This Well

CNN Senior Medical Correspondent Elizabeth Cohen is infamous among autism parents because of an August 2014 report she gave that included this line:

> *Vaccines are safe. Autism is not a side effect of autism. . . . Some people don't hear this well: Vaccines do not cause autism.*[3]

Ms. Cohen's condescension and dismissiveness, combined with what I would argue is a plain error, created the "Hear This Well" YouTube campaign. Parents of children with autism who had witnessed regression after vaccination were encouraged to make their own video lectures for Ms. Cohen, and to include the words "Hear This Well." Hundreds did.

An elderly father gave this heartbreaking account, holding up his son's baby picture:

> *This is my son. He was a normal baby. By the time he was eight months old he was well ahead of developmental expectations. He could walk and he could talk. . . . Then he got his shots. He could no longer crawl, let alone walk. He couldn't talk. Now he's in his bedroom, wearing a diaper. He's thirty-two years old. Vaccines do cause autism.*

A single father talked about his daughter:

> *She was born normal. When she was fifteen months old she received a round of vaccines. . . . She developed a high fever. . . . When the fever broke she lost everything. . . . We knew something was immediately wrong. . . . Vaccines destroyed my family, vaccines do cause autism, some people don't hear this too well.*

A young mother, her voice breaking:

> *My name's Mary. My daughter was typically developing until she suffered a vaccine injury at two years old and was subsequently diagnosed with autism. Some people choose to not hear this well; vaccines can and do cause autism.*

The videos overwhelm. Hundreds of parents. All saying the same thing. Honestly, I can't watch them all. It's too much. It's been thirteen years since Jamison's diagnosis. I've learned to bottle my pain. It sits, mostly untended, in the back of my brain. Mostly. It comes out once in a while, usually when I tell someone new about Jamison, about what happened to him. Sometimes it seeps out, but every once in a while it's a flood.

Just the other night, Jamison struck himself in the head, as hard as he could, with the back of his left hand. His hand swelled up, the size of a baseball, I was sure it was broken. He was in so much pain. He sat in the shower, trying to "wash off" the giant swelling. I lay on the bathroom floor near him and bawled my brains out, heaving sobs. Seeing him in pain, seeing him hit himself, seeing him not understand what his body was doing; it was just too much.

Then I got up, got dressed, and took him to the emergency room. Mercifully, it wasn't broken. If you're an autism parent, you're nodding, you understand. Shitty things happen, and you find a way to endure.

Can Parents Be Trusted?

Science has demonstrated that parents are accurate observers of their children's development. The most comprehensive review of parental reporting was published in 1999 in the *Journal of Paediatrics and Child Health*. Titled "The Value of Parents' Concerns to Detect and Address Developmental and Behavioural Problems," the study affirmed the accuracy of parental reporting about their child's development:

> *Parents, regardless of differences in education, socioeconomic status, and child-rearing experience, are able to raise concerns that accurately reflect children's developmental and behavioural status.*[4]

Yet parents are routinely second-guessed when they report their child's development regression after a vaccine appointment. In 2005 researchers at the University of Washington decided to test the autism regression phenomenon for themselves. In a study in *JAMA Psychiatry* titled, "Validation of the Phenomenon of Autistic Regression Using Home Videotapes," researchers viewed before and after video of children who had been developing normally and then regressed into autism, according to their parents. What did they find?

> *This study validates the existence of early autistic regression.*

The study's lead author, Dr. Geraldine Dawson, who later would lead the national organization Autism Speaks, also defended parental recollection, claiming her study "provides an important lesson that parents are good reporters on what is happening with their children. It underscores the importance of professionals to listen to parents." Yes, children regress into autism. Most parents I have met who witnessed a regression claim that happened immediately or soon after a vaccine appointment.

One Hell of a Coincidence

Katie Wright is gentle, warm, and polite. It's late fall, and I'm sitting in the kitchen of her family's sunny apartment on the Upper West Side of New York City. We're each holding a microphone, doing an interview for a new podcast show I've created. I surmise her manners are partly due to the influence of her father, Bob Wright, who was a high-ranking executive at General Electric when the company acquired NBC in 1986, putting Wright at the helm. During his tenure, Wright oversaw NBC's magical run at the top of the TV universe with shows like *Seinfeld* and *Cheers*, before the internet changed everything.

When Katie's son Christian regressed into autism, her parents didn't just step in to help; they used the experience to create the largest national organization dedicated to autism, Autism Speaks, in 2005. Bob and Suzanne Wright became, for a time, the faces of autism benefactors, and they have the humanitarian awards on their mantel to prove it. More than ten years later, Autism Speaks has another claim to fame: They've presided over an increase in the autism epidemic from 1 in 150 children to today's 1 in 36, and they've offered no plausible explanation for where all this autism is coming from. Hundreds of millions of dollars have been wasted on genetic research with nothing to show for it. For a parent like me, Autism Speaks is the ultimate parasitic nonprofit organization, feeding off a relentless epidemic while offering no real solutions for how to resolve it.

It wasn't supposed to be like this. In 2006, soon after Autism Speaks was formed, I was part of a large meeting at Autism Speaks's headquarters in New York City. The subject? How to steer some of Autism Speaks's research dollars towards the growing chorus of parents pointing the finger at vaccines. I asked Bob Wright a pointed question, "Bob, do you think vaccines caused Christian's autism?" Bob's answer to me, an answer I will never forget: "I don't know, but it's one hell of a coincidence."

I learned later that Katie's mom, Suzanne (who passed away in 2017), would tell people privately that Christian had been developing normally, talking a ton, behaving like a normal child, "until those damn vaccines."

I ask Katie about this, about her mother privately blaming vaccines for causing Christian's autism, while presiding over an autism organization that won't touch the issue. More than ten years have passed since that meeting at Autism Speaks, and not a dime has been allocated to look at vaccines. If vaccines are the primary driver of the autism epidemic, Autism Speaks wouldn't know, because they haven't looked. How can this be?

Katie struggles to explain. She lets on that she hasn't discussed vaccines with her parents in years and that the scientific advisory board at Autism Speaks was hijacked by a former pharmaceutical executive looking to find an autism pill (he didn't). None of her explanations make me feel any better.

This is only part of the story, though. While Katie struggles to explain her parents' inability to steer Autism Speaks toward researching the truth about autism, Katie herself has been relentless. Despite extreme pressure by Autism Speaks to keep her feelings to herself, Katie has never shut up about the thing that matters most: what happened to Christian, her oldest son.

While Katie's mom chose to only discuss what vaccines did to Christian in private, Katie has been public from day one. In fact, Katie has been so public she was the subject of a 2007 hit piece in the *New York Times* titled, "Autism Debate Strains a Family and Its Charity" after Katie appeared on the *Oprah Winfrey Show* and "described how her talkative toddler turned unresponsive and out-of-control after his vaccines."[5]

I'm rereading the *New York Times* article from 2007. Katie hadn't heard of Hannah Poling yet. She didn't know about the eighty-three cases of autism in vaccine court. And she certainly knew nothing about the emerging science implicating aluminum adjuvant in the development of autism, since none of it had been published. What she had was her own experience, her own observations, and she chose to courageously stand up, despite extreme pressure to sit down.

Hollywood Speaks. Sometimes

Actor Aidan Quinn is also the father of a child with autism, and his red-carpet interview caught an Access Hollywood reporter off guard when he asked Mr. Quinn if "autism ran in the family." Mr. Quinn responded:

> *I don't know if it runs in the family; there's one person in the family with autism, my daughter, my oldest daughter has autism. After she had an extreme reaction to a vaccination . . . she was a normal child. . . . The debate is from billions of billions of dollars of drug company money. . . . You're allowed to put in vaccines what you're not allowed to put in that carpet . . . all to increase the profits of drug companies.*[6]

Football star Doug Flutie is also an autism parent. On *Larry King Live* in 2008, he made clear that he felt his son had declined into autism after his vaccines:

> *There's two different groups out there. There's those that are genetically—that they're born with it and those that develop it. And I think they're two different animals there that, throughout the years—and a lot of parents are looking at immunizations. . . . I feel like my son developed it at around age two-and-a-half to three. So I think there's two different groups out there.*[7]

Actress Holly Robinson Peete, the wife of football star Rodney Peete, was sitting next to Mr. Flutie and agreed with him:

> *But don't you think, Doug, that most people—most stories I have heard and Rodney—that we've heard through our journey with autism is that people did see those milestones and hitting them, and then they abruptly stopped. Almost every story I know is like that.*

Grammy-award winning singer Toni Braxton, appearing on the same show, chimed in to corroborate Ms. Peete:

> *But I noticed a big difference in my son when he got his vaccines. He just, over time, he just started decreasing in his ability to become—to develop as he should. My oldest son was quite different. I think with any medication you ingest and put into your body, there's going to be side effects. And I think it affects some differently. And in my case, I feel it definitely affected my toddler.*

In 2004 actor Gary Cole explained that his daughter had "a very severe reaction" to a DTP shot at eighteen months old. According to a *Contra Costa Times* article, "her face swelled so much that her eyes were nearly shut. A short time later, her speech and eye contact began to regress, he said. His daughter, now age 11, has been diagnosed with autism spectrum disorder."[8]

Years later, in 2016, actor Robert De Niro would make the news, asserting that he and his wife felt their son's autism had been triggered by vaccines.[9] And Jenny McCarthy wrote a book, *Louder Than Words*, about her son's descent into autism after a vaccine appointment.[10]

These are a few celebrity parents of children with autism who have chosen to publicly comment about their ordeal. There are also celebrity parents who have sought help from Generation Rescue to help recover their children but are too afraid, for a variety of reasons, to speak out.

It's not a short list of names. And they all blame vaccines.

Our Stories Are Everywhere

A young, attractive couple videotapes a "Hear This Well" message. The husband starts, "We have two boys. One was vaccinated on schedule and reacted for over 30 days to his twelve-month vaccines." The wife takes her turn, "The other was not."

The husband adds, "One was diagnosed with autism spectrum disorder and experienced OCD, rages, and tics." Back to his wife, "The other was not."

"Hear this well," says the husband. It's now the wife's turn to speak. She covers her mouth with her hand, overcome with emotion; "Vaccines do cause autism," she says, her voice breaking.

We're everywhere. Our stories are everywhere. What should we do now? What we should have done all along: Listen to the parents.

PART THREE

A Reckoning to End the Epidemic

CHAPTER 8

They Would Have Told Us

A concealed truth, that's all a lie is. Either by omission or commission we never do more than obscure. The truth stays in the undergrowth, waiting to be discovered.

—Josephine Hart

We must always take sides. Neutrality helps the oppressor, never the victim. Silence encourages the tormentor, never the tormented.

—Elie Wiesel

At approximately 10:30 a.m. on March 10, 2015, Robert F. Kennedy Jr. stepped off a small plane and onto the tarmac at McNary Field in Salem, Oregon, just minutes from Oregon's state capitol. "Bobby," as he is called by his friends, was arriving at my invitation, a last-minute surprise to, I hoped, kill a newly introduced bill that would make vaccinations mandatory for all of Oregon's school-age children. The legislation, Senate Bill 442, had been introduced by Democratic state senator Elizabeth Steiner Hayward (herself a family physician) with great fanfare—it was covered nationally by CBS News.

The word at the capitol for weeks had been that the bill was a train barreling down the tracks. Mandatory vaccination had become a new legislative push at the state level, with more than a dozen states planning to introduce bills to make vaccination exemptions—which had existed in every state except West Virginia and Mississippi—a thing of the past. Making vaccinations mandatory had become a part of the progressive liberal agenda, which meant states controlled by Democrats (like Oregon, my home state) were the easiest states to create early legislative wins. Of course, the same industry was behind all these state bills, with many legislators explaining to me that they'd been visited, time and again, by representatives of Merck. The state legislative plan was simple: Start with Oregon, add Washington, and then California will fall. Once three Western states pass legislation, the dominos will keep falling, or so the theory went.

Bobby Kennedy was about to put an end to all of that. He climbed into the passenger side of my SUV in the tiny parking lot at McNary Field, and we were off to the capitol. Bobby and I had never met in person, but we'd communicated many times over the years. When you are in this fight as an activist, you feel like a member of the Rebel Alliance, as journalist Dan Olmsted often called our community. Anyone fighting Big Pharma and their paid minions becomes like family.

We all make personal sacrifices to speak up and challenge conventional wisdom on a topic so controversial, but very few have paid a bigger price than Bobby Kennedy. He is the son of former attorney general and presidential candidate Robert F. Kennedy—before he was assassinated in 1968, when Bobby was 14—and the nephew of John F. Kennedy. Bobby Kennedy's political bloodline is as close to royalty as any you can find in the United States. Before he jumped into the vaccine fight, he had lived up to his family's name as a well-known and very public environmentalist, cofounding Waterkeeper Alliance, serving as senior attorney for the Natural Resources Defense Council, and teaching environmental law at Pace University, where he continues to serve as a professor emeritus.

Kennedy first caught the attention of the autism community at a conference called Autism One in May of 2013. In an impassioned session, he vowed to demand answers from CHOP's Dr. Paul Offit on use of thimerosal in vaccines and vaccine safety in general. His book, *Thimerosal: Let the Science Speak* exposed the dirty underbelly of the vaccine safety debate.[1] And it cost Kennedy dearly. Speaking out on vaccine safety, even while emphasizing that his own children were vaccinated, had the same grim professional and economic consequences experienced by others, including Andrew Wakefield and Jenny McCarthy. Many of Kennedy's colleagues began to slink away, trying to steer clear of a target on his back that keeps growing. Influential family members have called him privately, asking him to tone it down. And yet Bobby Kennedy persists, telling many privately that this is the biggest issue of our lifetime and he's not about to give up the fight.

Bobby and I caught up briefly in my car on the plan for the day ahead. He's a quick study, and artful with words, he nails all of his talking points within minutes. More than a dozen meetings had been scheduled with Oregon elected officials on both sides of the aisle. In general, Bobby's requests for meetings had been met warmly, with many identifying Bobby's father as one of their heroes.

For me the last few weeks had been a whirlwind. Like every newly intro-duced bill in Oregon, SB 442 had a public hearing on February 18, soon after the CBS News coverage, and I was one of many who chose to speak out against the bill in front of the Oregon Senate Health Committee. Over the course of a long afternoon at the state capitol, a political movement quietly formed among many of us opposing the bill. Three weeks later, as Bobby Kennedy was on his way to the capitol, our movement had a name—Oregonians for Medical Freedom—a paid lobbyist, an active board, and a membership approaching two thousand. We were bombarding our elected officials with daily emails about the dangers of SB 442, and Mr. Kennedy was our latest attempt to kill the bill before it had a chance to be put up for a vote.

Rebecca Tweed was standing in front of the capitol, awaiting our arrival. In her early thirties with a slight build and bright red hair, Ms. Tweed was not your average lobbyist: She was a vegan (pretty common in Oregon) but also a right-wing Republican (extremely uncommon). Ms. Tweed was also a highly effective lobbyist, well known at the capitol, and her hiring two weeks earlier to support our effort to kill SB 442 was probably greeted with groans by the bill's advocates, all Democrats. Now, in one of the many ironic twists of this fight, Ms. Tweed would be escorting a Kennedy through the state capitol, to try to kill legislation supported by the progressive left.

As I dropped Bobby off with Ms. Tweed on the capitol's steps, State Senator Tim Knopp approached us for a quick photo. Senator Knopp, a Republican and a member of the Oregon Senate Health Committee, had emerged as one of our most important legislative allies. With a family member injured by the MMR vaccine, and a general distrust of government interference in medical decisions, Senator Knopp was doing everything he could to support our efforts to kill SB 442. In fact, some of our most important meetings had been set up by Senator Knopp and his staff. He smiled proudly in the picture with Bobby Kennedy, and the three of them headed inside for a full day of meetings.

One day after Bobby Kennedy's visit to the capitol, the bill was dead. Dead! It had lost the support of many legislators, including a number of Democrats. Senator Elizabeth Steiner Hayward, the bill's original sponsor, remained defiant in defeat, a statement from her office reading:

> *She is disappointed that the conversations have largely revolved around who is right or wrong about science and the benefits vs. risk of vaccines, rather than about the health and well-being of Oregon's children.*[2]

What really happened? In meetings with legislators, Bobby Kennedy had been remarkably candid. Yes, vaccines reduce certain infectious diseases. But they cause real harm, too, and the agency tasked with monitoring vaccine safety, the Centers for Disease Control and Prevention, is a "cesspool of corruption." Taking away a parent's right to choose to have his or her child vaccinated would remove a critical check and balance for a medical procedure that still had many unanswered questions.

Don't do it, Bobby warned; don't give them that power. This is the worst environmental disaster I have ever seen, Bobby explained, and the legislators of Oregon listened; they walked away from the bill—in droves. Senator Knopp later told me he'd never seen anything like it, the day Bobby Kennedy came to the capitol; he'd never seen a bill die such a swift death. Of the dozen similar bills being introduced in other states, only California would end up making vaccines mandatory in 2015, and no states have succeeded since. I'm told the topic is "dead" in Salem and that no legislators want to revisit what happened in 2015.

Fast-forward two years, and a presentation by Patrick Johnson, assistant director inside the American Academy of Pediatrics' Department of Federal Affairs shows that the concerns about Robert F. Kennedy Jr.'s potential to be disruptive to the vaccine program have only grown.[3] Titled "Vaccine Challenges in a New Administration," Mr. Johnson's presentation dealt with two interrelated topics: (1) President Trump's public statements about the link between vaccines and autism, and (2) the apparent connection between the president and Bobby Kennedy, made public in a January 10,

2017, a meeting between Bobby and the president-elect at Trump Tower, aligning two of the least likely bedfellows. President Trump's tweets about vaccines and autism don't leave much to the imagination:

August 2012: Massive combined inoculations to small children is the cause for big increase in autism.

March 2014: Healthy young child goes to doctor, gets pumped with massive shot of many vaccines, doesn't feel good and changes—AUTISM. Many such cases!

September 2014: I am being proven right about vaccinations—the doctors lied. Save our children & their future.

Behind the scenes, stories emerged within the activist community that Donald Trump had borne witness to an employee's child regressing after vaccination. Soon after, in one of the Republican primary debates hosted by CNN during the campaign, candidate Trump provided more insight about his motivation for raising this issue:

> *But you take this little beautiful baby, and you pump—I mean, it looks just like it's meant for a horse, not for a child, and we've had so many instances, people that work for me . . . just the other day, two years old, two and a half years old, a child, a beautiful child went to have the vaccine, and came back, and a week later got a tremendous fever, got very, very sick, now is autistic.*[4]

Mr. Johnson's April 2017 presentation at the AAP's national convention had an alarmist tone, recounting every action of Robert F. Kennedy Jr and President Trump, including the reported news that President Trump had recently asked Bobby to chair a Vaccine Safety Commission. Mr. Johnson emphasized that a "coordinated response is crucial" and that he was meeting regularly with "pro-vaccine organizations to share information, coordinate strategy and messaging." Every time I look at the tagline at the bottom of each page of the AAP's presentation—"dedicated to the health of all children"—I feel my blood boil.

At the same time, President Trump appears to have lost his energy for the issue. From the beginning, his opinions about this topic were viewed as a mixed blessing by the autism community, given his divisive nature. Soon after meeting with Bobby Kennedy, President Trump backed away from autism. It's fair to wonder if President Trump will do anything to end the autism epidemic. I'm not convinced, despite what he witnessed.

In a special feature in the *British Medical Journal* (*BMJ*) in late 2017, associate editor Dr. Peter Doshi revealed how the most influential pro-vaccine advocacy organizations are all funded by the pharmaceutical industry.[5] With their names being, for example, the Immunization Action Coalition, Every Child By Two, and even the American Academy of Pediatrics, Dr. Doshi explains, "How much funding the vaccine advocacy non-profits receive from vaccine manufacturers is hard to pin down, but it seems to be substantial," and he goes on to detail that, "in its most recent 2016 annual giving report, AAP lists numerous corporate donors, including vaccine manufacturers GlaxoSmithKline, MedImmune, Merck, Pfizer, Sanofi Pasteur, and Seqirus."

Dr. Doshi explains that many of these advocacy groups, who go to great lengths to appear like objective third parties, also receive funding directly from the CDC and appear to move in lockstep with the CDC's policy goals: "The *BMJ* asked IAC, ECBT, and AAP to point to an instance when they had questioned a CDC recommendation. None did." Barbara Mintzes, a University of Sydney lecturer and researcher on conflicts of interest, offered a strong critique of these faux-independent organizations:

> *These groups are so strongly pro-vaccination that the public is getting a one-sided message that all vaccines are created equal and vaccination is an important public health strategy, regardless of the circumstances.*

I'm reminded of the sordid history of so many profit-seeking industries that were ultimately shown to be causing real harm. While I've already recounted the Tobacco Playbook, the lead industry was equally vicious in prolonging the poisoning of so many not only through the use of lead in gasoline but also lead in paint, where it was particularly damaging to children. In 2013 *The Atlantic* took this topic on with an article titled "Why It Took Decades of Blaming Parents before We Banned Lead Paint."[6] The article explains:

> *Since the 1920s, the lead industry had organized to fight bans, restrictions, even warnings on paint-can labels. It had marketed*

the deadly product to children and parents, spreading the lie that lead paint was safe. For decades, paint ads appeared in the Saturday Evening Post, Good Housekeeping, National Geographic, *and other national magazines and local newspapers. Coloring books were handed out to children. The industry even sent Dutch Boy costumes to children on Halloween, and printed coloring books that showed children how to prepare it.*

The Atlantic explains how lead paint makers blamed parents who "failed to stop children from placing their fingers and toys in their mouths" and that children poisoned by lead had a disease that "led them to suck on 'unnatural objects' and thereby get poisoned."

It's all so hauntingly similar to many of the comments we hear from vaccine makers, CDC officials, and their paid spokespeople. Vaccine injury is "one in a million." The timing of regression into autism and vaccine appointments is a coincidence. The clear biological evidence linking vaccines to autism is the work of "anti-vaccine activists" and "debunked science" and can't be believed. Lead manufacturers followed a similar path:

> *But the industry wouldn't remove all lead from their products. It fought every attempt at regulation. Industry representatives threatened lawsuits against television stations such as CBS that aired popular shows like* Highway Patrol *in which the product was depicted as dangerous. . . . All this despite records that show that the industry knew that their product was poisoning children.*

This is what self-interested people do, unfortunately. They cover it up, deny, and prolong the inevitable.

A 1945 ad from Philip Morris reminds you that "an ounce of prevention is worth a pound of cure" and that "Philip Morris [cigarettes] are scientifically proved far less irritating to the nose and throat," reassuring consumers that "when smokers changed to Philip Morris, substantially every case of irritation of the nose and throat—due to smoking—either cleared up completely, or definitely improved." And they let you know that "findings [were] reported in a leading medical journal."[7] We read the ad today and laugh out loud. Which part of the "safe and effective" marketing message about vaccines will make future generations laugh just as hard?

There's a popular meme that's shared within the autism community on social media. With a picture of a sheep's face, the caption reads, "If vaccines caused autism, they would have told us." This is a common argument I hear, and I understand. It feels too huge to believe. Have people in the know really stood by and watched something so terrible happen to so many children and their families? In my early years of researching this topic, I shared this reservation. It's hard to wrap your brain around it: "Have they really let this happen?"

"In the financial world, the result of the pressure to manipulate numbers to provide the answers bosses want has a name—securities fraud," autism parent and author Mark Blaxill told Congress in 2012. "In medicine there are similar pressures: they're called special interest politics and peer review and what the CDC has given us is the medical equivalent of securities fraud. All to avoid the inconvenient reality of the autism epidemic."[8]

Identifying the "they" behind the enablement of the autism epidemic is confusing. Is it just the CDC? How much of a role has Big Pharma played? What about scientists who have published bogus, distracting, or misleading scientific studies? What about pediatricians who turn a blind eye to the complaints of parents. And what about the role of the AAP? I think it's really all of the above because the lines between CDC, Big Pharma, the AAP, and most pediatricians are very, very blurry. They are all profiting immensely from our giant vaccine program.

Dr. Paul Thomas is a pediatrician in my hometown of Portland, Oregon. He's not just any pediatrician; he has the single largest pediatric practice in the city, and he's also the best-selling coauthor (with Jennifer Margulis, PhD) of *The Vaccine-Friendly Plan*, published in 2016. Dr. Thomas is a member of the American Academy of Pediatrics, but his views on vaccines are decidedly not mainstream, and he's a harsh critic of his colleagues:

> *I debated the rise in autism endlessly with my colleagues. Though I believe they were as worried as I was, it was, sadly, easier for many of them to shrug their shoulders, adjust the stethoscopes around their necks, and deny the evidence in front of them.*[9]

So is it really that hard to imagine that a bunch of self-interested people could do their small part to obscure the reality of the autism epidemic? In

2017 *Huffington Post* reporter Martha Rosenberg answered this question with one of my all-time favorite headlines: "Vaccines Are Totally Safe Say the People Who Brought Us Vioxx, Bextra, Baycol, Trovan, Phen-Fen, Xarelto, Raxar and Seldane..."[10]

Ms. Rosenberg's article was promptly removed by the *Huffington Post*, causing Ms. Rosenberg to tweet: "#Huf has censored this factual, sourced piece by a credential reporter on #vaccines." Thinking back to that popular meme, couldn't we insert any man-made health catastrophe of the past century into the same statement? These only sound absurd in retrospect because we know how each of these stories ends:

"If the water in Flint, MI, had been full of lead, they would have told us."
"If asbestos caused mesothelioma, they would have told us."
"If lead paint caused brain damage, they would have told us."
"If Vioxx caused heart attacks, they would have told us."
"If thalidomide caused birth defects, they would have told us."
"If silicone breast implants leaked, they would have told us."
"If DDT destroyed ecosystems, they would have told us."

Do I need to keep going? Millions of children could be injured before the truth becomes common knowledge. I pray that the day of reckoning for vaccines is not still decades away. The internet, social media, a powerful Kennedy publicly shouting, and perhaps a sympathetic president might bring about the truth sooner. I'm hopeful. Personally, I think it's the science—and the admissions of key scientists—that will win the day, just like it did with tobacco.

A Brief Review of How We Got Here

I think we're very close to a reckoning of the autism epidemic. I know I've shared so much information with you in this book. I'd like to pause and revisit the major events and key takeaways.

In 1986 a new law indemnifies vaccine makers from liability, leading to a spike in the number of vaccines children receive. The 1986 law calls for the establishment of a "vaccine court," which means that if your child is injured, you have to sue the US government. In vaccine court, there's no jury, just a "special master." As vaccine makers shed their fear of lawsuits from vaccine injuries, the number of vaccines on the childhood schedule triples by the late 1990s.

Meanwhile, safety testing for vaccines takes place one vaccine at a time and for a short period of time. When vaccine makers test a vaccine for safety, they records adverse events for a week (or less). Side effects that take more than a week to manifest, which is most, are never recorded. Synergistic effects with previous or subsequent vaccines are also therefore never discovered. Once a vaccine is on the market, side effects, which can be extremely complex to identify, are rarely detected or recorded accurately. Most doctors don't know what to look for. The Vaccine Adverse Event Reporting System (VAERS), which is the public's recourse for reporting a vaccine injury, captures less than 1 percent of injuries because parents must know to actively seek it out. These factors—inadequate safety testing, near nonexistent doctor training, and a minuscule rate of reporting from the public—has allowed an emerging epidemic of vaccine injuries to hide in plain sight.

As more and more parents begin to report regression after vaccine appointments in the mid- to late 1990s, the CDC responds by publishing studies to quash concern. The emergence of the internet in the late 1990s allowed parents to start comparing stories—many of which sounded eerily similar—and mobilize in a new way. The CDC pushed back with epidemiological studies looking at a single ingredient (thimerosal) to "prove" that the vaccine schedule in its entirety was safe. CDC scientists also compared children who received some mercury in their vaccines to children who received slightly less mercury as more blanket evidence that vaccines do not cause autism. The study's author, Dr. Thomas Verstraeten, complained that the study's findings were misrepresented, but the messaging—that vaccines are safe and don't cause autism—sticks nevertheless.

When British doctor Andrew Wakefield raises concerns about the MMR vaccine in 1998, a kangaroo court strips him of his medical license, and the ensuing media frenzy morphs into a defense of the entire vaccine schedule and an attack on anyone who reasonably questions it. As scientists investigating the link between vaccines and autism begin to fear getting "Wakefielded," the CDC produces further epidemiological studies that are, once again, misrepresented to show that because certain studies claim MMR doesn't cause autism, no vaccine—or combination of vaccines—could possibly cause autism. Eight years later Dr. Wakefield coproduces a documentary, *Vaxxed*, about Dr. William Thompson, a CDC whistle-blower who confessed to publishing fraudulent data exonerating MMR in 2004 in a study he coauthored. As of this writing, attempts to have Dr. William Thompson testify before Congress have been unsuccessful.

In late 2004 the brains of persons with autism are studied for the first time. Dr. Carlos Pardo-Villamizar of Johns Hopkins discovers that the immune system in the brains of people with autism is in a permanent state of inflammation, leading to an obvious question: "What's causing the inflammation?"

In 2007 the most important discovery about the biological cause of autism emerges from Caltech scientist Dr. Paul Patterson. Patterson's foundational discovery that immune activation events, at critical phases of brain development, lead to the development of autism appears to tie together key findings: Vaccines are specifically intended to trigger immune activation events. Parents' reports of their children's injuries following vaccine appointments correspond to Patterson's immune activation event hypothesis. Autism brains are shown to be in a state of constant inflammation.

Meanwhile, the vaccine court turns out to be a treasure trove of information about how vaccines can cause autism. After Hannah Poling's case is publicly leaked to journalist David Kirby in 2008, Mary Holland and Lou Conte unearth more than eighty additional cases in which the vaccine court awarded damages to families with children who experienced regressive autism caused by vaccines. Many of the vaccine court's decisions provide medical details for how the vaccines caused brain damage and autism, according to Holland et al.'s 2011 study published in *Pace Environmental Law Review*, "Unanswered Questions from the Vaccine Injury Compensation Program."

International scientists begin to study the neurological risks of the widely used vaccine adjuvant, aluminum. The number of studies multiplies, and they consistently demonstrate that vaccine aluminum crosses the blood-brain barrier, resulting in immune activation events and serious neurological problems. Now the specific ingredient that appears to be triggering autism has been identified. In 2017 Professor Christopher

Exley discovers "shockingly high" levels of aluminum in the brains of people with autism. Exley urges extreme caution in administering aluminum-containing vaccines.

In late 2017 the CDC releases the latest figures on autism—1 in 36—showing that incidence continues to skyrocket. The autism rate was roughly 1 in 10,000 in the 1970s, based on thorough, large-scale studies in Wisconsin, Minnesota, and nationally. When my son was diagnosed in 2004, the rate was 1 in 150. Today, it's 1 in 36. A cottage industry has developed trying to explain away an epidemic. Books like *NeuroTribes* propagate myths that "autism has always been with us." No data supports this revisionist history. Evidence that we have an epidemic has been validated many times in published studies.

In early 2018 two of the most important expert witnesses in vaccine court—Dr. Andrew Zimmerman and Dr. Richard Kelley—switch sides in dramatic fashion, testifying on behalf of the family of Yates Hazlehurst, one of the three children used as a "test case" in the Omnibus Autism Proceedings (OAP) of 2009, that Yates's autism was caused by vaccines. Had they held this position in 2009, the vaccine court likely would have been compelled to favor the vaccine-autism connection, resulting in justice for more than five thousand claimants, possibly triggering the kind of reckoning needed to end this epidemic. Dr. Zimmerman states that many of his colleagues share his view that vaccines can trigger autism if there is "mitochondrial dysfunction," something Dr. Kelley estimates is true for 25 to 50 percent of children with autism.

And here we are: Scientists are speaking up, doctors are speaking up, and parents have always spoken up. I believe we are on the cusp of a reckoning. There is no way to end the autism epidemic without exposing the lies surrounding it and demanding accountability. The question now is, What will it take for us to get from point A to point B? In the following chapter I lay out a proposal for the steps I think could get us there.

CHAPTER 9

Next Steps:
A Twelve-Point Proposal

Truth is truth to the end of reckoning.
—William Shakespeare

These days special education numbers for children in the developed world are off the charts. Schools are drowning with discipline issues, deadly allergies, expulsions, budget shortfalls, and stressed-out teachers. It's an unmitigated disaster. Anne Dachel of Wisconsin is a published author and relentless advocate for the health of America's children. The mother of an adult son on the autism spectrum, Anne has been a teacher for three decades and has seen the stunning increase in the number of sick children (both mentally and physically) in America's schools. She writes:

> We keep looking for ways to explain what's happening to our children, while we pretend nothing has changed. I've heard lots of teachers say things like, "They come with so many issues from home," "They used to be kept at home," and "They used to be in institutions." Our schools are filled with disabled kids who weren't here 25 years ago. Look at the accommodations on IEPs for students just in regular ed. I've had students who are allowed to pace in the back of the classroom or walk out and sit in the hall if they feel overwhelmed. Large numbers of kids couldn't function in school if they weren't medicated. We modify

tests and assignments for kids who can't deal with regular work. And that's just what's happening in the mainstream classroom.[1]

In the United States 13 percent of children are in special education today, with many counties and schools reporting numbers of 25 percent or higher.[2] No matter where you look, the stories are the same: There is a massive physical and mental health deterioration happening in this generation of children. Rising special education, anxiety disorders, ADHD, autism, depression, anaphylactic food allergies, behavioral issues, and on and on. Name it, they have all exploded. Schools are breaking down, struggling to keep up. Teachers are stressed out, overworked, and in short supply.

And it's nearly impossible to find people in positions of power in the public health establishment asking the obvious question: Where in the world did all these sick children come from? I believe, with the benefit of history, we will call these kids something like the "aluminum generation." This book has shown you evidence that aluminum adjuvant can trigger autism. Science has also shown that vaccines can trigger autoimmune conditions, including asthma, deadly food allergies, diabetes, and eczema. Maybe this is just the tip of the iceberg. Could vaccines also be triggering learning disorders, anxiety, and other issues that are cropping up in such abundance in American classrooms?

Dr. Paul Thomas's Sensible Approach

"I have over 13,000 children in my pediatric practice and I have to say, as unpopular as this observation might be, my unvaccinated children are by far the healthiest," says Dr. Paul Thomas, a Dartmouth-trained pediatrician who has been practicing medicine for thirty years and also happens to be my children's pediatrician here in Portland.[3]

I'm sitting with Dr. Thomas now. It's October 2017. Paul, as I now call him, has become a close and trusted friend, as well as one of the most influential people in the autism community, and I'm interviewing him for my new podcast, How to End the Autism Epidemic. His recent best seller, *The Vaccine-Friendly Plan* (cowritten with Jennifer Margulis, PhD), has challenged the mainstream medical establishment at every turn, and Paul has emerged as a fearless voice.

Unfortunately, Paul is a rare doctor, a pediatrician who spent his career vaccinating kids who is now publicly stating that something is wrong, that too many children are sick, and that vaccines are more than likely the primary cause. I want to understand from Paul what triggered his awakening: How did he realize what was going on?

Paul explains, "What ended up happening for me was that some of my patients didn't seem to be doing as well neurologically, developmentally, as kids used to be, and I started wondering, what the heck is going on? I started seeking out alternative information and doing my own research."

He walks me through the research he did, the conferences he attended; he recounts that "once you start looking, you become more aware that there's actually something going on with what we're doing and the outcomes we're starting to see. Kids not developing, regressing into autism."

In the mid-2000s he started to see children who regressed into autism after being perfectly normal, something he had never seen before. Paul decided to change the way he doctored newborns. He reduced the number of vaccines he gave. He delayed certain vaccines, avoided antibiotics, and counseled parents on other ways to avoid toxins. The result was that among his more than two thousand patients, none developed autism. There should have been fifty.

> I've had a team compiling data for a research study that is now undergoing peer review—some of which is published in my new book. The data is surprising and counterintuitive, perhaps, but it shows very clearly that the incidence of chronic disease and brain abnormalities in the entirely unvaccinated children in my practice, even those with siblings with autism, is much, much lower than in children following the CDC's recommended schedule.

So one doctor changes the way he treats his pediatric population and sees no autism.

Could it be that easy?

A Simple Proposal to End the Autism Epidemic

What follows are my recommendations for how to end the autism epidemic. Consider it a twelve-point plan to dramatically reduce the rate of autism in the United States.

1. Immediately reduce the total number of vaccines given to American children.

The word "vaccinate" can mean so many different things, and not all vaccines are created equally. So it's time to get specific, and it's time to reduce the number of vaccines American children receive. First, if other developed countries haven't added a vaccine to their schedule, why should we give it to American children? Second, any vaccine added since the 1986 law removing liability from vaccine manufacturers is up for discussion. And third, if science exists implicating a vaccine or showing it's done more harm than good, that's a serious red flag.

In the United States there are thirteen separate vaccines currently on the US schedule, most given to children between two and four times each. They are: (1) hepatitis B, (2) rotavirus, (3) DTaP, (4) Hib, (5) PCV, (6) polio, (7) influenza, (8) MMR, (9) varicella, (10) hepatitis A, (11) meningococcal, (12) Tdap, (13) HPV.

Many developed countries don't give: hepatitis B (unless the mother is hepatitis B positive), rotavirus, influenza, varicella, hepatitis A, and HPV. So that simple exercise would remove six vaccines from the US schedule.

New since 1986 (and not already excluded): Hib, PCV, meningococcal. Hib is a potentially deadly bacteria. It's particularly dangerous for infants. That said, the Hib vaccine contains aluminum, so the risk/benefit equation is complex. I would leave it on the schedule. PCV (often called "prevnar") has too many questions associated with it, including the possibility that PCV vaccines are contributing to antibiotic resistance and the explosion in methicillin-resistant *Staphylococcus aureus* (MRSA) cases.[4] It should be removed. Meningococcal is a very new vaccine, only added to the schedule in 2012 for young children. Serious questions remain about its safety and efficacy. I would remove it.[5]

Conclusion: Reduce the vaccine schedule to the following vaccines: DTaP, Hib, polio, and MMR. Of course, this will be viewed by pro-vaccine talking heads as a radical and dangerous idea, despite the fact that until the late 1980s, the entire US vaccine schedule was DTaP, polio, and MMR. Furthermore, decisions need to be made about when, exactly, to give these vaccines. In general, first vaccines should be delayed until children have reached their first birthday and the MMR delayed until they are past three years old, as Dr. Paul Thomas does in his practice.

A Safer, Simpler Vaccine Schedule

Vaccinate for:

- DTaP
- Hib
- Polio
- MMR

Improve Safety by:

- Screening for risk factors before vaccinating
- Delaying all vaccines until 12 months or older
- Delaying the MMR vaccine until 36 months or older
- Establishing clear rules for when not to vaccinate (a child is sick, has eczema, is taking antibiotics, etc.)

What about aluminum? Of the four vaccines that the reduction exercise above keeps on the vaccine schedule—DTaP, Hib, polio, and MMR—two of them contain aluminum: DTaP and Hib. What's a parent supposed to do? This highlights one of the single biggest challenges with vaccine development. Right now, vaccines work by hyperstimulating the immune system, but this is the same process that can trigger immune activation events and cause autism in certain vulnerable children. Could it be that any vaccine adjuvant would pose a similar risk? We learned that Dr. Richard Kelley actually administers an anti-inflammatory when he vaccinates children to try to offset the immune activation events. It's my own belief that twenty years from now, pediatricians will be vigilant about avoiding anything that might trigger immune activation events in children under the age of three as the understanding of the risks becomes more common knowledge. In the meantime, parents are left to try to make the proper risk/benefit decision, as scientists like Dr. Christopher Exley caution against any aluminum-containing vaccines. There's not a simple answer.

2. With the remaining vaccines, have the CDC and AAP institute an immediate policy change for when and how the vaccines are administered.

Children in the United States are routinely vaccinated while they are sick and when they are taking antibiotics. While the CDC website discourages these practices, American pediatricians violate these guidelines every day, as they did with my son and the children of so many parents I know. The communication from the AAP and CDC needs to be much stronger to reduce the likelihood that children will be vaccinated at their most vulnerable moments.

3. Make the MMR available as three separate shots.

The MMR vaccine is a "triple live virus" vaccine that may be creating too heavy a burden for some children's immune systems to process all at once. I have heard so many stories of regression and seizures immediately after the MMR. In the United States parents cannot access separate vaccines for measles, mumps, and rubella, but in Japan that's exactly how they are given: as separate shots. Why? Because Japanese health authorities were worried about the MMR's side effects, as *Japan Today* reported in 2016:

> In 1993, Japan stopped using the combination vaccine for mumps, measles and rubella (MMR) in routine immunisations. The Health Ministry said the triple vaccine was linked to side effects, notably non-viral meningitis. Of the 1.8 million children who were administered it, some had adverse reactions and three children reportedly died. Japan, as a result, remains the only developed country to have banned the MMR combination vaccine, and use separate jabs for measles and rubella [they don't give the mumps vaccine].[6]

Why can't Americans get the M, M, and R shots singularly? My understanding is that Merck has a patent on the MMR that gives them 100 percent of the market; I guess we know who would fight against this change the hardest.

4. Substitute titer tests for booster shots.

Booster shots are provided for most vaccines. For example, the DTaP vaccine is typically given four separate times before a baby's fifteen-month birthday. Many of these shots are unnecessary, as immunity has already been conferred through the first vaccine, which titer tests—which measure antibodies in the blood—can reveal. A blood test carries far fewer risks than a vaccine, so the AAP should recommend that titer tests be performed prior to giving booster shots. For babies who have already developed the desired immunity, no booster shots are needed.

5. Screening for vulnerable children needs to be implemented immediately.

As Drs. Zimmerman and Kelley discussed in their depositions, screening tools need to be rolled out through the CDC and AAP immediately. Some vulnerabilities are genetic or based on health conditions of the parents. Some vulnerabilities are the product of how the child presents physically. Eczema, persistent ear infections, diarrhea, dark circles under the eyes—any of these could serve as a warning that vaccines may cause further harm. We need a clear, explicit screening system.

6. The IACC needs to be scrapped and reconstituted.

The Department of Health and Human Services created a committee, the Interagency Autism Coordinating Committee, which coordinates "federal efforts and provides advice to the Secretary of Health and Human Services on issues related to autism spectrum disorder."[7] The IACC has been a disaster and has stood by as the autism rate has jumped from 1 in 166 when it was formed to 1 in 36 today. None of the scientists I quoted in chapter 5 have ever had the chance to address the IACC, and environmental causes of autism are never discussed. The IACC embodies the mainstream denialism of the autism epidemic and does more harm than good. As I mentioned in chapter 3, Dr. Joshua Gordon, the chair of the IACC, lacks any perspective on vaccine-autism science.

7. Vaccine safety must be removed from the CDC.

Ten years ago two members of Congress, Representatives Dave Weldon and Carolyn Maloney, tried to pass a bill to separate vaccine safety from the CDC. From a press release:

> At a press conference Wednesday morning, U.S. Reps. Dave Weldon, M.D. (R-FL) and Carolyn Maloney (D-NY) introduced a bill that would give responsibility for the nation's vaccine safety to an independent agency within the Department of Health and Human Services, removing most vaccine safety research from the Centers for Disease Control (CDC). Currently, the CDC has responsibility for both vaccine safety and promotion, which is an inherent conflict of interest increasingly garnering public criticism.[8]

At the time Congressman Weldon was quoted as saying, "There's an enormous inherent conflict of interest within the CDC and if we fail to move vaccine safety to a separate independent office, safety issues will remain a low priority and public confidence in vaccines will continue to erode." Congresswoman Maloney added, "We need adequate, unbiased research on vaccines, and this legislation would deliver that. I applaud Dr. Weldon for his tremendous commitment to and leadership on this issue. He is truly dedicated to protecting our children and the public at large." Alas, like every bill intended to reduce the power and influence of the CDC, the bill never passed, but it sits there as a template for how to make this separation of the fox from the henhouse happen.

8. Scientists who understand the relationship between immune activation events, vaccines, and autism need to speak as one.

Will Autism Speaks ever step up and bring all this science and all these scientists together? If not, these scientists producing all this compelling science on how vaccines and autism are related need to join forces and speak as one. We have a Nobel Prize winner on our side! It's time to share the complete understanding of the biological basis for autism with the world.

9. The congressional hearing that never happened in 2013 needs to be held and Drs. Zimmerman, Kelley, and Poling need to be compelled to speak.

The House of Representatives' Oversight and Government Reform Committee almost held a hearing in November 2013 about the National Vaccine Injury Compensation Program following Mary Holland's paper detailing the eighty-three cases of vaccine-induced autism and Rolf Hazlehurst's memo detailing apparent corruption during the OAP hearings—until industry influences were brought to bear and the hearing was canceled. The hearing needs to take place, and Drs. Zimmerman, Kelley, and Poling need to be compelled to testify.

10. Dr. William Thompson needs to be compelled to testify.

A CDC whistle-blower is hiding in plain sight. Dr. Thompson has alleged fraud at CDC on a critical study assessing the relationship between vaccines and autism, yet no one in Congress has compelled Dr. Thompson to testify.

11. Suramin trials should be accelerated and prioritized.

We have a prestigious researcher from UC San Diego claiming that in a small, double-blind placebo trial, an infusion of the drug suramin dramatically improved the symptoms of autism in participants (see chapter 10). This potentially game-changing outcome needs to be replicated immediately in a larger trial.

12. The AAP needs to listen to the biomedical doctors who are recovering children.

The AAP has shown no interest in stories about children with autism recovering through biomedical intervention. The reason for this is obvious: If recovery implicates vaccines, then the AAP's pediatricians are implicated in the autism epidemic. This concern about self-protection needs to be overcome for the sake of the children the AAP claims they are organized to protect.

Right now, thousands of American children, every single day, are having their lives unnecessarily and permanently altered by a reckless, poorly tested, and poorly monitored vaccine program that puts industry profits ahead of children's safety. My son and millions of other children are being stricken with a mental disability that reduces their ability to pursue a life of liberty and happiness. This is a man-made disaster that needs to end now, and it should be treated like a national emergency.

Of course, the clock is ticking for kids with autism. While our public health establishment spends its energy and effort trying to convince parents that there's nothing amiss, parents are struggling everyday to meet the needs of their kids, often with little or no support. There is support out there, however—biomedical doctors, nutritionists, and most especially a massive community of autism parents dedicated to helping one another and recovering kids.

Just as people deny that there's an autism epidemic, many people deny that kids can recover from autism. Recovery is real. Many more children need to be treated appropriately to give them the best chance at it. Recovery is part of the reckoning process because when we treat children for vaccine injury and they recover, it exposes what caused the injury in the first place. More importantly, it gives innocent children the chance to lead the life they were meant to have. The following chapter offers a road map for recovery.

CHAPTER 10

Treatment and Recovery

There is today a tremendous disconnect between obtainable knowledge
and implemented treatment for autism. There is an ever-widening gap
between what parents know and what physicians know. The parents
have made themselves experts in complex biochemistry, immunology,
and gastroenterology. They know what is happening on the cutting
edge of autism treatment because their kids need them to know. This
kind of parent overtakes their pediatrician's expertise very quickly.[1]

—Dr. Julie Buckley, author,
Healing Our Autistic Children

Children are recovering from autism every day. Typically, their parents
implement biomedical intervention, the symptoms that defined the
autism disappear, and the children go on to lead a normal life. In 2008 Lisa
and I produced a twenty-six-minute documentary called *Autism Yesterday*.
It told the story of five children and their families recovering from autism.
Today three of those children are either in college or on that path!

When people lie about or obfuscate the cause of autism, they impair
the important work of recovery. Recovered children are proof that autism
is an environmental condition that has a cause and a treatment. Epidemic
denialists, in particular, hinder the willingness of some parents to seek
treatment, if they're led to believe that their children's autism was inevitable
and genetic. Recovery is real.

Does that mean all children recover? Sadly, no. Many parents try biomedical
intervention and don't see their children recover. It can be a long, frustrating,
and exhausting road, full of hope and disappointment. Certain therapies are

expensive, and few at this point are covered by insurance. Most mainstream doctors don't know anything about them, so you have to forge your own path, find other families in the same boat, and educate yourself beyond belief. No autism parents should ever have to feel like failures—on top of all the other daily struggles—if their child doesn't recover. This is one of the great injustices of the autism tragedy: The failure is on the part of our public health establishment, and yet parents—often with other children to care for and other responsibilities and stresses in their lives—are left to shoulder it all on their own.

That said, I think it's fair to say that almost all children who are treated improve, and some recover. So where have others experienced success? Where should an autism parent turn first? What are the most promising options on the horizon?

What Is Biomedical Intervention?

The best book ever written on this topic is *Healing and Preventing Autism: A Complete Guide* by Dr. Jerry Kartzinel and Jenny McCarthy.[2] I highly recommend you get this book and read it.

Remember Dr. Lynne Mielke, our original DAN! doctor that I talked about in the introduction to this book? You will need someone like her—a physician trained in the biomedical recovery of autism who can design an individualized program for your child. Like many of the original DAN! doctors, Dr. Mielke continues to treat children today. Most autism biomedical doctors are now part of the Medical Academy of Pediatric Special Needs (MAPS). Their website offers a clinician directory with doctors available in almost every state.

Of course, I'm not a doctor, but these are some of the basic therapies of a biomedical program that might be included in your child's individualized treatment plan:

Special diet. Children with autism typically suffer from a wide range of food allergies. Removing offending foods can have a profound impact on behavior. The high-impact food categories to remove include gluten, dairy, soy, and sugar. Children have recovered from the removal of gluten alone. There are two diets that deserve special mention. They are much harder to implement, but both have many success stories: the GAPS diet and the ketogenic diet.

Gut healing. The guts of children with autism are often severely impaired. Diet will improve gut function, as does the removal of artificial colors and flavors. Many children also take probiotics and supplements to regulate candida, a form of yeast that is typically overgrown in the intestines of children with autism.

Nutrition. Because of their compromised guts and general ill health, children with autism often benefit from targeting vitamins and minerals. For some, vitamin B12 can be an immediate boost. For others, magnesium will alleviate many symptoms. Other doctors specialize in "mitochondrial cocktails" that are formulated to address the mitochondrial dysfunction Drs. Zimmerman and Kelley discussed in their depositions and in Hannah Poling's case.

Detoxification. Far-infrared saunas, ionic footbaths, magnetic clay, chlorella, and cilantro are a few of the many ways to support the body in detoxification. Many parents report remarkable results once a detox program has been implemented.

Advanced therapies. Stem cells, hyperbaric oxygen, and intravenous immunoglobulin (IVIG) infusions are just a few examples of treatments that have helped children recover.

Where do you start? Read a lot, and find a MAPS doctor near you. Those two actions will be your best chance for an optimal recovery.

The Suramin Study

In 2016 UCSD professor Dr. Robert Naviaux published a study that had done a trial of a single drug, suramin, on ten children with autism.[3] The results were promising, with all of the children who received suramin showing improvement, including a few "miracles." The trial was done as a double-blind study, making the results more robust and credible. Even more interesting, Dr. Naviaux put forth his own theory about what was causing autism, and why suramin seemed to help:

> *Our research is leading us to the conclusion that autism is caused by a treatable metabolic syndrome in many children. The exact percentage is currently unknown. Metabolism is the language the brain, gut and immune system use to communicate. These three systems are*

linked. You can't change one without changing the other. Each of these systems works differently in autism, but more specifically, the communication between these systems is changed in autism. Such changes occur both during and after the pregnancy. Suramin can only improve metabolic functions once a child is treated. While anti-purinergic therapy (APT) with suramin may not directly change some aspects of abnormal brain development that were present before treatment, APT may improve the function of many brain systems, even if brain structure does not change. And in children and teens whose brains are still developing, the course or trajectory of brain development might also be changed by treatment.[4]

I'm fascinated by Dr. Naviaux's hypothesis. Note that Dr. Naviaux is identifying the same phenomenon that Drs. Zimmerman and Kelley are seeing. Dr. Naviaux also coined a new term—cell danger response (CDR)—that sounds like the state of cells after an immune activation event:

The metabolic syndrome that underlies the dysfunction is caused by the abnormal persistence of the cell danger response or CDR. Aspects of the CDR are also known to scientists as the "integrated stress response." Both genes and environment contribute to the CDR, so even genetic causes of autism lower the threshold for CDR activation and produce the metabolic syndrome. Ultimately, if the symptoms of autism are caused by a metabolic syndrome, the hopeful message is that the symptoms can be treated, even though we can't change the genes.[5]

I've talked to several of the parents of children who were in Dr. Naviaux's study. They told me it was like someone turned the lights on in their child. Unfortunately, after about six weeks, the improvements began to fade. Because suramin is not yet licensed to be used for children with autism outside of the study, the parents aren't able to get ongoing infusions. Let's hope that will change. In the meantime, the suramin trial raises what I think are the most important questions we need answers to about autism: Is autism permanent brain damage or is the brain "locked" in an inflamed or hyperstimulated state? And therefore, if it's "unlocked" can a child return to normal?

Dr. Naviaux's study would imply that if you can turn off the cell danger response, normal brain function can resume. This is potentially earth-shattering news and corroborates stories I have heard from recovered children: They were always aware of the world but felt as if they were "locked" from expressing themselves. We pray that Dr. Naviaux's research continues and that the FDA approves suramin for use in children. It could change everything.

By the way, Dr. Naviaux never mentions vaccines. He often mentions that the environment can cause the cell danger response. I won't put words in his mouth, but I know what thing in the environment at least some of the parents in the trial believe caused their child's autism.

What about Aluminum, Specifically?

The recent science demonstrating that aluminum is triggering immune activation events raises an obvious question: Does this new information change the nature of biomedical intervention? Is it time to get the aluminum out or find some other method to turn off the permanent immune system activation in the brains of children with autism that is causing inflammation and impairing brain function? Here are some of the better ideas I have heard for how to do that:

Drink silica mineral water. Dr. Christopher Exley, the scientist who discovered high levels of aluminum in autism brains, claims that mineral waters with high natural silica are the best way to remove aluminum from the brain. The two brands he recommends that are available in the United States are Vittel and Fiji water. Specifically, he says to drink 1.5L (51 oz) of the mineral water in a one-hour time period every day, something he feels we should all do to keep the aluminum out of our bodies.

Adopt the ketogenic diet. In 2017 a study called "Ketogenic Diet Improves Behaviors in a Maternal Immune Activation Model of Autism Spectrum Disorder" discussed the impact a ketogenic diet had on suppressing immune activation in mice.[6] The scientists wrote:

> *Here we show that metabolic therapy with a KD* [ketogenic diet] *improves and can even reverse ASD-like behaviors in the MIA mouse model.*

It's worth noting that the ketogenic diet has been used for years to help reduce seizures. Ketogenics are going through a bit of a revolution, with "exogenous ketones" now being made available as supplement products to put a body into ketosis more quickly. Could these exogenous ketones accelerate recovery? I have no idea, but this study alone seems to show it's worth far more exploration.

Heal the microbiome. We know that aluminum adjuvant can contribute to gastrointestinal distress. A 2013 study—"The Microbiota Modulates Gut Physiology and Behavioral Abnormalities Associated with Autism"—highlights the relationship between the gut microbiota, immune activation, and autism:

> *Our findings provide a novel mechanism by which a human commensal bacterium can improve ASD-related GI deficits and behavioral abnormalities in mice, possibly explaining the rapid increase in ASD prevalence by identifying the microbiome as a critical environmental contributor to disease. We propose the transformative concept that autism is, at least in part, a disease involving the gut that impacts the immune, metabolic and nervous systems, and that microbiome-mediated therapies may be a safe and effective treatment for ASD.[7]*

The scientists used a particular strain of probiotic, *Bacteroides fragilis*, and found that the probiotic "corrects gut permeability, alters microbial composition and ameliorates ASD-related defects in communicative, stereotypic, anxiety-like and sensorimotor behaviors."

Vitamin D. The Vaccine Papers website discusses the role vitamin D can play in reducing immune activation:

> *Vitamin D favorably regulates the immune system, simultaneously improving its effectiveness at eliminating pathogens, and reducing inflammation. . . . Vitamin D is consumed by the immune system when it's activated. It is a nutrient that is metabolized at a faster rate during infection or inflammation. Consequently, people with inflammatory conditions need greater amounts of vitamin D. They must supplement*

at a higher dose to achieve healthy blood levels. Since chronic immune activation is always present in autism, autistics require higher vitamin D intake than normal people.

A 2015 study from China supported the role of vitamin D: "Core Symptoms of Autism Improved after Vitamin D Supplementation."[8] The authors noted that "we report on a 32-month-old boy with ASD and vitamin D3 deficiency. His core symptoms of autism improved significantly after vitamin D3 supplementation."

Selenium. A study titled, "Selective Induction of IL-6 by Aluminum-Induced Oxidative Stress Can Be Prevented by Selenium" in the *Journal of Trace Elements in Medicine and Biology* in 2012 concluded the potentially restorative effects of the mineral selenium:

> *Therefore it was concluded that short-term exposure to Al [aluminum] causes adverse effects on the intracellular oxidative stress processes in the liver, as reflected by the selective increase in the IL-6 concentration. This process can be restored by co-administration of the trace element Se [selenium] as a part of the glutathione redox system.*[9]

Do the interventions that remove aluminum from the body or reduce the impact of immune activation events work to recover children? I don't think we have enough data yet to know, but I hope you can see how important it is to understand how our children's autism was caused. We use causation as a road map for how to treat and, we hope, recover our children.

Epilogue

Find a place inside where there's joy, and the joy will burn out the pain.
—Joseph Campbell

It's late November 2017, and Jamison and I are playing hooky from life for an unplanned trip to Hawaii. Jamison is fifteen now. He's six feet two, nearly a grown man, an inch or two taller than his dad. Autism is still a part of his life, although biomedical intervention gave him back the ability to speak—an incredible gift—and removed almost all of his frustration. We remain hopeful that his symptoms will keep improving, "recovery" remains our goal, and he's surrounded by a group of doctors who continue to help his body heal. Travel is now a breeze. We're on a long hike, turning the corner on a path to find an amazing ocean view. Jamison's at his happiest outside, a true nature boy. He's a self-taught swimmer, and watching him navigate the waves with his giant smile is a sublime joy for me. Our frequent family trips here are largely spent in the water.

Everything about my life changed because of Jamison's diagnosis. My career began to hold less and less interest for me. Business travel became unbearable—I was needed at home. In 2013 I retired from the firm I founded and dedicated my time to caring for the well-being of my kids. For my older son and my youngest child, my daughter, I've had the privilege of being the head coach of more than a dozen of their sports teams. For Jamison it means that I drop him off and pick him up from school most days, and our evenings and afternoons are often spent together. He creates a perspective on life that no one else can. He loves the simple things: nature, waves, hugs, a great meal. He smiles when he's surrounded by family, never tells a lie, and never judges anyone. He reminds you of everything that really matters, and he makes most things seem as trivial as they really are.

Lisa and I are closer than ever. Autism puts an incredible strain on all marriages, but it's made our bond stronger. When you feel like you are living "behind the matrix," it helps to have a running mate. She's mine, and her wisdom and perspective are sprinkled throughout this book.

A friend recently listened to my story about Jamison and commented that it sounded as though I felt guilty about what had happened to him. Of course I feel guilty! And at times writing this book took me back to my darkest moments. Spelling out so clearly what happens to children as they slide into autism forced me to relive the horrors of that time nearly fifteen years ago with Jamison when he was just a little baby. Those moments we entrusted him to our pediatrician, only to have him returned to us sicker than ever. I'm haunted by the words of Dr. Andrew Zimmerman, writing about vaccines triggering Hannah Poling's autism:

> *Thus, if not for this event [a vaccine appointment], Hannah may have led a normal full productive life.*[1]

I feel the same way about Jamison. My friend is hurting for me; he tries to alleviate my guilt. "Dude, you couldn't have known; you were trying to keep him safe and healthy." I've heard this argument before because I say the same things to parents of newly diagnosed kids. But for me it's the fire that still burns. Guilt is the fuel that wrote this book. I've realized there are really only two things that lessen my guilt: (1) helping prevent autism in other families, and (2) anytime Jamison shows cognitive improvement. I don't know how else to make it up to Jamison but to do everything I can to help him recover.

Recently, Jamison's ability to read has taken a major uptick. This book would still be too much for him, but perhaps one day it won't be. Jamie, if you're reading this now, please know that I love you more than any words can ever express, I'm so sorry for what happened to you; I'm so grateful you're here—you've helped so many by being the amazing guy you are. You are my best friend. I love you, bud.

Acknowledgments

My son Jamison inspires me every day. Faced with the daunting prospect of navigating the world with autism, he does so with a beautiful smile on his face. His calm presence and warmth make him a beloved friend to many. Every moment I have ever spent fighting for the truth about the autism epidemic is in honor of him. I tell him every day that he's my best friend. I hope I'm his.

The autism community is filled with amazing parents and people, many of whom have had a profound impact on me. My list could take up ten pages, but I'm particularly indebted to Jenny McCarthy, Candace MacDonald, Brian Hooker, Bobby Kennedy, Kevin Barry, Mark Blaxill, Polly Tommey, Kent Heckenlively, Mary Holland, Becky Estepp, Del Bigtree, Dr. Paul Thomas, Dan Olmsted, and Dr. Bernard Rimland. I consider you all fellow warriors, and I'd gladly join you in any fight. A special shout out to mother-warrior Kim Stagliano, editor of the *Age of Autism* blog, who helped edit my writing. And Jennifer Margulis, thank you for connecting me with my amazing publisher, Chelsea Green, and for being a great mentor and cheerleader. Brianne Goodspeed and Margo Baldwin, thank you for your unqualified support of this book and expertise in creating the finished product—I'm grateful beyond words.

I'm grateful to my parents, who taught me to never trust authority and always believed me when I told them what happened to Jamison, and my big sister for always having my back.

More than anyone, I'm indebted to my wife Lisa. A fellow Stanford grad, she's the brains and the heart of everything I do. She's endured autism with me, and she's been at my shoulder every step of the way. We've never fallen out of sync, and I could never find words to tell her how grateful I am that she's with me. She's also the proud parent alongside me of two other beautiful children, Jamison's older brother Sam and younger sister Quinlan, who have shown courage, grace, empathy, and love in dealing with their middle sibling's plight. I'm extremely lucky to have the family I have, and I love them dearly.

Notes

Introduction

1. "Is Autism Genetic or Environmental?" *Greater Boston*, WGBH TV, Boston, MA.
2. Dr. Russell Blaylock, "The Deadly Impossibility of Herd Immunity through Vaccination," *International Medical Council on Vaccination* (blog), February 18, 2012, https://globalfreedommovement.org/the-deadly-impossibility-of-herd -immunity-through-vaccination/.
3. This website provides details of vaccine protection duration, listed by vaccine: http://www.immune.org.nz/vaccines/efficiency-effectiveness.
4. "Vaccination Coverage Among Adults in the United States, National Health Interview Survey, 2015," Centers for Disease Control and Prevention, https:// www.cdc.gov/vaccines/imz-managers/coverage/adultvaxview/coverage -estimates/2015.html.
5. Andrew Buncombe, "One in Three Donald Trump Supporters Believe Vaccines Cause Autism—So Does the President-Elect," *The Independent*, December 29, 2016, http:// www.independent.co.uk/life-style/health-and-families/health-news/donald-trump -supporters-believe-anti-vaxxers-autism-vaccines-president-elect-a7500701.html.
6. Chris Exley, "Aluminum Adjuvants in Vaccines," The Hippocratic Post (blog), April 12, 2017, https://www.hippocraticpost.com/infection-disease/aluminium -adjuvants-vaccines/.

Chapter 1: "There Is No Autism Epidemic"

1. Dan Olmsted and Mark Blaxill, *Denial: How Refusing to Face the Facts about Our Autism Epidemic Hurts Children, Families, and Our Future* (New York: Skyhorse Publishing, 2017), inside cover.
2. Steve Silberman, *Neurotribes: The Legacy of Autism and the Future of Neurodiversity* (New York: Penguin, 2015): 470.
3. Steve Silberman, "Neurodiversity Rewires Conventional Thinking about Brains," *Wired*, April 16, 2013.
4. Silberman, "Neurodiversity."
5. Steve Phelps, "Before Autism Had a Name," *The Atlantic*, August 24, 2015.
6. Silberman, "Neurodiversity."

7. Anne Dachel, "Robert Kennedy Jr. at DC Rally," *Age of Autism* (blog), April 14, 2017, http://www.ageofautism.com/2017/04/robert-kennedy-jr-at-dc-rally.html.

8. Graham Slaughter, "Group Homes for Adults with Autism Unaffordable and Inaccessible, Parents Say," *CTVNews*, June 8, 2016, https://www.ctvnews.ca/health/group-homes -for-adults-with-autism-unaffordable-and-inaccessible-parents-say-1.2937838.

9. Olmsted and Blaxill, *Denial*, 38.

10. Olmsted and Blaxill, *Denial*, xvii.

11. Olmsted and Blaxill, *Denial*, xvii.

12. Olmsted and Blaxill, *Denial*, xiii.

13. Data sourced from the California Department of Education's Diagnostic Center of Central California's website: http://www.dcc-cde.ca.gov/af/afbasic.htm.

14. Gnakub N. Soke et al., "Brief Report: Prevalence of Self-Injurious Behaviors among Children with Autism Spectrum Disorder—A Population-Based Study," *Journal of Autism and Developmental Disorders* 46, no. 11 (2016): 3607–3614.

15. Keydra L. Phillips et al., "Prevalence and Impact of Unhealthy Weight in a National Sample of US Adolescents with Autism and Other Learning and Behavioral Disabilities," *Maternal and Child Health Journal* 18, no. 8 (2014): 1964–1975.

16. Paul T. Shattuck et al., "Postsecondary Education and Employment among Youth with an Autism Spectrum Disorder," *Pediatrics* 129, no. 6 (2012): 1042–1049.

17. Ariane V. S. Buescher et al., "Costs of Autism Spectrum Disorders in the United Kingdom and the United States," *JAMA Pediatrics* 168, no. 8 (2014): 721–728.

18. Laura A. Scheive et al., "Concurrent Medical Conditions and Health Care Use and Needs among Children with Learning and Behavioral Developmental Disabilities, National Health Interview Survey, 2006–2010," *Research in Developmental Disabilities* 33, no. 2 (2012): 467–476.

19. Joseph Shapiro, "The Sexual Assault Epidemic No One Talks About," *National Public Radio*, January 8, 2018, https://www.npr.org/2018/01/08/570224090/ the-sexual-assault-epidemic-no-one-talks-about.

20. *Autism and Health: A Special Report by Autism Speaks* (New York: Autism Speaks, 2017), https://www.autismspeaks.org/sites/default/files/docs/facts_and_figures _report_final_v3.pdf.

21. "Personal Tragedies, Public Crisis," Autistica, 2016, https://www.autistica.org.uk /downloads/files/Personal-tragedies-public-crisis-ONLINE.pdf.

22. *1 in 88 Children: A Look into the Federal Response to Rising Autism Rates, Before the House Comm. on Oversight and Government Reform*, 112th Cong. (2012); complete summary of the hearing available at: http://oversight.house.gov/wp-content/ uploads/2013/04/2012-11-29-Ser-No-112-194-FC-Hearing-on-Autism.pdf.

23. Robert F. Kennedy Jr., "Is the Autism Epidemic Real?," *EcoWatch* (blog), April 6, 2016, https://www.ecowatch.com/is-the-autism-epidemic-real-1891078228.html.

24. Olmsted and Blaxill, *Denial*, 143.

25. Dan Olmsted and Mark Blaxill, "Voting Himself Rich: CDC Vaccine Adviser Made $29 Million or More after Using Role to Create Market," *Age of Autism* (blog), February 16, 2009, http://www.ageofautism.com/2009/02/voting-himself-rich-cdc- vaccine-adviser-made-29-million-or-more-after-using-role-to-create-market.html.

26. Dan Olmsted, "Age of Autism Awards 2010: Dr. Paul Offit, Denialist of the Decade," *Age of Autism* (blog), December 29, 2010, http://www.ageofautism.com/2010/12/age-of-autism-awards-2010-dr-paul-offit-denialist-of-the-decade.html.

27. Justine van der Leun, "AOL Health: Autism Experts Offit and Dawson on Causes, Cures and Controversies," *Autism Science Foundation* (blog), March 9, 2010, https://autismsciencefoundation.wordpress.com/2010/03/09/aol-health-autism-experts-offit-and-dawson-on-causes-cures-and-controversies/.

28. Peter Hotez, "Russian–United States Vaccine Science Diplomacy: Preserving the Legacy," *PLoS Neglected Tropical Diseases* 11, no. 5 (2017); competing interest section spells out that Dr. Hotez is a patent holder for hookworm, schistosomiasis, and "several other" vaccines.

29. Dr. Fombonne's paper, "Pervasive Developmental Disorders in Montreal, Quebec, Canada: Prevalence and Links with Immunizations" in *Pediatrics* 118, no. 1 (2006), included this disclosure: "Since June 2004, Dr. Fombonne has been an expert witness for vaccine manufacturers in US thimerosal litigation."

30. Orac, "Well, That Didn't Take Long: The Knives Come Out for Paul Shattuck," *Respectful Insolence* (blog), April 5, 2006, https://respectfulinsolence.com/2006/04/05/well-that-didnt-take-long-the/.

31. Olmsted and Blaxill, *Denial*, 144–145.

32. Dr. Bernard Rimland, "The Autism Epidemic, Vaccinations, and Mercury," *Journal of Nutritional and Environmental Medicine* 10 (2000): 261–266.

33. Rimland, "The Autism Epidemic, Vaccinations, and Mercury," 261.

34. Darold Treffert et al., "Epidemiology of Infantile Autism," *Archives of General Psychiatry* 22, no. 5 (1970): 431–438.

35. Darold Treffert, "The Autism 'Epidemic' in Perspective," *Wisconsin Medical Society* (blog), https://www.wisconsinmedicalsociety.org/professional/savant-syndrome/archive/2015-archive/whats-new-2015-private/the-autism-epidemic-in-perspective/.

36. Larry Burd et al., "A Prevalence Study of Pervasive Developmental Disorders in North Dakota," *Journal of the American Academy of Child & Adolescent Psychiatry* 26, no. 5 (1987): 700–703.

37. Larry Burd et al., "A Prevalence Methodology for Mental Illness and Developmental Disorders in Rural and Frontier Settings," *International Journal of Circumpolar Health* 59, no. 1 (2000): 74–86.

38. Olmsted and Blaxill, *Denial*, 123.

39. The entire study and all the data is available on the website of the National Archives at: https://www.archives.gov/research/electronic-records/nih.html.

40. Accessible through the website of the National Archives at: https://catalog.archives.gov/search?q=*:*&rows=20&tabType=all&facet=true&facet.fields=oldScope,level,materialsType,fileFormat,locationIds,dateRangeFacet&highlight=true&f.parentNaId=606622&f.level=fileUnit&sort=naIdSort%20asc.

41. Dachel, "Robert Kennedy Jr. at DC Rally."

42. L. E. Sever et al., *Volume I: An Introduction to the History, Scope, and Methodology of the Project* (Columbus, OH: Battelle, prepared for the National Institute of

Neurological and Communicative Disorders and Stroke, 1983); available via the National Archives.

43. E. Fuller Torrey et al., "Early Childhood Psychosis and Bleeding during Pregnancy—A Prospective Study of Gravid Women and Their Offspring," *Journal of Autism and Childhood Schizophrenia* 5, no. 4 (1975): 287–297.

44. Phone interview with Dr. Torrey, October 18, 2017.

45. Olmsted and Blaxill, *Denial*, 126.

46. *Changes in the Population of Persons with Autism and Pervasive Developmental Disorders in California's Developmental Services System: 1987 through 1998, A Report to the Legislature* (Sacramento: California Department of Developmental Services, 1999).

47. Olmsted and Blaxill, *Denial*, 128.

48. Lisa A. Croen et al., "The Changing Prevalence of Autism in California," *Journal of Autism and Developmental Disorder* 32, no. 3 (2002): 207–215.

49. Lisa A. Croen and Judith K. Grether, "Response: A Response to Blaxill, Baskin, and Spitzer on Croen et al. (2002), 'The Changing Prevalence of Autism in California," *Journal of Autism and Developmental Disorders* 33, no. 2 (2003): 227–229.

50. Robert S. Byrd et al., *Report to the Legislature on the Principal Findings from the Epidemiology of Autism in California: A Comprehensive Pilot Study* (Davis: MIND Institute, University of California, Davis, 2002), http://www.dds.ca.gov/autism/docs/study_final.pdf.

51. James G. Gurney et al., "Analysis of Prevalence Trends of Autism Spectrum Disorder in Minnesota," *Archives of Pediatrics & Adolescent Medicine* 157, no. 7 (2003): 622–627.

52. Craig Newschaffer et al., "National Autism Prevalence Trends from United States Special Education Data," *Pediatrics* 115, no. 3 (2005): 277–282.

53. Olmsted and Blaxill, *Denial*, 117.

54. Ira Hertz-Picciotto and Lora Delwiche, "The Rise in Autism and the Role of Age at Diagnosis," *Epidemiology* 20, no. 1 (2009): 84–90.

55. David Kirby, "UC Davis Study Authors: Autism Is Environmental (Can We Move On Now?)," *Huffington Post*, February 7, 2009, https://www.huffingtonpost.com/david-kirby/uc-davis-study-autism-is_b_156153.html.

56. Cynthia D. Nevison, "A Comparison of Temporal Trends in United States Autism Prevalence to Trends in Suspected Environmental Factors," *Environmental Health* 13, no. 73 (2014), 1–16.

57. Cynthia D. Nevison, "Empirical Data Show Autism Is on the Rise. Is It Logical to Blame the Toxins of the 1970s?" *SafeMinds* (blog), September 10, 2014, https://safeminds.org/blog/2014/09/10/empirical-data-show-autism-rise-logical-blame-toxins-1970s/.

58. James Lyons-Weiler, "Why Are the Same People Who Failed at Science on Agent Orange in Charge of Vaccine Safety and Developmental Disorders at the CDC?," World Mercury Project, February 27, 2018, https://worldmercuryproject.org/news/why-are-the-same-people-who-failed-at-science-on-agent-orange-in-charge-of-vaccine-safety-and-developmental-disorders-at-the-cdc/.

59. "CDC Estimates 1 in 68 School-Aged Children Have Autism; No Change from Previous Estimate," Centers for Disease Control and Prevention, March 31, 2016, https://www.cdc.gov/media/releases/2016/p0331-children-autism.html.

60. "Principal Investigator for CDC Utah Autism Data Filed Whistleblower Lawsuit," *AHRP* (blog), April 10, 2016, http://ahrp.org/lawsuit-by-principal-investigator -for-cdc-utah-autism-data-filed-whistleblower-lawsuit/.

61. "Utah Whistleblower Lawsuit Alleges Data Errors and Research Misconduct as CDC Report Releases U.S. Autism Rate of 1.5%," *HealthChoice* (blog), March 31, 2016, http://healthchoice.org/2016/03/31/utah-whistleblower-lawsuit-alleges-data -errors-and-research-misconduct-as-cdc-report-releases-u-s-autism-rate-of-1-5/.

62. Dr. Judith Pinborough-Zimmerman, Facebook post, December 1, 2017.

63. Brita Belli, "The Search for Autism's Missing Piece: Autism Research Slowly Turns Its Focus to Environmental Toxicity," *The Environmental Magazine*, January– February 2010, https://emagazine.com/autism-clue/.

Chapter 2: "Vaccines Are Safe and Effective"

1. Interview with Dr. Paul Thomas, pediatrician in Portland, OR, with more than 13,000 patients, December 6, 2016.

2. Emmanuel Stamatakis, Richard Weiler, and John P. A. Ioannidis, "Undue Industry Influences That Distort Healthcare Research, Strategy, Expenditure and Practice: A Review," *European Journal of Clinical Investigation* 43, no. 5 (2013): 469–475.

3. Bourree Lam, "Vaccines Are Profitable, So What?," *The Atlantic*, February 10, 2015, https://www.theatlantic.com/business/archive/2015/02/vaccines-are-profitable -so-what/385214/.

4. "Vaccine Market by Technology (Inactivated, Subunit, Conjugate, Live Attenuated, Toxoid, and Dendritic Cell Synthetic), Type (Therapeutic, Preventive), Indication (Allergy, Infectious Disease, Tumors and Others) for Infants, Early Aged, and Post Aged: Global Industry Perspective, Comprehensive Analysis, Size, Share, Growth, Segment, Trends and Forecast, 2014–2020," Zion Research, 2016, http:// www.marketresearchstore.com/news/vaccine-market-218.

5. Jay P. Sanford et al., *Vaccine Supply and Innovation* (Washington, DC: National Academies Press, 1985), Table 4.5, p. 55.

6. Glen Nowak, *Increasing Awareness and Uptake of Influenza Immunization* (Atlanta: Centers for Disease Control and Prevention, 2015), http://nationalacademies.org /hmd/~/media/Files/Activity%20Files/PublicHealth/MicrobialThreats/Nowak.pdf.

7. Mr. Johnson's presentation is available on the website of the National Adult and Influenza Immunization Summit at https://www.izsummitpartners.org/content /uploads/2008/NIVS/Johnson_2008.pdf.

8. Peter Doshi, "Are US Flu Death Figures More PR than Science?" *British Medical Journal* 331 (2005): 1412.

9. Tom Jefferson, "Influenza Vaccination: Policy versus Evidence," *British Medical Journal* 333 (2006): 912.

10. Peter Doshi, "Influenza: Marketing Vaccine by Marketing Disease," *British Medical Journal* 346 (2013): f3037.

11. Jon Cohen, "Why Flu Vaccines So Often Fail," *Science*, September 20, 2017. http://www.sciencemag.org/news/2017/09/why-flu-vaccines-so-often-fail.

12. Bernard Guyer et al., "Annual Summary of Vital Statistics: Trends in the Health of Americans during the 20th Century," *Pediatrics* 106, no. 6 (2000), 1307–1317.

13. Suzanne Humphries and Roman Bystrianyk, *Dissolving Illusions: Disease, Vaccines, and the Forgotten History* (CreateSpace Independent Publishing Platform, 2013), foreword.

14. J. T. Biggs, *Leicester: Sanitation versus Vaccination* (London: The National Anti-Vaccination League, 1912), 72.

15. Dr. Andrew Weil, *Health and Healing: The Philosophy of Integrative Medicine and Optimum Health* (New York: Mariner Books, 2004), 82.

16. Taryn Luna, "California Vaccine Rates Increase after Legislature Toughens Rules for Children," *Sacramento Bee*, April 12, 2017, http://www.sacbee.com/news/politics-government/capitol-alert/article144271694.html.

17. Stanley Plotkin, *Plotkin's Vaccines, 7th Edition* (Philadelphia: Elsevier, 2018); key information from the book can be found at http://www.immune.org.nz/vaccines/efficiency-effectiveness.

18. Walter W. Williams et al., "Surveillance of Vaccination Coverage Among Adult Populations—United States, 2015," *Morbidity and Mortality Weekly Report* 66, no. 11 (2017): 1–28, https://www.cdc.gov/mmwr/volumes/66/ss/ss6611a1.htm.

19. Gretchen Dubeau, "If Only Half of America Is Properly Vaccinated, Where Are the Epidemics?," *The Hill*, September 13, 2016, http://thehill.com/blogs/congress-blog/healthcare/295562-if-only-half-of-america-is-properly-vaccinated-where-are-the.

20. This table is maintained by the Centers for Disease Control and Prevention and available on their website at https://www.cdc.gov/vaccines/pubs/pinkbook/downloads/appendices/G/coverage.pdf.

21. Marlene Cimons, "Vaccine Injury Fund Bill Approved but Faces Veto," *Los Angeles Times*, October 20, 1986, http://articles.latimes.com/1986-10-20/news/mn-6535_1_vaccine-manufacturers.

22. Robert Pear, "Reagan Signs Bill on Drug Exports and Payment for Vaccine Injuries," *New York Times*, November 15, 1986, http://www.nytimes.com/1986/11/15/us/reagan-signs-bill-on-drug-exports-and-payment-for-vaccine-injuries.html.

23. Alan R. Hinman, "DTP Vaccine Litigation," *American Journal of Diseases of Children* 140 (1986): 528–530.

24. Cimons, "Vaccine Injury Fund Bill."

25. Pear, "Reagan Signs Bill."

26. From the National Vaccine Injury Compensation website, maintained by the Department of Health and Human Services; payouts are available through this link: https://www.hrsa.gov/sites/default/files/hrsa/vaccine-compensation/monthly-website-stats-2-01-18.pdf.

27. "Vaccine Market by Technology."

28. Sanford et al., *Vaccine Supply and Innovation*.

29. Elisabeth Rosenthal, "The Price of Prevention: Vaccine Costs Are Soaring," *New York Times*, July 2, 2014, https://www.nytimes.com/2014/07/03/health/Vaccine -Costs-Soaring-Paying-Till-It-Hurts.html.

30. The Danish Health and Medicines Authority provides the Danish vaccine schedule at: https://www.sst.dk/en/disease-and-treatment/~/media/B74655FEA6DF477 1998A6BDEA96A374A.ashx.

31. The National Health Service website addresses the chickenpox vaccine at https:// www.nhs.uk/chq/Pages/1032.aspx?CategoryID=62.

32. The Oregon Health Authority lists reportable diseases through this website: http:// www.oregon.gov/oha/ph/DiseasesConditions/CommunicableDisease/Reporting CommunicableDisease/Pages/reportable.aspx.

33. "8 Ways to Improve Your Child's Immune System," *Ask Dr. Sears* (blog), https:// www.askdrsears.com/topics/health-concerns/vaccines/more-vaccine-articles/boost -childs-immune-system.

34. Mike Stobbe, "Whooping Cough Vaccine May Not Halt Spread of Illness," *NBC News*, November 25, 2013, https://www.nbcnews.com/health/cold-flu/whooping -cough-vaccine-may-not-halt-spread-illness-f2D11655363.

35. Don Thea, "Resurgence of Whooping Cough May Owe to Vaccine's Inability to Prevent Infections," *Boston University School of Public Health* (blog), September 21, 2017, https://www.bu.edu/sph/2017/09/21/resurgence-of-whooping-cough-may -owe-to-vaccines-inability-to-prevent-infections/.

36. Julia Belluz, "Harvard Has a Mumps Outbreak. Here's Why the Virus Can Have a Field Day on Campus," *Vox* (blog), April 28, 2016, https://www.vox.com/2016/4/28 /11520670/mumps-virus-outbreak-harvard.

37. Mike Stobbe, "U.S. Vaccine Panel to Discuss Waning Effectiveness, New Shots," *USA Today*, October 24, 2017, https://www.usatoday.com/story/news/2017/10/24 /u-s-vaccine-panel-discuss-waning-effectiveness-new-shots/797446001/.

38. Ed Silverman, "Merck Is Accused of Stonewalling Over Effectiveness of Mumps Vaccine," *Wall Street Journal*, June 8, 2015, https://blogs.wsj.com/pharmalot/2015 /06/08/merck-is-accused-of-stonewalling-over-effectiveness-of-mumps-vaccine/.

39. The IPOL vaccine package insert can be found at the FDA's website here: https:// www.fda.gov/downloads/biologicsbloodvaccines/vaccines/approvedproducts/ ucm133479.pdf.

40. The Recombivax HB vaccine package insert can be found at the FDA's website here: https://www.fda.gov/downloads/biologicsbloodvaccines/vaccines/approved- products/ucm110114.pdf.

41. Dr. Harold E. Buttram, "Response: Superficial and Misleading Critique," *British Medical Journal*, October 4, 2004, http://www.bmj.com/ rapid-response/2011/10/30/superficial-and-misleading-critique.

42. Ross Lazarus et al., *Electronic Support for Public Health–Vaccine Adverse Event Reporting System (ESP:VAERS)* (Rockville, MD: The Agency for Healthcare Research and Quality, prepared by Harvard Pilgrim Health Care, Inc., 2010), 6, https://healthit.ahrq.gov/sites/default/files/docs/publication/r18hs017045 -lazarus-final-report-2011.pdf.

43. Available on the Vaccine Adverse Events Reporting System website maintained by the CDC: https://vaers.hhs.gov/data/datasets.html.

44. Lazarus et al., *Electronic Support for Public Health*, 6.

45. Institute of Medicine, *Adverse Effects of Pertussis and Rubella Vaccines* (Washington, DC: The National Academies Press, 1991), https://doi.org/10.17226/1815.

46. Institute of Medicine, *Adverse Effects of Vaccines: Evidence and Causality* (Washington, DC: The National Academies Press, 2012), https://doi.org/10.17226/13164.

47. Gary Goldman and Neil Miller, "Relative Trends in Hospitalizations and Mortality among Infants by the Number of Vaccine Doses and Age, Based on the Vaccine Adverse Event Reporting System (VAERS), 1990–2010," *Human and Experimental Toxicology* 31, no. 10 (2012): 1012–1021.

48. Available on the American Academy of Pediatrics website: https://www.aap.org /en-us/advocacy-and-policy/aap-health-initiatives/immunizations/Pages /Common-Parental-Concerns.aspx.

49. Peter Aaby et al., "The Introduction of Diphtheria-Tetanus-Pertussis and Oral Polio Vaccine among Young Infants in an Urban African Community: A Natural Experiment," *EBiomedicine*, 17 (2017): 192–198, http://www.ebiomedicine.com /article/S2352-3964(17)30046-4/fulltext.

50. Tetyana Obukhanych, *Vaccine Illusion: How Vaccination Compromises Our Natural Immunity* (Amazon Digital Services LLC, 2012), introduction.

51. Karen Lema, "Philippine President Vows to Get to the Bottom of Dengue Vaccine 'Health Scam,'" *Reuters*, December 3, 2017, https://fr.reuters.com/article/company News/idFRL3N1O307Z.

52. Michaeleen Doucleef, "Vaccine Safety Concerns Shut Down Immunization Campaign in Philippines," *National Public Radio*, December 5, 2017, https://www .npr.org/sections/goatsandsoda/2017/12/05/568368515/vaccine-safety-concerns -shut-down-immunization-campaign-in-philippines.

53. Stephanie Soucheray, "Contrary Dengue Vaccine Response Hints at Possible Problems with Zika," *CIDRAP NEWS*, July 28, 2016, http://www.cidrap.umn.edu /news-perspective/2016/07/contrary-dengue-vaccine-response-hints-possible -problems-zika.

54. Heather Yourex-West and Sage McIntosh, "Canadian Study Finds Flu Shot Could Increase Risk of Getting Sick," *Global News*, January 30, 2015, https:// globalnews.ca/news/1804162/canadian-study-finds-flu-shot-could-increase -risk-of-getting-sick/.

55. Jing Yan et al., "Infectious Virus in Exhaled Breath of Symptomatic Seasonal Influenza Cases from a College Community," *PNAS* 115, no. 5 (2018): 1081–1086, https://doi.org/10.1073/pnas.1716561115.

56. Merck has a press release of 2016 results on its company website: http://investors. merck.com/news/press-release-details/2017/Merck-Announces-Fourth-Quarter -and-Full-Year-2016-Financial-Results/default.aspx.

57. Julia Belluz, "Why Japan's HPV Vaccine Rates Dropped from 70% to Near Zero," *Vox*, December 1, 2017, https://www.vox.com/science-and-health/2017 /12/1/16723912/japan-hpv-vaccine.

58. The entire report can be found at the Medwatcher Japan website: http://www
.yakugai.gr.jp/topics/file/en/Refutation%20of%20GACVS%20Statement%20
on%20Safety%20of%20HPV%20Vaccines_17%20December%202015.pdf.

59. Paul Cullen, "The HPV Propaganda Battle: The Other Side Finally Fights Back,"
The Irish Times, September 16, 2017, https://www.irishtimes.com/life-and-style/
health-family/the-hpv-propaganda-battle-the-other-side-finally-fights-back
-1.3221166.

60. M. Martínez-Lavín and L. Amezcua-Guerra, "Serious Adverse Events after HPV
Vaccination: A Critical Review of Randomized Trials and Post-Marketing Case
Series," *Clinical Rheumatology* 39, no. 10 (2017): 2169.

61. Scott P. Commins et al., "Alum-Containing Vaccines Increase Total and Food
Allergen-Specific IgE, and Cow's Milk Oral Desensitization Increases Bosd4
IgG4 While Peanut Avoidance Increases Arah2 IgE: The Complexity of Today's
Child with Food Allergy," *The Journal of Allergy and Clinical Immunology* 137, no. 2
(2016): AB151.

62. Margarida Castell et al., "Development and Characterization of an Effective Food
Allergy Model in Brown Norway Rats," *PLOS One* 10, no. 4 (2015), https://doi
.org/10.1371/journal.pone.0125314.

63. Yehuda Shoenfeld et al., *Vaccines and Autoimmunity* (Hoboken, NJ: Wiley
Blackwell, 2015).

64. David J. Spencer et al., "Epidemiological Basis for Eradication of Measles in 1967,"
Public Health Reports 82, no. 3 (1967): 253–256.

65. Roger M. Barkin, "Measles Mortality: A Retrospective Look at the Vaccine Era,"
American Journal of Epidemiology 2, no. 4 (1975): 341–349.

66. David M. Mannino et al., "Surveillance for Asthma—United States, 1960–1995,"
Morbidity and Mortality Weekly Report 47, no. 1 (1998): 1–27, https://www.cdc
.gov/mmwr/preview/mmwrhtml/00052262.htm.

67. Stuart Blume and Jan Hendricks, "Measles Vaccination before the Measles-
Mumps-Rubella Vaccine," *American Journal of Public Health* 103, no. 8 (2013):
1393–1401.

68. Available on the Physicians for Informed Consent website: https://physiciansfor
informedconsent.org/measles/vrs/.

69. Morton S. Biskind, "Public Health Aspects of the New Insecticides," *American
Journal of Digestive Diseases* 20, no. 11 (1953): 331–41.

70. Biskind, "New Insecticides," 334.

71. Biskind, "New Insecticides," 334.

72. Humphries and Bystrianyk, *Dissolving Illusions*.

73. Statement on the website of the Centers for Disease Control in a section titled
"Polio Elimination in the United States" can be found at https://www.cdc.gov
/polio/us/.

74. Stephen Mawdsley, "Polio Provocation—the Health Debate That Refused to Go
Away," *University of Cambridge Research* (blog), September 3, 2013, http://www
.cam.ac.uk/research/features/polio-provocation-the-health-debate-that-refused
-to-go-away.

75. M. Gromeier and E. Wimmer, "Mechanism of Injury-Provoked Poliomyelitis," *Journal of Virology* 76, no. 6 (1998): 5056–5060.
76. Seven-part series at *The Age of Autism* blog available at http://www.ageofautism .com/2011/09/the-age-of-polio-how-an-old-virus-and-new-toxins-triggered-a -man-made-epidemic-1.html.
77. Daniel W. Cramer et al., "Mumps and Ovarian Cancer: Modern Interpretation of an Historic Association," *Cancer Causes & Control* 21, no. 8 (2010): 1193–1201.
78. Hans-Ulrich Albonico et al., "Febrile Infectious Childhood Diseases in the History of Cancer Patients and Matched Control," *Medical Hypotheses* 51, no. 4 (1998): 315–320.
79. F. E. Alexander et al., "Risk Factors for Hodgkin's Disease by Epstein-Barr Virus (EBV) Status: Prior Infection by EBV and Other Agents," *British Journal of Cancer* 82, no. 5 (2000): 1117–1121.
80. Stephen A. Hoption Cann et al., "Acute Infections as a Means of Cancer Prevention: Opposing Effects to Chronic Infections?," *Cancer Detection and Prevention* 30, no. 1 (2006): 83–93.
81. E. Susan Amirian et al., "History of Chickenpox in Glioma Risk: A Report from the Glioma International Case–Control Study," *Cancer Medicine* 5, no. 6 (2016): 1352–1358.
82. Robert Mendelsohn, "The Medical Time Bomb of Immunization against Disease," *East West Journal*, November 1984, 48.
83. Mendelsohn, "Medical Time Bomb," 48.
84. Priyanka Boghani, "Dr. Robert W. Sears: Why Partial Vaccinations May Be an Answer," *PBS Frontline*, March 23, 2015, https://www.pbs.org/wgbh/frontline /article/robert-w-sears-why-partial-vaccinations-may-be-an-answer/.
85. Joseph Mercola, "Vaccination: The Neurological Poison So Common Your Doctor Probably Pushes It," *Mercola.com*, April 11, 2012, https://articles.mercola.com /sites/articles/archive/2012/04/11/vaccination-impact-on-childrens-health.aspx.
86. Suzanne Humphries, "Smoke, Mirrors, and the 'Disappearance' of Polio," *International Medical Council on Vaccination*, November 17, 2011, http://drsuzanne .net/wp-content/uploads/2012/07/Smoke-Mirrors-and-the-"Disappearance" -Of-Polio-_-International-Medical-Council.pdf.
87. Rachael Ross, "Vaccines, Vaccine Injury, & My Perspective as a Doctor & Mom," *Dr. Rachael*, July 1, 2016, http://drrachael.com/vaccines-vaccine-injuries -my-perspective-as-a-doctor-and-mom/.
88. Daniel Neides, "Make 2017 the Year to Avoid Toxins (Good Luck) and Master Your Domain: Words on Wellness," Cleveland *Plain Dealer*, January 6, 2017, http://www.cleveland.com/lyndhurst-south-euclid/index.ssf/2017/01 /make_2017_the_year_to_avoid_to.html.

Chapter 3: "The Science Is Settled"

1. Olmsted and Blaxill, "Voting Himself Rich."
2. Maggie Fox, "Asked and Answered: Yes, Vaccines Are Safe," *Today* (blog), January 10, 2017, https://www.today.com/health/are-vaccines-safe-answer-clear-yes-t106904.

3. Julia Belluz, "Robert De Niro and RFK Jr. Have Joined Forces to Push Vaccine Nonsense," *Vox* (blog), February 15, 2017, https://www.vox.com/2017/2/15/14622632/robert-de-niro-rfk-jr-vaccine-press-conference.

4. Paul A. Offit, "Vaccine History: Developments by Year," *Children's Hospital of Philadelphia* (blog), http://www.chop.edu/centers-programs/vaccine-education-center/vaccine-history/developments-by-year.

5. Offit, "Vaccine History."

6. Available on the Centers for Disease Control and Prevention's website at: https://www.cdc.gov/vaccines/schedules/hcp/imz/child-adolescent.html.

7. David Kirby, "New Study: Hepatitis B Vaccine Triples the Risk of Autism in Infant Boys," *Huffington Post*, November 17, 2011, https://www.huffingtonpost.com/david-kirby/new-study-hepatitis-b-vac_b_289288.html.

8. J. D. Grabenstein, *ImmunoFacts: Vaccines and Immunologic Drugs—2013 (38th revision)* (St. Louis: Wolters Kluwer Health, 2012).

9. Thomas Verstraeten, "Safety of Thimerosal-Containing Vaccines: A Two-Phased Study of Computerized Health Maintenance Organization Databases," *Pediatrics* 112, no. 5 (2003): 1039–1048.

10. Thomas Verstraeten, "Thimerosal, the Centers for Disease Control and Prevention, and GlaxoSmithKline," *Pediatrics* 113, no. 4 (2004): 932.

11. Alberto Eugenio Tozzi, "Neuropsychological Performance 10 Years After Immunization in Infancy with Thimerosal-Containing Vaccines," *Pediatrics* 123, no. 2 (2009): 475–482.

12. Carla K. Johnson, "Study Adds to Evidence of Vaccine Safety," *Associated Press*, January 26, 2009.

13. J.B. Handley, "Feeding the Hungry Lie, Italian Style," *Age of Autism* (blog), January 27, 2009, http://www.ageofautism.com/2009/01/feeding-the-hungry-lie-italian-style.html.

14. Vincenzo Miranda, "This Study Is Not Methodologically Correct," *Pediatrics* 123, no. 2 (2009), published comments to Tozzi et al., "Neuropsychological Performance 10 Years after Immunization in Infancy with Thimerosal-Containing Vaccines."

15. Anjali Jain et al., "Autism Occurrence by MMR Vaccine Status among US Children with Older Siblings with and without Autism," *JAMA* 313, no. 15 (2015): 1534–1540.

16. Press release on the JAMA Network website can be found here: https://media.jamanetwork.com/news-item/no-association-found-between-mmr-vaccine-and-autism-even-among-children-at-higher-risk/.

17. Dr. Gordon's biography page on the NIMH website: https://www.nimh.nih.gov/about/director/index.shtml.

18. Private email correspondence from Dr. Joshua Gordon, May 31, 2017.

19. L. E. Taylor et al., "Vaccines Are Not Associated with Autism: An Evidence-Based Meta-analysis of Case-Control and Cohort Studies," *Vaccine* 32, no. 29 (2014): 3623–3629.

20. Private email correspondence between autism parent and Dr. Joshua Gordon, July 10, 2017.

21. Private email correspondence from Dr. Joshua Gordon, September 1, 2017.
22. Definition from Wikipedia: https://en.wikipedia.org/wiki/Biological_plausibility.
23. Definition from Wikipedia: https://en.wikipedia.org/wiki/Encephalopathy.
24. James Surowiecki, *The Wisdom of Crowds* (New York: Anchor Books, 2005), back cover.
25. From the CDC's website, addressing the Vaccine Adverse Events Reporting System: https://wonder.cdc.gov/wonder/help/vaers/reportable.htm.
26. Fugitive "profiles" on the website of the Office of Inspector General website: https://oig.hhs.gov/fraud/fugitives/profiles.asp.
27. Debra Goldschmidt, "Journal Questions Validity of Autism and Vaccine Study," CNN, August 28, 2014, https://www.cnn.com/2014/08/27/health/irpt-cdc-autism-vaccine-study/index.html.
28. David Lewis, "Mistrust of Government Drives Public Concerns Regarding Vaccine Safety," *The Oconee Enterprise*, December 3, 2015, A6.
29. Eric Hurwits et al., "Effects of Diphtheria-Tetanus-Pertussis or Tetanus Vaccination on Allergies and Allergy-Related Respiratory Symptoms," *Journal of Manipulative and Physiological Therapeutics* 23, no. 2 (2000): 81–90.
30. Carolyn Gallagher et al., "Hepatitis B Triple Series Vaccine and Developmental Disability in US Children Aged 1–9 Years," *Toxicological & Environmental Chemistry* 90, no. 5 (2008): 997–1008.
31. Carolyn M. Gallagher et al., "Hepatitis B Vaccination of Male Neonates and Autism Diagnosis," *Journal of Toxicology and Environmental Health* 73, no. 24 (2010): 1665–1677.
32. Anthony R. Mawson et al., "Pilot Comparative Study on the Health of Vaccinated and Unvaccinated 6- to 12-Year-Old U.S. Children," *Journal of Translational Science* 3, no. 3 (2017): 1–12.
33. Neides, "Make 2017 the Year."
34. Anthony R. Mawson et al., "Preterm Birth, Vaccination and Neurodevelopmental Disorders: A Cross-Sectional Study of 6- to 12-Year-Old Vaccinated and Unvaccinated Children," *Journal of Translational Science* 3, no. 3 (2017): 1–8.

Chapter 4: "The Reward Is Never Financial"

1. Anne Dachel, "Dr. Halvorsen on Wakefield, Witch Hunts and Vaccine Safety," *Age of Autism* (blog), February 8, 2011, http://www.ageofautism.com/2011/02/dr-halvorsen-on-wakefield-witch-hunts-and-vaccine-safety.html.
2. From the *Business Wire* website; a press release announcing the 7th edition of *Plotkin's Vaccines*: https://www.businesswire.com/news/home/20170523006047/en/Plotkins-Vaccines-Edition-No.-7-2017--.
3. "Who Are the Most Influential People in Vaccines?" poll conducted by the Vaccine Nation Blog can be found at: http://www.vaccinenation.org/2013/02/19/influential-people-vaccines/.
4. The 2009 Maxwell Finland Award for Scientific Achievement Award includes an extensive biography of Dr. Plotkin at: http://www.nfid.org/awards/plotkin.pdf.
5. Dan Olmsted and Mark Blaxill, "Voting Himself Rich."

6. "Second Michigan Mom in Court over Refusal to Vaccinate Child," *Fox News*, October 10, 2017, http://www.foxnews.com/health/2017/10/10/second-michigan -mom-in-court-over-refusal-to-vaccinate-child.html.

7. Email correspondence between Dr. Paul Offit and David Brown, August 18, 2009, http://www.rescuepost.com/files/offit-disclosures.pdf.

8. Comm. on Government Reform, Conflicts of Interest in Vaccine Policy Making, H.R. Doc (2000), https://worldmercuryproject.org/wp-content/uploads/conflicts -of-interest-government-reform-2000.pdf.

9. Olmsted and Blaxill, "Voting Himself Rich."

10. Marc Santora, "New York City's Flu Shot Mandate for Young Children Is Struck Down," *New York Times*, December 17, 2015.

11. Paul A. Offit, "Vaccine Exemptions? Call Them What They Really Are," Medscape, August 10, 2012, https://www.medscape.com/viewarticle/768746.

12. Ernest L. Wynder, Evarts A. Graham, and Adele B. Croninger, "Experimental Production of Carcinoma with Cigarette Tar," *Cancer Research* 13, no. 12 (1953): 855–864.

13. Jim Estes, "How the Big Tobacco Deal Went Bad," *New York Times*, October 6, 2014, opinion section.

14. Myron Levin, "Big Tobacco Is Guilty of Conspiracy," *Los Angeles Times*, August 18, 2006.

15. Oreskes and Conway, *Merchants of Doubt*, 16–17.

16. Oreskes and Conway, *Merchants of Doubt*, 16.

17. Jaimy Lee, "Pharma's $6 Billion Annual Ad Spend Targeted by Media Publishers," *Medical Marketing & Media*, August 21, 2017, https://www.mmm-online.com /media-news/pharmas-6-billion-annual-ad-spend-targeted-by-media-publishers /article/683050/.

18. Chris McGreal, "How Big Pharma's Money—and Its Politicians—Feed the US Opioid Crisis," *The Guardian*, October 19, 2017, https://www.theguardian.com /us-news/2017/oct/19/big-pharma-money-lobbying-us-opioid-crisis.

19. Reuters Staff, "Former CDC Head Lands Vaccine Job at Merck," *Reuters*, December 21, 2009, https://www.reuters.com/article/us-merck-gerberding /former-cdc-head-lands-vaccine-job-at-merck-idUSTRE5BK2K520091221.

20. "Vaccine Market by Technology."

21. Sanford et al., *Vaccine Supply and Innovation*.

22. The Centers for Disease Control and Prevention lists childhood vaccination schedules; historical vaccination schedules were sourced through Learntherisk.org.

23. Benjamin Zablotsky, "Estimated Prevalence of Children with Diagnosed Developmental Disabilities in the United States, 2014–2016," *NCHS Data Brief* no. 291 (2017), https://www.cdc.gov/nchs/data/databriefs/db291.pdf.

24. NCL Communications, "Survey: One-Third of American Parents Mistakenly Link Vaccines to Autism," National Consumers League, April 2014, http:// www.nclnet.org/survey_one_third_of_american_parents_mistakenly_link_ vaccines_to_autism.

25. Oreskes and Conway, *Merchants of Doubt*, 15–16.

26. Ameet Sarpatwari et al., "The Opioid Epidemic: Fixing a Broken Pharmaceutical Market," *Harvard Law & Policy Review* 11, no. 2 (2017): 463–484.

27. Ron Unz, "Chinese Melamine and American Vioxx: A Comparison," *The American Conservative*, April 18, 2012, http://www.theamericanconservative.com/articles /chinese-melamine-and-american-vioxx-a-comparison/.

28. Jim Edwards, "Merck Created Hit List to 'Destroy,' 'Neutralize' or 'Discredit' Dissenting Doctors," CBS News, *MoneyWatch*, May 6, 2009, https://www.cbs news.com/news/merck-created-hit-list-to-destroy-neutralize-or-discredit -dissenting-doctors/.

29. Amy James, "Lawsuit Reveals Merck Maintained Hit List of Doctors Critical of Vioxx," *The Bitter Pill* (blog), April 23, 2009, https://uniteforlife.wordpress .com/2009/04/23/lawsuit-reveals-merck-maintained-hit-list-of-doctors -critical-of-vioxx/.

30. Ariane Buescher et al., "Costs of Autism Spectrum Disorders in the United Kingdom and the United States," *JAMA Pediatrics* 168, no. 8 (2014): 721–728.

31. Rebecca Robbins, "Drug Makers Now Spend $5 Billion a Year on Advertising. Here's What That Buys," *STAT News*, March 9, 2016, https://www.statnews.com /2016/03/09/drug-industry-advertising/.

32. Aimee Picchi, "Drug Ads: $5.2 Billion Annually—and Rising," CBS News, March 11, 2016, https://www.cbsnews.com/news/drug-ads-5-2-billion-annually-and -rising/.

33. Dana O. Sarnak et al., "Paying for Prescription Drugs Around the World: Why Is the U.S. an Outlier?" *The Commonwealth Fund, Issue Brief*, October 2017, http:// www.commonwealthfund.org/~/media/files/publications/issue-brief/2017/oct /sarnak_paying_for_rx_ib_v2.pdf.

34. Sharyl Attkisson, "How Independent Are Vaccine Defenders?" CBS News, July 25, 2008, https://www.cbsnews.com/news/how-independent-are-vaccine-defenders/.

35. Dylan Byers, "Sharyl Attkisson Resigns from CBS News," *Politico*, March 10, 2014, https://www.politico.com/blogs/media/2014/03/sharyl-attkisson-resigns-from -cbs-news-184836.

36. Sharyl Attkisson, *Stonewalled: My Fight for Truth against the Forces of Obstruction, Intimidation, and Harassment in Obama's Washington* (New York: Harper Collins, 2015), 146.

37. Attkisson, *Stonewalled*, 147.

38. Allan M. Brandt, "How a PR Firm Helped Establish America's Cigarette Century," *AlterNet* (blog), April 15, 2017, https://www.alternet.org/story/50359/ how_a_pr_firm_helped_establish_america%27s_cigarette_century.

39. Oreskes and Conway, *Merchants of Doubt*, 16.

40. Andrew Wakefield et al., "Ileal-lymphoid-nodular Hyperplasia, Non-specific Colitis, and Pervasive Developmental Disorder in Children," *The Lancet* 351, no. 9103 (1998): 637–641.

41. "Dr. Wakefield: Govt. Experts Have Conceded that MMR Vaccine Caused Autism," *The Refusers* (blog), April 17, 2013, https://therefusers.com/dr-wakefield -govt-experts-have-conceded-that-mmr-vaccine-caused-autism/.

42. Simon Much et al., "Retraction of an Interpretation," *The Lancet* 363, no. 9411 (2004): 750.

43. "MMR Doctor Wins High Court Appeal," BBC News, March 7, 2012.

44. Isabelle Thomas, "Dr Andrew Wakefield, The Lancet Study and My Two Boys— Isabella Thomas," *Miss Eco Glam* (blog), April 16, 2013, http://www.missecoglam .com/health/vaccines/item/5446-dr-andrew-wakefield-the-lancet-study-and-my -two-boys-isabella-thomas.

45. Dr. Andrew Wakefield, "That Paper," *The Autism File* no. 33 (2009): 12–17.

46. Kevin Barry, *Vaccine Whistleblower* (New York: Skyhorse Publishing, 2015), 15.

Chapter 5: Emerging Science and Vaccine-Induced Autism

1. Daniel Niven, "Closing the 17-Year Gap between Scientific Evidence and Patient Care," *University Affairs*, January 17, 2017, https://www.universityaffairs.ca /opinion/in-my-opinion/closing-17-year-gap-scientific-evidence-patient-care/.

2. "Brain's Immune System Triggered in Autism," John Hopkins Medicine, November 15, 2004, https://www.hopkinsmedicine.org/Press_releases/2004/11_15a_04.html.

3. Carlos A. Pardo, "Neuroglial Activation and Neuroinflammation in the Brain of Patients with Autism," *Annals of Neurology* 57, no. 1 (2005): 67–81.

4. Paul H. Patterson, "Pregnancy, Immunity, Schizophrenia, and Autism," *Engineering and Science* 69, no. 3 (2006): 14.

5. K. Suzuki, et al., "Microglial Activation in Young Adults with Autism Spectrum Disorder," *JAMA Psychiatry* 70, no. 1 (2013): 49–58.

6. "Brain's Immune System Triggered in Autism," John Hopkins Medicine.

7. Jessica Stoller-Conrad, "Noted Neuroscientist Paul Patterson Dies," *Caltech* (blog), June 30, 2014.

8. Patterson, "Pregnancy, Immunity, Schizophrenia, and Autism."

9. Paul Patterson, "Maternal Immune Activation Yields Offspring Displaying Mouse Versions of the Three Core Symptoms of Autism," *Brain, Behavior, and Immunity* 26, no. 4 (2012): 607–616.

10. Melissa Bauman et al., "Activation of the Maternal Immune System during Pregnancy Alters Behavioral Development of Rhesus Monkey Offspring," *Biological Psychiatry* 75, no. 4 (2014): 332–341.

11. Paul Patterson et al., "Maternal Immune Activation Alters Fetal Brain Development through Interleukin-6," *The Journal of Neuroscience : The Official Journal of the Society for Neuroscience* 27, no. 40 (2007): 10695–10702.

12. Xiaochong Li et al., "Brain IL-6 Elevation Causes Neuronal Circuitry Imbalances and Mediates Autism-like Behaviors," *Biochimica et Biophysica Acta* 1822, no. 6 (2012): 831–842.

13. William Carlezon et al., "Perinatal Immune Activation Produces Persistent Sleep Alterations and Epileptiform Activity in Male Mice," *Neuropsychopharmacology* 43, no. 3 (2018): 482–491.

14. Christopher Shaw et al., "Aluminum Adjuvant Linked to Gulf War Illness Induces Motor Neuron Death in Mice," *Neuromolecular Medicine* 9, no. 1 (2007): 83–100.

15. From an interview Dr. Shaw provided in the documentary *The Greater Good*.

16. "Flu Vaccination Coverage among Pregnant Women—United States, 2015–16 Flu Season," Centers for Disease Control and Prevention, September 29, 2016, https://www.cdc.gov/flu/fluvaxview/pregnant-coverage_1516estimates.htm.

17. Christopher Shaw et al., "Aluminum Vaccine Adjuvants: Are They Safe?," *Current Medicinal Chemistry* 18, no. 17 (2011): 2630–2637.

18. Christopher Shaw et al., "Mechanisms of Aluminum Adjuvant Toxicity and Autoimmunity in Pediatric Populations," *Lupus* 21, no. 2 (2012): 223–230.

19. Zakir Kahn et al., "Slow CCL2-Dependent Translocation of Biopersistent Particles from Muscle to Brain," *BMC Medicine* 11, no. 1 (2013): 99.

20. "CCL2," April 11, 2017, https://en.wikipedia.org/wiki/CCL2.

21. Romain Gherardi et al., "Biopersistence and Brain Translocation of Aluminum Adjuvants of Vaccines," *Frontiers in Neurology* 6 (2015): Article 4.

22. Guillemette Crepeaux et al., "Non-linear Dose-Response of Aluminium Hydroxide Adjuvant Particles: Selective Low Dose Neurotoxicity," *Toxicology* 375 (2017): 48–57.

23. Robert J. Mitkus et al., "Updated Aluminum Pharmacokinetics Following Infant Exposures through Diet and Vaccination," *Vaccine* 29, no. 51 (2011): 9538–9543.

24. Romain K. Gherardi et al., "Critical Analysis of Reference Studies on the Toxicokinetics of Aluminum-Based Adjuvants," *Journal of Inorganic Biochemistry* 181 (2018): 87–95.

25. Gherardi et al., "Critical Analysis of Reference Studies."

26. Zhibin Yao et al., "Neonatal Vaccination with Bacillus Calmette–Guérin and Hepatitis B Vaccines Modulates Hippocampal Synaptic Plasticity in Rats," *Journal of Neuroimmunology* 288 (2015): 1–12.

27. Zhibin Yao et al., "Neonatal Hepatitis B Vaccination Impaired the Behavior and Neurogenesis of Mice Transiently in Early Adulthood," *Psychoneuroendocrinology* 73 (2016): 166–176.

28. Christopher Exley et al., "Aluminium in Brain Tissue and Autism," *Journal of Trace Elements in Medicine and Biology* 46 (2018): 76–82.

29. Exley et al., "Aluminium in Brain Tissue."

30. Heather Hazlett et al., "Early Brain Development in Infants at High Risk for Autism Spectrum Disorder," *Nature* 542, no. 7641 (2017): 348–351.

31. From an interview of Professor Exley available on YouTube: https://www.youtube.com/watch?v=r0TahxmLBnw.

32. From an interview of Professor Exley available on YouTube: https://www.youtube.com/watch?v=SmkVv8pcVhc.

33. From a biography of Ms. Croninger on the Gauss' Children website at this link: http://www.gausschildren.org/genwiki/index.php?title=CRONINGER,_Adele_Bullen_(1920_-_1968).

34. Ernest L. Wynder, Evarts A. Graham, and Adele B. Croninger, "Experimental Production of Carcinoma with Cigarette Tar," *Cancer Research*, December 1953, 855–864.

35. Katie Forster, "France to Make Vaccination Mandatory from 2018 as It Is 'Unacceptable Children Are Still Dying of Measles,'" *The Independent*, July 5, 2017, https://www

.independent.co.uk/news/world/europe/france-vaccination-mandatory-2018-next
-year-children-health-measles-dying-anti-vaxxers-edouard-a7824246.html.

36. Carolyn Patterson, private email correspondence with the author, February 28, 2017.

Chapter 6: The Clear Legal Basis That Vaccines Cause Autism

1. Dr. Richard Kelley, written affidavit, January 24, 2016.

2. The PRNewswire press release from the National Autism Association titled, "Court Awards Over \$20 Million for Vaccine-Caused Autism" can be found at https://www.fiercebiotech.com/biotech/court-awards-over-20-million-for-vaccine-caused-autism.

3. Wendy Davis, "The Immune Response," *ABA Journal*, October 2010, http://www.abajournal.com/magazine/article/the_immune_response.

4. A running total is maintained on the Vaccine Injury Compensation Fund website; this link shows a total payout amount of \$3,844,512,784.45, last updated on February 2, 2018: https://www.hrsa.gov/sites/default/files/hrsa/vaccine-compensation/monthly-website-stats-2-01-18.pdf.

5. "Memorandum Regarding Misconduct by the United States Department of Justice and the United States Department of Health and Human Services during the Omnibus Autism Proceeding as to the Expert Opinions of Dr. Andrew Zimmerman," written by Rolf Hazlehurst, can be found at: http://www.rescuepost.com/files/rh-memo-1.pdf.

6. This table of historical vaccination rates is maintained by the Centers for Disease Control and Prevention and is available on their website: https://www.cdc.gov/vaccines/pubs/pinkbook/downloads/appendices/G/coverage.pdf.

7. Myron Levin, "Vaccine Injury Claims Face Grueling Fight," *Los Angeles Times*, November 29, 2004, http://articles.latimes.com/2004/nov/29/business/fi-vaccinecourt29.

8. "Compensating Vaccine Injuries: Are Reforms Needed?" September 28, 1999, Statement of the National Vaccine Information Center, Barbara Loe Fisher, Co-founder & President, Hearing of the House Subcommittee on Criminal Justice, Drug Policy and Human Resources, can be found here: https://www.gpo.gov/fdsys/pkg/CHRG-106hhrg66079/html/CHRG-106hhrg66079.htm.

9. Lazarus et al., *Electronic Support for Public Health*, 6.

10. Available at the website of Richard Gage & Associates: http://www.richardgage.net.

11. Mary Holland et al., "Unanswered Questions from the Vaccine Injury Compensation Program: A Review of Compensated Cases of Vaccine-Induced Brain Injury," *Pace Environmental Law Review* 28, no. 2 (2011): Article 6.

12. *Vaccine Injury Compensation: Most Claims Took Multiple Years and Many Were Settled through Negotiation, Report to the Chairman, Comm. on Oversight and Government Reform* (2014) (Prepared by the United States Government Accountability Office), https://www.gao.gov/assets/670/667136.pdf.

13. Rolf Hazlehurst, "Memorandum Regarding Misconduct."

14. Arthur Allen, "Shots in the Dark," *Washington Post Magazine*, August 30, 1998, http://www.washingtonpost.com/wp-srv/national/longterm/sunmag/shots/shot1.htm.

15. "Autism General Order #1," Office of Special Masters, July 3, 2002, https://www.uscfc.uscourts.gov/sites/default/files/autism/Autism+General+Order1.pdf.

16. Wayne Rohde, *The Vaccine Court: The Dark Truth of America's Vaccine Injury Compensation Program* (New York: Skyhorse Publishing, 2014), chapter 10.

17. Letter from Dr. Andrew Zimmerman to attorney Clifford Shoemaker, November 30, 2007.

18. Deposition of Richard Kelley, MD, in the matter of Rolf H. Hazlehurst vs. E. Carlton Hays, November 7, 2016.

19. Andrew Zimmerman et al., "Developmental Regression and Mitochondrial Dysfunction in a Child with Autism," *Journal of Child Neurology* 21, no. 2 (2006): 170–172.

20. Jon Poling, "Dr. Jon Poling to Dr. Steven Novella: Don't Attack the Moms," *Age of Autism* (blog), July 22, 2008, http://www.ageofautism.com/2008/07/dear-dr-novella.html.

21. Thomas Hafemeister, "Government Agrees to Compensate Family That Claims Childhood Vaccinations Caused Autism; Implications of Settlement Are Contested," *Developments in Mental Health Law* 27, no. 2 (2008), https://www.questia.com/magazine/1G1-219451047/government-agrees-to-compensate-family-that-claims.

22. David Kirby, "The Vaccine-Autism Court Document Every American Should Read," *Huffington Post*, February 26, 2008, https://www.huffingtonpost.com/david-kirby/the-vaccineautism-court-d_b_88558.html.

23. David Kirby, "The Vaccine-Autism Court Document Every American Should Read."

24. "Vaccine Case Draws New Attention to Autism Debate," CNN.com, March 7, 2008, http://www.cnn.com/2008/HEALTH/conditions/03/06/vaccines.autism/index.html.

25. Poling, "Don't Attack the Moms."

26. The interview is available on YouTube: https://www.youtube.com/watch?v=YxfgqsZ8BV0.

27. David Kirby, "The Next Big Autism Bomb: Are 1 in 50 Kids Potentially at Risk?" *Huffington Post*, November 17, 2011, https://www.huffingtonpost.com/david-kirby/the-next-big-autism-bomb-_b_93627.html.

28. Sharyl Attkisson, "Vaccines, Autism and Brain Damage: What's in a Name?" CBS News, September 14, 2010, https://www.cbsnews.com/news/vaccines-autism-and-brain-damage-whats-in-a-name/.

29. *Diagnostic and Statistical Manual of Mental Disorders, Fourth Edition (DSM-IV)* (Washington, DC: American Psychiatric Association, 1994).

30. Robert F. Kennedy Jr. and David Kirby, "Vaccine Court: Autism Debate Continues," *Huffington Post*, March 27, 2009, https://www.huffingtonpost.com/robert-f-kennedy-jr-and-david-kirby/vaccine-court-autism-deba_b_169673.html.

31. Kennedy and Kirby, "Vaccine Court."

32. Holland et al., "Unanswered Questions."

33. Lou Conte and Tony Lyons, *Vaccine Injuries: Documented Adverse Reactions to Vaccines* (New York: Skyhorse Publishing, 2014), 113–114.

34. You can find the broadcast on the Fox News website: http://video.foxnews.com /v/4687300/?#sp=show-clips.

35. Mark Blaxill and Jennifer Larson, "OGR Chairman Issa 'Delays' Hearings on Vaccine Injury Compensation Program. Affected Families Stunned," *Age of Autism* (blog), November 20, 2013, http://www.ageofautism.com/2013/11/ogr-chairman-issa-delays-hearings-on-vaccine-injury-compensation-program -affected-families-stunned.html.

36. Conte and Lyons, *Vaccine Injuries,* chapter 9.

37. Louis Conte, "Postponing VICP Hearing: Who Is Afraid and of What?" *Age of Autism* (blog), November 25, 2013, http://www.ageofautism.com/2013/11 /postponing-vicp-hearing-who-is-afraid-and-of-what.html.

38. Deposition of Andrew Zimmerman, MD, in the matter of Rolf H. Hazlehurst vs. E. Carlton Hays, November 9, 2016.

39. Deposition of Richard Kelley, MD, in the matter of Rolf H. Hazlehurst vs. E. Carlton Hays, November 7, 2016.

40. World Mercury Project, "CDC Blocks Testimony by Vaccine Whistleblower in Medical Malpractice Case," *EcoWatch*, October 19, 2016, https://www.ecowatch .com/cdc-vaccines-autism-2051536402.html.

41. World Mercury Project, "CDC Blocks Testimony."

42. Deposition, Andrew W. Zimmerman, MD, McCarthy Reporting Service. Circuit Court of Madison County, Tennessee. December 15, 2016; Deposition, Richard Kelley, MD, Esquire Solutions. Circuit Court of Madison County, Tennessee. November 7, 2016.

43. Jon Poling, "Mitochondrial Dysfunction Not Rare in Autism," *Atlanta Journal-Constitution*, April 11, 2008, http://adventuresinautism.blogspot.com/2008/04 /jon-poling-mitochondrial-dysfunction.html.

44. "Bernadine Healy Speaks on Vaccines," World Mercury Project, June 13, 2017, https:// worldmercuryproject.org/resource-directory/bernadine-healy-speaks-vaccines/.

45. Sarah Landry et al., "Addressing Parents' Concerns: Do Multiple Vaccines Overwhelm or Weaken the Infant's Immune System?" *Pediatrics* 109 (2002): 124–129.

Chapter 7: The Critical Mass of Parents All Saying the Same Thing

1. Lisa Shulman, "Why Pediatricians Need to Listen to Parents," *Albert Einstein College of Medicine* (blog), December 17, 2015, http://blogs.einstein.yu.edu/why -pediatricians-need-to-listen-to-parents/.

2. J.B. Handley, Facebook video, posted on November 23, 2016.

3. CNN Senior Medical Correspondent Elizabeth Cohen's "hear this well" video link can be found on YouTube: https://www.youtube.com/watch?v=WsLuR3X6cpg.

4. F. P. Glascoe, "The Value of Parents' Concerns to Detect and Address Developmental and Behavioural Problems," *Journal of Paediatrics and Child Health* 35, no. 1 (1999): 1–8.

5. Jane Gross, "Autism Debate Strains a Family and Its Charity," *New York Times*, June 18, 2007, https://www.nytimes.com/2007/06/18/us/18autism.html.

6. A video of the interview with Aidan Quinn can be found on YouTube: https://www
.youtube.com/watch?v=XRB2TLFvc3s.

7. "Autism: Is There Hope?," CNN, *Larry King Live*, Transcripts, http://transcripts.cnn
.com/TRANSCRIPTS/0802/27/lkl.01.html.

8. Sandy Kleffman, "Ban on Mercury in Vaccines Gets Push," *Contra Costa Times*,
August 19, 2004.

9. "Robert De Niro Debates Autism's Link to Vaccines on TODAY Show,"
Today (blog), April 15, 2016, https://www.today.com/popculture/
robert-deniro-debates-autism-s-link-vaccines-today-show-t86136.

10. Jenny McCarthy, *Louder Than Words: A Mother's Journey in Healing Autism* (New
York: Dutton, 2007).

Chapter 8: They Would Have Told Us

1. Robert F. Kennedy Jr., *Thimerosal: Let the Science Speak: The Evidence Supporting the
Immediate Removal of Mercury, a Known Neurotoxin, from Vaccines* (New York:
Skyhorse Publishing, 2014).

2. Lydia O'Connor, "Mandatory Vaccine Bill Fails in 2 States," *Huffington Post*, March
16, 2015, https://www.huffingtonpost.com/2015/03/16/vaccine-bills-fail-oregon
-washington_n_6882196.html.

3. Presentation available at the Immunization Action Coalition website: https://www
.immunizationcoalitions.org/content/uploads/2017/04/IZCoalitions_April_2017
_AAP.pdf.

4. Amanda Marcotte, "Donald Trump Uses GOP Debate to Push Anti-
Vaccination Myths," *Slate*, September 16, 2015, http://www.slate.com/blogs/xx
_factor/2015/09/16/donald_trump_suggested_vaccines_cause_autism_during
_the_cnn_gop_debate_he.html.

5. Peter Doshi, "The Unofficial Vaccine Educators: Are CDC Funded Non-profits
Sufficiently Independent?," *British Medical Journal* 359 (2017), 1–6.

6. David Rosner and Gerald Markowitz, "Why It Took Decades of Blaming Parents
before We Banned Lead Paint," *The Atlantic*, April 22, 2013, https://www
.theatlantic.com/health/archive/2013/04/why-it-took-decades-of-blaming
-parents-before-we-banned-lead-paint/275169/.

7. Philip Morris, "An Ounce of Prevention Is Worth a Pound of Cure," advertisement (circa
1945), as found at https://www.flickr.com/photos/93468786@N00/5006372117.

8. Mr. Blaxill's complete testimony is available on the Committee on Oversight
and Government Reform's website: https://oversight.house.gov/wp-content
/uploads/2012/11/Blaxill-Testimony-Bio-TnT.pdf.

9. Paul Thomas and Jennifer Margulis, *The Vaccine-Friendly Plan: Dr. Paul's Safe and
Effective Approach to Immunity and Health-from Pregnancy through Your Child's Teen
Years* (New York: Ballantine Books, 2016), xiii.

10. Martha Rosenberg, "Vaccines Are Totally Safe Say the People Who Brought Us
Vioxx, Bextra, Baycol, Trovan, Phen-Fen, Xarelto, Raxar and Seldane...," *Huffington
Post*, January 24, 2017, https://www.march-against-monsanto.com/huffpo
-censored-and-deleted-anti-pharma-vaccine-post-from-their-website-read-it-here/.

Chapter 9: Next Steps: A Twelve-Point Proposal

1. Anne Dachel, email correspondence with the author, July 12, 2017.
2. "Children and Youth with Disabilities," National Center for Education Statistics, May 2017, https://nces.ed.gov/programs/coe/indicator_cgg.asp.
3. Thomas and Margulis, *The Vaccine-Friendly Plan*, 151.
4. Birgitta Henriques-Normark et al., "Bacterial Vaccines and Antibiotic Resistance," *Upsala Journal of Medical Sciences* 119, no. 2 (2018): 205–208.
5. Joseph Mercola, "Perhaps One of the Most Unnecessary Vaccines Ever," *Mercola.com*, July 14, 2011, https://articles.mercola.com/sites/articles/archive/2011/07/14 /barbara-loe-fisher-on-the-meningococcal-vaccine.aspx.
6. David McNeill, "Japan's National Immunisation Program Still Trails Europe," *Japan Today*, January 23, 2016, https://japantoday.com/category/features/health/japans -national-immunisation-program-still-trails-behind-europe.
7. The Interagency Autism Coordinating Committee website can be found here: https://iacc.hhs.gov.
8. "Weldon, Maloney Introduce Vaccine Safety Bill," website of Congresswoman Carolyn B. Maloney, July 26, 2006, https://maloney.house.gov/media-center /press-releases/weldon-maloney-introduce-vaccine-safety-bill.

Chapter 10: Treatment and Recovery

1. Julie Buckley, *Healing Our Autistic Children: A Medical Plan for Restoring Your Child's Health* (New York: St. Martin's Griffin, 2010), 20.
2. Jerry Kartzinel and Jenny McCarthy, *Healing and Preventing Autism: A Complete Guide* (New York: Plume, 2010).
3. Robert Naviaux et al., "Low-Dose Suramin in Autism Spectrum Disorder: A Small, Phase I/II, Randomized Clinical Trial," *Annals of Clinical and Translational Neurology* 4, no. 7 (2017): 491–505.
4. "Q&A: Suramin Autism Treatment-1 (SAT-1) Trial," UC San Diego Health, https://health.ucsd.edu/news/topics/Suramin-Autism/Pages/Q-and-A.aspx.
5. "Q&A: Suramin Autism Treatment-1."
6. David Ruskin, "Ketogenic Diet Improves Behaviors in a Maternal Immune Activation Model of Autism Spectrum Disorder," *PLoS ONE* 12, no. 2 (2017), 1–14.
7. Elaine Hsiao et al., "The Microbiota Modulates Gut Physiology and Behavioral Abnormalities Associated with Autism," *Cell* 155, no. 7 (2013): 1451–1463.
8. Feiyong Jia et al., "Core Symptoms of Autism Improved after Vitamin D Supplementation," *Pediatrics* 135, no. 1 (2015): e196–198.
9. Dale Viezeliene et al., "Selective Induction of IL-6 by Aluminum-Induced Oxidative Stress Can Be Prevented by Selenium," *Journal of Trace Elements in Medicine and Biology* 27, no. 3 (2013): 226–229.

Epilogue

1. Letter from Dr. Andrew Zimmerman to attorney Clifford Shoemaker, November 30, 2007.

Index

A

AAP. *See* American Academy of Pediatrics
acute disseminated encephalomyelitis, 186
ADDM. *See* Autism and Developmental
  Disabilities Monitoring Network
ADEM, 186
ADHD, 7, 20, 83, 103, 204, 234
adults, prevalence of autism (US), 17–18, 20,
  33–34
adverse effects, 63, 69. *See also* Vaccine
  Adverse Event Reporting System
    1% reported, 63–64, 79, 79f, 114, 174, 230
    and adjuvants, 71
    of aluminum, 152, 155, 248
    arthritis, 62, 64, 65
    asthma, 20, 69, 70, 72, 82, 100–101, 234
    and autoimmune conditions, 42, 65, 70–71
    and DTaP vaccine, 121
    and HPV vaccine (Gardasil), 70
    and Hazlehurst, 192
    identification of, 79, 175, 192, 230
    and immune activation, 149, 159
    and MMR vaccine, 73, 238
    possible (not tested), 65
    and preterm birth, 103
    safety testing, 62–63, 112
    symptoms (Medwatcher Japan), 69,
      230
    timing, 62, 159
Advisory Committee on Immunization
  Practices (CDC), 62, 107
    on vaccine efficacy, 62
age of onset (autism), 19, 26, 92

Allen, Arthur, on vaccine court and vaccine
  safety, 176
allergies, 4, 5, 7, 20, 42, 70–71, 100–101, 103,
  205, 234, 243
aluminum adjuvant
    and Alzheimer's, 158
    and behavior changes, 149–50
    and biomedical intervention, 246–48
    and biopersistence, 153–55, 205
    Cadusseau on, 153–55
    Exley on, 10, 157–58, 159–61, 163, 166,
      231–32, 237
    and gastrointestinal problems, 247
    Gherardi on, 153–55, 157, 166
    and immune activation, 141, 150–51, 158,
      162, 164, 165, 231–32, 237, 246
    Joyeux on, 167–68
    low dose, 154–55
    and MMR vaccine as a stimulant, 164–65
    Shaw on, 150, 151–52, 165–66
    as a trigger for autism, 161f, 231–32, 237,
      246
    and vaccine safety testing, 151
Alzheimer's and aluminum adjuvant, 158
American Academy of Pediatrics, 4, 9, 42, 55,
  170, 198, 199, 206
    and biomedical intervention, 241
    and CDC, 226
    Department of Federal Affairs, 224
    and GlaxoSmithKline, 226
    and MedImmune, 226
    and Merck, 226
    on multiple vaccines, 65, 203

American Academy of Pediatrics (*continued*)
    Johnson, Patrick, presentation (2017),
        224–25
    Kelley on, 198–99
    and Pfizer, 226
    public relations, 91, 238
    recommended vaccine schedule, 58, 237
    and Sanofi Pasteur, 226
    and Seqirus, 226
    support from Big Pharma, 42, 226, 228
    in support of Big Pharma, 42, 54, 130, 228
    and vaccine–autism connection, 198–99
    and vaccine safety, 199
    and vulnerable children screening, 239
    Zimmerman on, 199–200
American Medical Association, 44, 49f, 92
American Public Health Association annual
    meeting (1966), 71
antipurinergic therapy (APT), 245
"anti-vaccine" label, 10–11
    and Vaxxed Bus, 210
    and vaccine–autism connection, 227
Aquino, Corazon, 68
arthritis, 62, 64, 65
Asperger's in *DSM*-IV, 37
asthma, 20, 69, 70, 72, 82, 234
    and DTP, 100–101
    and tetanus, 100–101
attention-deficit/hyperactivity disorder, 7, 20,
    83, 103, 204, 234
Attkisson, Sharyl, 129–31
    on Big Pharma, 130–31
    on Department of Health and Human
        Services (US), 130–31
Autism and Developmental Disabilities
    Monitoring Network, 39
Autism Education Summit, 8
Autism Epidemiology Study, 35
Autism Research Institute, 5, 25
Autism's False Prophets (Offit), 23
Autism Science Foundation, 88
autism and siblings, 91–93, 235
Autism Society of America, 25
Autism Speaks, 20, 126, 214–16, 240
Autism Yesterday (movie), 242
autoimmune conditions
    and aluminum adjuvant, 70–71, 152, 154
    and autism, 101
    and Gardasil, 112
    and hepatitis B, 102, 113
    and vaccines, 7, 42, 65, 70–71, 79, 204, 234

Vaccines and Autoimmunity (Shoenfeld and
    Agmon-Levin), 71

B
Bacillus Calmette–Guérin, 158
    and immune activation, 159
Bandim Health Project, 66
Banks, Bailey, 186
behavior effects (autism), 19, 27, 145, 146,
    168, 186–88
    cessation of speech, 2, 146, 148
    and gut microbiome, 247
    head banging, 162, 213
    and hepatitis B vaccine, 160
    and ketogenic diet, 246
    repetitive behaviors, 146, 148
    running, 2
    self-injury, 20
    social interaction decrease, 148
    spinning, 2
Biggs, John Thomas, 49–50
    Leicester: Sanitation versus Vaccination
        (1912), 49
Big Pharma, 9, 58, 125. *See also* Offit, Paul;
    Plotkin, Stanley; Tobacco Playbook
    Attkisson on, 130–31
    and autism epidemic, 21, 228
    and dengue vaccine safety, 67–68
    Doshi on, 226
    ethics, 117, 122–23
    Every Child By Two, 130, 190, 226
    and feigned exasperation, 85, 104, 110
    fraud, 128
    and Gardasil safety, 69–70
    GlaxoSmithKline, 45, 90, 109, 128, 226,
        228
    Hill & Knowlton (PR firm), 131
    Immunization Action Coalition, 226
    influence, 42–43, 47, 103, 125
    Kennedy on, 21
    and liability, 53–55, 129
    MedImmune, 226
    Merck, 23, 24, 62, 69–70, 106, 107, 109,
        112–13, 125, 128–30, 222, 226, 238
    and Oversight and Government Reform
        Committee hearing on vaccine court, 190
    Pfizer, 109, 226
    and polio vaccine, 74–77
    profit motivation, 43, 43f, 106–107
    and safety testing of vaccines, 112, 123
    Sanofi Pasteur, 67–68, 109, 168, 226

Seqirus, 226
    Task Force for Global Health, 110
    and vaccine–autism connection, 85, 89–91
    and vaccine court, 174, 177, 180, 190–91
    Vioxx, 55, 128–29
    and Wakefield, 127–28, 136–37, 168, 230
biological plausibility, 75, 89, 96, 100, 125
biomedical intervention (autism), 5, 8, 197,
    241, 242–44
    advanced therapies, 244
    and aluminum, 246–48
    and the American Academy of Pediatrics,
        241
    Autism Yesterday (movie), 242
    definition, 243–44
    detoxification, 5, 39, 244
    diet, 5, 211, 243, 246–47
    Generation Rescue, 8
    gut healing, 3, 5, 132, 244, 247
    ketogenic diet, 243, 246–47
    Medical Academy of Pediatric Special
        Needs, 243
    microbiome, 247
    and Mielke, Lynn, 3, 243
    nutrition, 4, 5, 211, 241, 244
    recovery, 3–6, 8, 25, 186, 201, 217, 241–43,
        246, 248
    as placebo, 2
    and Rimland, Bernard, 25, 211–12
    selenium, 248
    silica mineral water, 246
    treatment plan, 243–48
    vitamin B12, 244
    vitamin D, 247–48
biomedical research, 8
biopersistence, aluminum, 153–55, 205
Biskind, Morton S., 74–75
    on DDT and polio, 75
Blaylock, Russell, on herd immunity, 7
Blaxill, Mark, 4, 35
    on Asperger's in *DSM*-IV, 37
    on better diagnosis, 33–34, 35
    on culpability, 22, 24
    on cause of autism, 4, 15, 34
    Denial, 18
    on deniers, 18
    on fraud, 228
    on Offit and rotavirus vaccine, 107
    on polio, 77
    on prevalence, 18–19, 29, 34
    on prognosis, 19

on *NeuroTribes* (Silberman), 18
Bolton, John R., 53
booster shots, 57, 238
Bowman, David, 184–85
    on encephalopathy, 184
Boyle, Coleen, 21, 32–33
    on better diagnosis, 32
Braxton, Toni, 217
Buckley, Julie, 242
Buttram, Harold E., on vaccine safety
    testing, 63

C

Cadusseau, Josette
    on aluminum adjuvant safety, 153–55
    on low-dose aluminum adjuvant, 155
California State Assembly, 66
Camerota, Alisyn, 189
Campbell, Joseph, 249
cause of autism. *See also individual causes*
    aluminum adjuvant, 161f, 231–32, 237, 246
    Blaxill on, 4, 15, 34
    genetics, 3, 4, 5, 22, 37–39, 207, 215, 216,
        242
    environment, 3, 4, 15, 22–23, 27, 33,
        38–39, 40, 77, 179, 203, 239, 242,
        245–46, 247
    immune activation event, 122, 141,
        147–48, 158, 161, 196–97, 231, 240
    influenza (flu), 149
    mitochondrial dysfunction, 178–79, 181,
        184, 191–92, 194, 201, 205, 232
    Olmsted on, 15, 34
    vaccines, 3, 8, 161–62, 181–84, 188–89,
        205
CCL-2 (cytokine), 153
CDC, 9, 42, 90, 170, 171, 183, 197
    on adverse events, 63–64
    Advisory Committee on Immunization
        Practices, 62, 107
    and aluminum adjuvant, 155–58
    Autism and Developmental Disabilities
        Monitoring Network, 39
    and autism epidemic, 21, 83f, 198
    and autism prevalence, 16f, 32, 39–40,
        83f, 232
    and better diagnosis, 33
    and Big Pharma, 44
    on brain development and vaccines, 151f
    and conflict of interest, 10, 91, 97–99, 107,
        199, 224, 226, 239

CDC (*continued*)
 and cost of vaccination, 58
 Doshi on, 45
 fear tactics, 44
 and fraud, 200–201, 206, 210, 228, 231
 Freidan, Thomas, 193
 Gerberding, Julie, 125, 183
 implementation of national vaccine
  program, 10
 on infectious disease mortality trends and
  vaccines, 49f
 on influenza vaccine, 47
 Kelley on, 200–201
 Kennedy on, 224
 Maloney on, 240
 and measles, 72
 and mitochondrial dysfunction, 194
 and multiple vaccines, 59f, 203
 National Influenza Vaccine Summit
  (2004), 44
 Nowak and media relations, 44
 Pinborough-Zimmerman on, 39–40
 Poling case, position, 171, 186, 195
 and prevalence of autism, 232
 as Public Health Service, 72
 Shaw on, 165–66
 in support of vaccine advocacy groups, 226
 on thimerosal, 165, 230
 Thompson, William, 193
 tracking children with autism, 10, 32,
  39, 63–64
 and vaccine–autism connection, 83f,
  197, 198
 vaccine coverage rates (adults), 51–52
 vaccine coverage rates (children), 52f, 53
 on vaccine effectiveness, 62
 on vaccine ingredients, 86–87f
 vaccine policy, 45–46, 107, 226, 237–38
 on vaccines and brain development, 151f
 on vaccines and mortality, 49f
 and vaccine safety testing, 63, 65, 239–40
 vaccine schedule, 55, 56–57f, 57–58,
  59f, 86, 95, 109, 151f, 176, 230,
  235, 237
 vaccine studies, 230–231
 and vulnerable children screening, 239
 Zimmerman on, 197–98
CDR. *See* cell danger response
Cedillo, Michelle, 181, 203
cell danger response, 245–46
 Naviaux on, 245

Centers for Disease Control and Prevention.
 See CDC
chickenpox vaccine, 52f, 56, 57f, 59, 86, 87f,
 88, 136, 181, 206, 236
children, prevalence of autism (US), 18,
 28–29, 32, 35, 36, 38, 40, 207
 Minnesota, 36
 North Dakota, 27
 Wisconsin, 26, 207
Cochrane Collaboration, 45, 73
Cohen, Elizabeth, and Hear This Well, 212
Cole, Gary, 217
Colin, Lisa, 187
colitis, 20, 132
Committee on Appropriations (US House),
 30–31
Committee on Oversight and Government
 Reform (US House), 20–21
 and Big Pharma, 190
 on conflicts of interest, 107
 on National Vaccine Injury Compensation
  Program, 190–91, 240
conflicts of interest (vaccine policy), 107–12
Conte, Lou, 185, 187, 231
 on autism epidemic and vaccine court,
  190–91
 on compensated vaccine court cases,
  188–89
 on vaccine–autism connection, 188–89
 Vaccine Injuries, 185, 188
Conway, Erik
 Merchants of Doubt, 124, 141
Crepeaux, Guillemette, 157
Crichton, Michael, 84
Croen, Lisa, 35
Croninger, Adele B., on tobacco and cancer,
 73, 78, 99, 124, 126, 163, 168
cytokines, 143
 CCL-2 (cytokine), 153
 definition, 143
 interleukin-6, 122, 147–48, 158–60, 161,
  161f, 248

D
Dachel, Anne, 233
DAN! doctors, 4–6, 211–12, 243
DAN! Protocol, 5
Dawson, Geraldine, 214
DDT and polio prevalence, 74–75, 77
 Biskind on, 74–75
Defeat Autism Now!. *See* DAN!

dengue fever vaccine (Dengvaxia), 67–68
Dengvaxia (dengue fever vaccine), 67–68
Denial (Olmsted and Blaxill), 15
denialism, 15–40, 242. *See also* Offit, Paul;
  Silberman, Steven
  Interagency Autism Coordinating
    Committee, 239
  Blaxill on, 18
  Kennedy on, 21
  Maloney on, 21
  Merzenich on, 40
  Olmsted and Blaxill on, 18
  Rimland on, 24–25
  and vaccine court compensation, 189
  Vaccine Injury Circle of Denial, 78–79,
    79f
Denialist of the Decade, 23
De Niro, Robert, 85, 217
Department of Developmental Services
  (California), 34, 38
Department of Education (California), 20
Department of Education (US), 35, 36, 38
Department of Federal Affairs (AAP), 224
Department of Health and Human Services
  (US). *See also* CDC, vaccine court, Vaccine
  Injury Table
  Attkisson, Sharyl, on, 130–31
  on compensation for injury, 184
  on encephalopathy, 97, 184
  Fisher on, 174
  Hazlehurst, Rolf, on, 190
  and Interagency Autism Coordinating
    Committee (IACC), 94, 239
  on Poling case, 183
  and vaccine court, 172
  and vaccine safety, 239
Department of Justice (US), 171
detection (autism). *See* diagnosis (autism)
detoxification, 5, 39, 244
diagnosis (autism), 19–21, 177
  Asperger's, 37
  behavioral, 19–20, 185
  Blaxill on, 33–34, 35
  Boyle on, 32
  and Committee on Oversight and
    Government Reform, 21–22, 32–33
  and compensation, 187
  Hazlehurst, Yates, 194
  and hepatitis B vaccination, 101–2
  Hertz-Picciotto on, 37
  improved, 26, 27–34, 35

loosening criteria, 35–38
  Maloney on, 32
  MIND Institute on, 35, 37
  Nevison on, 38
  Olmsted on, 33–34, 35
  Poling, Hannah, 181, 185
*Diagnostic and Statistical Manual of Mental
  Disorders*, 36–37, 185
  DSM-III, 27
  DSM-IV, 37
diarrhea, 2, 20, 69, 239
Dickinson, Jim, 68
diet, 5, 211, 243, 246–47
diphtheria-tetanus-pertussis vaccine. *See* DTP
  vaccine
Dissolving Illusions (Humphries), 81
Division of Vaccine Injury Compensation,
  181
domino effect ideology, 137, 163, 222
Donegan, Jayne, 48
Doshi, Peter
  on influence of Big Pharma, 226
  on influenza death statistics, 45
  on influenza vaccine, 46
DTP (diphtheria-tetanus-pertussis) vaccine,
  49f, 52f, 53, 56, 56f, 63, 81, 86
  Institute of Medicine on, 64
  Plotkin on, 114–15, 120–21
  studies, 64, 100–101, 113, 123
  and vaccine injuries, 54, 64, 66, 100–101,
    173, 174, 176, 217
DuBeau, Gretchen, on herd immunity, 52
Dull, Bruce, 72
Duterte, Rodrigo, on dengue fever vaccine, 67

E

ear infections, 2, 5, 20, 181, 193, 207
eczema, 1, 70, 205, 234, 237, 239
Emory University, 50
encephalopathy
  acute, 64
  and autistic behavior, 184
  Bowman on, 184
  chronic, definition, 97
  definition, 96
  National Vaccine Injury Compensation
    Program on, 97, 188–89
  and Poling, Hannah, 178, 181, 183, 184
  as regressive autistic symptom, 185
  and vaccine court, 185–89
  as vaccine injury, 64, 97, 187, 188

enterocolitis, 20, 132
environmental cause (autism), 3, 4, 15, 22–23, 27, 33, 38–39, 40, 77, 179, 203, 239, 242, 245–46, 247
epidemic (autism). *See* denialism
epidemic denialism. *See* denialism
epidemiology vs. biology, 99–100, 201–2
epilepsy, 20
Evans, Geoffrey, on National Vaccine Injury Compensation Program, 176
Every Child By Two, 130, 190, 226
Exley, Christopher
    on aluminum adjuvants and autism, 10, 157–58, 159–61, 163, 166, 231–32, 237
    on aluminum in brain tissue, 160–61
    and removal of aluminum from the brain, 246
    on vaccine–autism connection, 162
eye contact, 2, 5, 217

F

FDA Modernization Act, 165
First, Lewis, 90
Fisher, Barbara Loe, 174
Flutie, Doug, 216
Fombonne, Eric, 24
food allergies, 5, 20, 42, 70, 71, 234, 243
France, mandatory vaccination (2017), 167
Friedan, Thomas, 193

G

Gallagher, Carolyn, 101–2
    and hepatitis B vaccine and autism study, 101–2
    on hepatitis B vaccine and special education study, 101
Gardasil. *See* human papilloma virus vaccine
gastrointestinal problems, 3, 4, 5, 20, 132, 244
    and aluminum adjuvant, 247
Gerberding, Julie
    and CDC, 47, 125, 183
    and Merck, 47, 125
Generation Rescue, 8, 217
Generation Rescue Grants, 8
genetic cause (autism), 3, 4, 5, 22, 37–39, 207, 215, 216, 242
    Lyons-Weiler on, 39
    "missing" cases, 18–19, 28, 30
Gherardi, Romain, 141
    on aluminum adjuvant and autism, 166

on aluminum adjuvant safety, 153–55, 157, 166
    on low-dose aluminum adjuvant, 155
Gill, Christopher J., 61
GlaxoSmithKline, 45, 90, 109, 128, 226, 228
Golkiewicz, Gary, 177
Good Doctor, The (TV show), 19
Goodman, Melody, 101–2
    and hepatitis B vaccine and autism study, 101–2
    on hepatitis B vaccine and special education study, 101
Gordon, Joshua, 93–95
    and Interagency Autism Coordinating Committee, 94
    and National Institute of Mental Health, 93
    and vaccine–autism science, 94–95, 239
Government Accountability Office (US), 175
Guillain-Barré syndrome, 62, 65
Gulf War syndrome and vaccines, 149–50
Gupta, Sanjay, 183–84
gut healing, 3, 4, 5, 132, 244, 247

H

Halstead, Scott, 68
Halvorsen, Richard, 105
Hart, Josephine, 221
Hayward, Elizabeth Steiner, 221, 224
Hazlehurst, Rolf
    on Department of Health and Human Services (US), 190
    on Kelley, 207–208
    on Poling settlement, 182
    on vaccine court, 173, 175–76, 190
    and Yates's case, 192–93
    on Zimmerman, 207–8
Hazlehurst, Yates
    and civil suit, 172, 191–93, 232
    and mitochondrial dysfunction, 191–92, 193–94
    and vaccine reaction, 192
    Zimmerman on, 193–94
headaches, 20, 65, 69, 145
head banging, 162, 213
Health Committee (Oregon Senate), 223–24
Healing and Preventing Autism (Kartzinel and McCarthy), 243
Healy, Bernadine, 202
Hear This Well campaign, 212–13, 218
hepatitis A vaccine, 51, 52f, 56, 59, 65, 86, 88, 150, 236

hepatitis B vaccine, 6, 51, 52f, 55n, 56, 59, 62, 65, 86, 88, 101–2, 113, 118, 119, 150, 157, 158–60, 173, 236
  and autism diagnosis, 101–102
  Gallagher on, 101
  and immune activation, 158–59
  Plotkin on, 113
herd immunity, 7, 41, 50
  Blaylock on, 7
  DuBeau on, 52
  and mandatory vaccination, 51
  myth, 7, 50–53, 108
  Pan on, 51
  SB 277, 51
Hertz-Picciotto, Irva, 37
  on loosening diagnostic criteria (autism), 37
  on environmental factors, 38
Hib vaccine, 52f, 56, 56f, 57f, 63, 86, 87f, 88, 136, 150, 173, 181, 236, 237. *See also* influenza vaccine
Hill & Knowlton (PR firm), 127, 131
Holland, Mary, 185, 187, 231, 240
  on compensated vaccine court cases, 188–89
  on vaccine–autism connection, 188–89
Hooker, Brian, 22
Hotez, Peter, 24, 85, 90, 99
human papilloma virus (HPV) vaccine (Gardasil), 69–70, 112–13
  adverse events, 69–70
  and autoimmune conditions, 112
  and aluminum adjuvant, 70
  in Ireland, 70
  and "Regret" (Irish parent group), 70
  safety, 69–70
Humphries, Suzanne, 81
  Dissolving Illusions (2013), 81
  and vaccine safety, 81–82

I

IACC, 94, 239
IL-6, 122, 147–48, 158–60, 161, 161f, 248
immune activation. *See also* inflammation
  and aluminum adjuvant, 141, 150–51, 158, 162, 164, 165, 231–32, 237, 246
  as autism trigger, 32, 122, 141, 147–48, 158, 161, 196–97, 231, 240
  behavior changes, 145, 147, 148
  after birth (postnatal), 148–49, 160
  and brain development, 159

  and brain enlargement, 162
  and cytokines, 143, 147
  and hepatitis B vaccine, 158–59
  and interleukin-6 (IL-6), 122, 147–48, 158–60
  maternal infection and, 145–47, 149, 246
  MIND Institute on, 146–47
  and mitochondrial disorder, 179
  and MMR vaccine, 164
  Patterson on, 145–47
  Plotkin on, 121–22
  postnatal, 148
  and schizophrenia, 32, 144, 146, 159
  synergistic effect of illness, 78
  and vaccination of children, 9, 121–22, 240
  and vaccination of pregnant women, 151
  and vitamin D, 247–48
Individuals with Disabilities Education Act (IDEA), 38
infantile autism, 26–27
Infantile Autism (Rimland), 24
inflammation. *See also* immune activation
  ADEM, 186
  and aluminum, 152, 154, 155, 205, 246
  CCL-2, 153
  and MMR vaccine, 186
  neural inflammation and autism, 142–43, 144, 154, 162, 186, 195–97, 203, 231, 246
  and polio, 75
  and vitamin D, 247–48
influenza vaccine, 44–47, 56, 57f, 206, 236. *See also* Hib vaccine
  coverage, 46, 51, 59, 86
  Dickenson on, 68
  Doshi on, 46
  efficacy, 47, 68–69
  Jefferson on, 45–46
  mandate (NYC, 2015), 108
  and pregnant women, 146–47, 151
informed consent, 11, 66, 192
Institute of Medicine, 64–65, 118, 137
  on DTaP/Tdap and autism, 120–21, 123
  on DTP side effects, 64
  on lupus cause, 119
  on most common reported vaccine injuries, 64–65
  on side effects (general vaccination), 120, 206
Interagency Autism Coordinating Committee, 94, 239

interleukin-6, 122, 147–48, 158–60, 161, 161f, 248
    Plotkin on, 122
intervention. *See* treatment
Issa, Darrell, 190
    on autism epidemic, 21

J

Jackson State University, 102
Jefferson, Tom, on influenza vaccine, 45–46
Johns Hopkins University, 142–143, 170
    Kennedy Krieger Institute, 170–71, 178–80, 191
Johnson, Mitch, 45
Johnson, Patrick, 224–25
Joyeux, Henri, on aluminum adjuvant, 167–68

K

Kaiser Permanente, 34
Kartzinel, Jerry, 243
    Healing and Preventing Autism, 243
Kelley, Richard, 169
    on CDC, 200–201
    as expert witness (Hazlehurst), 171–72, 191–92, 193, 232
    Hazlehurst, Rolf, on 207–8
    on Hazlehurst, Yates, 170, 191
    on multiple vaccines, 203
    on mitochondrial dysfunction, 194, 232
    on vaccine–autism connection, 198–99
Kennedy, Robert F. Jr., 30, 44, 85
    on denialism, 21
    on CDC corruption, 224
    on neurodiversity, 22
    on *NeuroTribes* (Silberman), 22
    on prevalence of autism (adults), 17
    and Senate Bill 442 (Oregon), 221–24
    on Silberman, 21–22
    Thimerosal: Let the Science Speak (2014), 222
    on vaccine court, 186–87
    and vaccine safety, 222, 224–25
Kennedy Krieger Institute, 170–71, 178–80, 191
Kessler, Gladys E., 124
ketogenic diet, 243, 246–47
King, Bryan, 92
Kirby, David
    on mitochondrial dysfunction, 184
    and Poling, Hannah, 180, 231
    on vaccine–autism science, 87–88, 102
    on the vaccine court, 186–87

Knopp, Tim, 223–24
Krakow, Robert, 187

L

Lamott, Anne, 1
Lancet study, 131–36
Langmuir, Alexander, 72
Lazarus, Ross, on VAERS, 64
lead industry, 226–27
Leicester: Sanitation versus Vaccination (Biggs), 49
Lewin Group, The, 92
Louder Than Words (McCarthy), 217
Lyons, Tony, 188
    Vaccine Injuries, 185, 188
Lyons-Weiler, James, 39

M

Maloney, Carolyn, 32, 239–40
    on autism epidemic, 21
    on better diagnosis, 32
    on CDC conflict of interest, 240
    on vaccine–autism connection, 33
mandatory vaccination
    Senate Bill 277 (California), 51, 58
    Senate Bill 442 (Oregon), 221, 223–24
MAPS. *See* Medical Academy of Pediatric Special Needs
Margulis, Jennifer, 228
    Vaccine-Friendly Plan, The, 228, 234
Master Settlement Agreement (tobacco), 124, 126
maternal immune activation, 145–47, 246
McCarthy, Jenny, 8, 222
    Healing and Preventing Autism, 243
    Louder Than Words (2007), 217
McDonald, Candace, 8
McLean Hospital, 148
measles and Hodgkin's disease, 78
measles-mumps-rubella vaccine. *See* MMR vaccine
measles vaccine, 71–74, 238
    efficacy, 73
    history, 72–73
    safety, 73
Medical Academy of Pediatric Special Needs, 243
MedImmune and American Academy of Pediatrics, 226
Medwatcher Japan, 69
Mendelsohn, Robert, on mass immunization, 80

meningococcal vaccine, 52f, 86, 88, 236
Merchants of Doubt (Oreskes and Conway),
  124
Merck, 23, 24, 47, 62, 109, 125, 130, 222
  and American Academy of Pediatrics, 226
  and HPV vaccine (Gardasil), 69–70,
    112–13
  MMR vaccine, 238
  and mumps vaccine efficacy, 62
  pain reliever (Vioxx), 128–29
  rotavirus vaccine, 106, 107
  and safety testing of vaccines, 112, 123
  Vioxx, 128–29
mercury. *See* thimerosal
Merkel, Tod, 61
Merzenich, Michael, 40
microbiome, 247
Mielke, Lynne, 3, 243
MIND Institute (UC Davis)
  on diagnosis (autism), 35, 37
  on maternal immune activation, 146–47
Mintzes, Barbara, 226
Miranda, Vincenzo, on Tozzi study, 91
misclassification (autism), 35
Mitkus, Robert J., 156–57
mitochondrial disease. *See* mitochondrial
  dysfunction
mitochondrial dysfunction, 39, 178–80,
  183–84, 194, 205, 244
  as autism trigger, 178–79, 181, 184,
    191–92, 194, 201, 205, 232
  definition, 178–79
  and Hazlehurst, Yates, 191–92, 193–94
  Healy on, 202
  and immune activation, 179
  Kelley on, 194, 232
  Kirby on, 184
  and nutrition, 244
  Poling, Jon, on, 194
  and Poling, Hannah, 179, 181, 183, 194
  prevalence in autism cases, 179, 194, 207
  as risk for regressive autism, 179
  and vaccines, 205, 232
  Zimmerman on, 193–94, 196, 201, 232
MMR (measles-mumps-rubella) vaccine, 23,
  24, 49f, 52f, 53, 55n, 56, 56f, 57f, 73, 78, 87f,
  181, 236–38
  and aluminum adjuvant, 164–65
  autism studies, 86, 88–89, 91–93, 94–95,
    98, 102, 132–35, 193, 210, 231
  and Banks, Bailey, 186
  and immune activation, 164
  in Japan, 238
  as three separate shots, 238
  and vaccine court, 173
Montagnier, Luc, on aluminum adjuvant,
  167–68
Moore, Martin, 50
multiple vaccines
  American Academy of Pediatrics on,
    65, 203
  Kelley on, 203
mumps and ovarian cancer, 78

N
National Childhood Vaccine Injury Act
  (1986), 54, 172
National Collaborative Perinatal Project
  (NCPP), 29–32
National Influenza Vaccine Summit
  (2004), 44
National Institute of Mental Health, 93, 161
National Institutes of Health, 30, 63, 165, 202
National Vaccine Information Center, 174
National Vaccine Injury Compensation
  Program. *See also* vaccine court
  on encephalopathy, 97, 188–89
  Evans on, 176
  fairness of, 175, 187–88
  Oversight and Government Reform
    Committee on, 190–91, 240
  and Poling, Hannah, 131, 180–85
  and use of the word *autism*, 185–89
  and Vaccine Injury Table, 174
Naviaux, Robert, 244
  on cell danger response, 245
  on suramin and autism, 244–45
NCPP (National Collaborative Perinatal
  Project), 29–32
Neides, Daniel, on vaccine safety, 83
neural inflammation, 142–43
neurodiversity, 15, 19
  Kennedy on, 22
  and resilience, 16
  Silberman on, 16
NeuroTribes (Silberman), 15, 201
  Blaxill on, 18
  Kennedy on, 22
Nevison, Cynthia
  on environmental factors, 39
  on loosening diagnostic criteria, 38
  on prevalence (autism), 38

Newschaffer, Craig, 36
nonspecific effects (NSEs), 66, 67
Nowak, Glen
  on media relations at CDC, 44
  on scare tactics, 44
nutrition, 4, 5, 211, 241, 244

O

obesity, 20, 39
Obukhanych, Tetyana, 66–67
  on vaccination and immunity, 67
  Vaccine Illusion (2012), 66
Office of Inspector General (US), 97
Offit, Paul, 22–24, 90, 96, 108
  on autism epidemic, 23
  and conflicts of interest, 107
  Denialist of the Decade, 23
  and Merck, 23, 130
  Olmsted on, 107
  on prevalence of autism, 23
  and religious objection to vaccines, 117–18
  and rotavirus vaccine patent, 23, 85
  and vaccine industry, 99, 106–7, 129–30
OHA (Oregon Health Authority), 60
Olmsted, Dan, 222
  on Asperger's in *DSM*-IV, 37
  on better diagnosis, 33–34, 35
  on culpability, 22, 24
  on cause of autism, 15, 34
  Denial, 18
  on deniers, 18
  on Offit and rotavirus vaccine, 107
  on polio, 77
  on prevalence of autism, 18–19, 29, 34
  on prognosis of autism, 19
  refuting *NeuroTribes* (Silberman), 18
Omnibus Health Bill (S. 1744), 54
Omnibus Autism Proceeding (2002–2009),
  177–91
  Poling test case, 178
  Poling settlement, 180–81
O'Neill, Tip, 53
Oregon Health Authority (OHA), 60
Oregonians for Medical Freedom, 223
Oregon Senate Health Committee, 223
Oreskes, Naomi
  Merchants of Doubt, 124, 141
Oversight and Government Reform
  Committee (US House), 20–21
  and Big Pharma, 190
  on conflicts of interest, 107

on National Vaccine Injury Compensation
  Program, 190–91, 240

P

Palevsky, Lawrence, on vaccine safety, 81
Pan, Richard, on herd immunity, 51–52
Pardo-Villamizar, Carlos, 141, 149, 154
  and neural inflammation and autism,
    142–44, 231
  and microglial activation, 143
Patterson, Carolyn, 168–69
Patterson, Paul, 141, 144
  on cytokines and autism, 147
  on immune activation, 145
  on immune activation and autism, 146,
    154, 162, 231
  on maternal vaccination, 145–46
  on neural inflammation and autism, 142
  and vaccine–autism connection, 145–46
PCV vaccine, 51, 52f, 56, 56f, 57f, 63, 86, 87f,
  88, 150, 236
PDD. See pervasive developmental disorders.
Peete, Holly Robinson, 217
pervasive developmental disorders, 27, 29, 34,
  186, 233–34
Pfizer and American Academy of Pediatrics,
  226
Philippe, Édouard, 167
Physicians for Informed Consent, 73, 77
Pinborough-Zimmerman, Judith, on CDC
  data (autism), 39–40
Pisani, Amy, 190
Playbook, Lead, 226–27
Playbook, Tobacco, 84, 104, 124–27, 227
Plotkin, Stanley, 105–123. *See also* Big
  Pharma
  and Big Pharma, 110–12
  on causation (vaccine injuries), 118–21
  and conflict of interest, 107–12
  on DTaP vaccine, 114–15, 120–21
  and ethics, 115–17
  on hepatitis B vaccine science, 113
  on immune activation, 121–22
  on interleukin-6, 122
  and Merck, 109, 112–13
  and GlaxoSmithKline, 109
  and Pfizer, 109
  Plotkin's Vaccines (7e, 2017), 105
  on religious objections (vaccines), 117–18
  and rotavirus vaccine, 106
  as vaccine expert witness, 106

on VAERS, 114
and Voices for Vaccines, 109
pneumococcal (PCV), 51, 52f, 56, 56f, 57f, 63,
   86, 87f, 88, 150, 236
Poling, Hannah, 171
   and encephalopathy, 178, 181, 183, 184
   and mitochondrial disorder, 179, 181,
      183, 194
   and post-settlement news coverage,
      182–83
   settlement, 171, 180–81
   and vaccine–autism connection, 183–84
Poling, Jon, 171
   and gag order, 171, 180
   on mitochondrial disfunction, 194
   on post-settlement news coverage, 183
   on Omnibus Autism Proceeding
      settlement, 180
   on vaccine–autism connection and
      Hannah, 183–184
poliomyelitis
   Biskind on, 75
   Blaxill on, 77
   and DDT, 74–77
   Gromeier on, 76
   and US DDT ban, 75
   in India, 75
   Olmsted on, 77
   in Philippines, 75
polio provocation, 75–77
polio vaccine, 52f, 74–78, 82, 86, 88, 136, 173,
   236, 237
   and DDT, 74–77
   Gromeier on, 76
   and provocation, 75–77
   Wimmer on, 76
Posey, Bill, 98
prevalence (autism), 16f, 22
   1931, 18–19
   1987, 27–28
   adults (US), 17–18, 20, 33–34
   analysis (2002), 35
   analysis (2003), 36
   analysis (2005), 36
   baseline, 26
   Blaxill on, 18–19, 29, 34
   and CDC, 32, 40, 232
   and changing diagnostic criteria, 38
   children (US), 18, 28–29, 32, 35, 36, 38,
      40, 207
   children (Minnesota), 36

children (North Dakota), 27
children (Wisconsin), 26, 207
and environmental factors, 38, 247
Kennedy on (adults), 17
methodology, 29
NCPP data, 29–32
Nevison on, 38
Offit on, 23
Olmsted on, 18–19, 29, 34
and vaccines, 207
prevalence (mitochondrial disorder), 179, 194,
   207
prevalence (polio and DDT), 74–75, 77
"pro-vaccine" label
   and American Academy of Pediatrics,
      225, 226
   Every Child By Two, 226
   Immunization Action Coalition, 226
   and Kelley, 206
   Voices for Vaccines, 106
   and Zimmerman, 206

Q
Quinn, Aidan, 216

R
Reagan, Ronald, on Omnibus Health Bill (S.
   1744), 54, 55
Reagan administration on vaccine injury,
   53–55
reclassification (autism), 26, 34–36
recovery (autism), 3–6, 8, 25, 186, 201, 217,
   241–43, 246, 248
   and Generation Rescue guidance, 8
Recombivax (hepatitis B vaccine), 62
regressive autism and mitochondrial
   dysfunction, 179
regressive autism and parents, 211–14
Research Center for Vitamins and Vaccines
   (Denmark), 66
revenues (vaccine), 43, 43f, 69, 128
Richard Gage & Associates, 175
Rimland, Bernard, 24
   on autism epidemic, 25
   and biomedical intervention, 25
   and Defeat Autism Now!, 211–12
   Silberman on, 24
Rohde, Wayne, 177
risk/reward calculation, 11, 23, 66, 74, 83, 174
Rosenberg, Martha, 229
Ross, Rachel, on vaccine schedule, 83

rotavirus vaccine, 23, 52f, 56, 56f, 59, 63, 85, 86, 87f, 88, 106, 107, 206, 236
rubella vaccine, 238

S

"safe and effective" message, 41–43, 66, 78, 80, 114, 123, 132, 137, 227
  and CDC, 199
  Humphries on, 81–82
  Mendelsohn on, 80
  Neides on, 83
  Palevsky on, 81
  Ross on, 82
  Sears on, 80–81
  Zimmerman on, 199–200
sanitation, 48–50
Sanofi Pasteur, 67–68, 109, 168
  and American Academy of Pediatrics, 226
Sarton, George, 41
SB 277 (California), 51, 58
SB 442 (Oregon), 221, 223–24
scare tactics (vaccines), 42–44, 95, 168
schizophrenia, 26, 32, 144, 145, 146, 159
Sears, Bob
  on healthy immune system, 60
  Vaccine Book, The (2008), 80
  on vaccine safety, 80
selenium, 248
Senate Bill 277 (California), 51, 58
Senate Bill 442 (Oregon), 221, 223–24
Sencer, David J., 71
Seqirus and American Academy of Pediatrics, 226
Shakespeare, William, 233
Shattuck, Paul, 24,
  Infantile Autism, 24
Shaw, Christopher, 149
  on aluminum adjuvant and behavior change, 150, 166
  on aluminum adjuvant safety, 151–52, 166
  on aluminum adjuvants and autism, 165–66
  and Gulf War syndrome and vaccines, 149–50
shock, 64
Shoemaker, Clifford, 178
Shoenfeld, Yehuda, 71
  Vaccines and Autoimmunity, 71
Shulman, Lisa, 209
siblings and autism, 91–93, 235

side effects, vaccines, 42, 55, 71, 79, 97, 120, 175, 230
  DTP, 64, 81
  Gardasil, 69–70
  Institute of Medicine on, 120, 206
  MMR, 135, 238
Silberman, Steven, 18, 28, 33, 201
  and cause of autism, 19, 21–22, 26
  Kennedy, Robert F. Jr., on, 21–22
  NeuroTribes (2015), 15, 201
  on neurodiversity, 16
  on normalizing autism, 15–16
  on Rimland, 24
silica mineral water, 246
Sinclair, Upton, 105
Singer, Judy, 15
sleeplessness, 1, 2, 4, 5, 70
Smith, Bryan, 193
Stratton, Kathleen, 137
suramin
  Naviaux on, 244–45
  trials, 240–41, 244–46
symptoms
  decreased eye contact, 2, 5, 217
  ear infections, 2, 5, 20, 181, 207
  eczema, 1, 70, 205, 234, 237, 239
  food allergies, 5, 20, 42, 70, 71, 234, 243
  gut distress, 3, 4, 5, 132, 244, 247
  head banging, 162, 213
  malnutrition, 4, 5, 244
  sleeplessness, 1, 2, 4, 5, 70
synergistic relationship
  illness and immunity, 78
  adverse effects of multiple vaccines, 230
  adverse effects of premature birth and vaccination, 103

T

Task Force for Global Health, 110
  and Voices for Vaccines, 109
Tesla, Nikola, 15
tetanus vaccine, 100–101, 120, 157
thimerosal, 165
  and FDA Modernization Act, 165
  and Kennedy, 222
  Kirby on, 102
  vaccine studies, 86–91, 87f, 94–95, 163
  Verstraeten study, 89–90
  Zimmerman on, 200
Thimerosal: Let the Science Speak (Kennedy), 222

Thomas, Isabelle, on MMR vaccine and Wakefield, 135
Thomas, Paul, 228, 234, 236
    on vaccine–autism connection, 235
    Vaccine-Friendly Plan, The, 228, 234
Thompson, William
    and science fraud, 193, 200–201, 210, 240
    on vaccine–autism science fraud, 98
    and *Vaxxed* (2006), 231
Thorsen, Poul
    and embezzling from the CDC, 97–98
    and vaccine–autism science, 98
titer tests, 238
Tobacco Industry Research Committee, 124, 127
Tobacco Playbook, 84, 104, 124–27, 227
    Master Settlement Agreement (1998), 124, 126
Tomljenovic, Lucija, 151–52
Tommey, Polly, 209–11
Torrey, E. Fuller, on autism prevalence (1975), 31–32
Tozzi study, 90–91
treatment (autism)
    biomedical, 3–6, 8, 25, 39, 132, 186, 197, 201, 211–12, 241–48
    diet, 5, 211, 243, 246–47
    institutionalization, 2
    nutritional supplements, 5, 244, 247
    probiotics, 5, 244, 247
Treffert, Darol
    on autism epidemic, 27
    on autism prevalence, 16f, 26–27, 83f
    on gender and autism, 26
    on schizophrenia, 26
triggers (autism). *See* cause of autism
Trump, Donald, and vaccine–autism connection, 224–26
Tweed, Rebecca, 223

U
US Court of Federal Claims. *See* vaccine court

V
vaccinated vs. unvaccinated children, 102–103
vaccination coverage rates
    US (1973), 53
    US (1985), 52f, 53
    US (2015), 51
Vaccine Adverse Event Reporting System. *See* VAERS

vaccine–autism connection, 3, 6, 8, 9, 82, 91, 97, 123, 161–62, 168, 171, 181–84, 188–89, 201, 205, 232
    and CDC, 83f, 198
    Conte on, 188–89
    Exley on, 162
    Flutie on, 216
    and feigned exasperation, 85, 104
    and Hazlehurst depositions (Zimmerman and Kelley), 204–208
    Holland on, 188–89
    Kelley on, 198–99
    and lies, 84, 132, 201, 210, 225, 228, 232
    Maloney on, 33
    and neurodevelopmental disorders, 103
    and Poling case, 179
    Poling, Jon, on, 183–84
    studies, 94, 98, 99, 101, 102–103, 145, 198, 201
    and vaccine schedule, 82, 97
    and Wakefield, 135
    Wright, Katie, on, 216
    Wright, Suzanne, on, 215
    Zimmerman on, 178, 179, 193–94, 201, 250
vaccine–autism science, 84–104, 87f, 163, 234, 239
    fraud, 98, 193, 200–201, 210, 231
    Kirby on, 87–88, 102
Vaccine Book, The (Sears), 80
vaccine court, 10, 170–76, 185, 229–30. *See also* National Vaccine Injury Compensation Program
    and Banks case, 186–87
    and Big Pharma, 174
    compensated claims, 58, 173, 185, 188–89, 231
    and Conte, Lou, 185, 187–89, 190–91, 231
    and due process, 172
    funding of, 55
    and Hazlehurst case, 192–93, 232
    Hazlehurst, Rolf, on, 173, 175–76, 190
    and Holland, Mary, 185, 187–89, 231, 240
    and Kelley, Richard, 169, 206, 232
    Kennedy &s Kirby on, 186–87
    on MMR vaccine as cause of autism, 186
    and National Childhood Vaccine Injury Act (1986), 172
    Omnibus Autism Proceeding (OAP, 2002–2009), 177–82, 185

vaccine court (*continued*)
  and Poling case 131, 171, 178–85
  and the pharmaceutical industry, 55, 131
  purpose, 172, 173, 176, 180, 204
  settlements, 171, 180, 189, 231
  statute of limitations, 175–76
  and use of the word *autism*, 185–89, 206
  Vaccine Court, The (Rohde), 177
  Vaccine Injury Table, 174–76
  Vaccine Injury Table amendment (1995),
    174
  and Zimmerman, Andrew, 169, 170,
    178–82, 191, 195, 232
Vaccine Court, The (Rohde), 177
vaccine efficacy
  dengue fever vaccine, 67–68
  influenza vaccine, 47, 68–69
  mumps vaccine, 61–62
  pertussis (whooping cough) vaccine, 61, 114
  and thimerosal, 165
  vaccines (general), 48–49, 49f, 51, 61, 81–82
Vaccine-Friendly Plan, The (Thomas and
  Margulis), 228, 234
vaccine industry. *See* Big Pharma
Vaccine Injuries (Conte and Lyons), 185, 188
vaccine injury, 5, 42, 53–55, 187. *See also*
  adverse events, National Vaccine Injury
  Compensation Program, vaccine court,
  VAERS
  "accepted," 174
  arthritis, 62, 64, 65
  circle of denial, 79f
  compensation, 6, 55, 58, 97, 131, 172,
    174–75, 180–89
  deniers, 15–40, 242
  encephalopathy, 64, 97, 187, 188
  Institute of Medicine on, 64–65
  liability, 6, 54–55
  National Childhood Vaccine Injury Act,
    54, 172
  recognition of, 78–79, 123, 174, 230
  reporting, 63–64, 114
  residual seizure disorder, 187
  shock, 64
  and Kelley testimony, 172, 194, 198–99,
    200, 202–3
  and Zimmerman testimony, 172, 193–98,
    199–200, 201–2, 203
  timing, 159, 227
  trial (medical negligence, *Hazlehurst vs.
    Hays*), 171–72, 192–204

Vaccine Injury Circle of Denial, 79f
Vaccine Injury Table, 174–76
  and vaccine schedule, 82, 83f, 96, 239
Vaccine Injury Table, 174–76
vaccine policy conflicts of interest, 107–12
vaccine revenues, 43, 43f, 69, 128
vaccines. *See also* Plotkin, Stanley
  and autoimmunity, 70–71
  common cold, 50
  dengue fever , 67–68
  DTP (diphtheria-tetanus-pertussis),
    49f, 52f, 53, 56, 56f, 63, 64, 66, 81, 86,
    100–101, 113, 123, 173, 174, 176, 217
  hepatitis A, 51, 52f, 56, 59, 65, 86, 88,
    150, 236
  hepatitis B, 6, 51, 52f, 55n, 56, 59, 62, 65,
    86, 88, 101–2, 113, 118, 119, 150, 157,
    158–60, 173, 236
  Hib, 52f, 56, 56f, 57f, 63, 86, 87f, 88, 136,
    150, 173, 181, 236, 237
  human papilloma virus (HPV), 69–70,
    112–13
  influenza, 44–47, 56, 57f, 108, 146–47,
    151, 206, 236
  measles, 71–74, 238
  meningococcal, 52f, 86, 88, 236
  and mitochondrial dysfunction, 205, 232
  MMR, 23, 24, 49f, 52f, 53, 55n, 56, 56f,
    57f, 73, 78, 86, 87f, 88–89, 91–93, 94–95,
    98, 102, 132–35, 164–65, 173, 181, 186,
    193, 210, 231, 236–38
  pneumococcal (PCV), 51, 52f, 56, 56f, 57f,
    63, 86, 87f, 88, 150, 236
  polio, 52f, 74–78, 82, 86, 88, 136, 173,
    236, 237
  rotavirus, 23, 52f, 56, 56f, 59, 63, 85, 86,
    87f, 88, 106, 107, 206, 236
  rubella, 238
  side effects, 42, 55, 64, 69–70, 71, 79, 81,
    97, 120, 135, 175, 230, 238
  studies, 86, 87f, 230
  tetanus, 100–101, 120, 157
  and thimerosal, 86–91, 87f, 94–95, 163,
    165
  varicella, 52f, 56, 57f, 59, 86, 87f, 88, 136,
    181, 206, 236
Vaccine Safety Commission (US), 225
vaccine safety testing, 6, 62–63, 79, 113–14,
  123, 230
  and aluminum, 151
  Buttram on, 63

and multiple vaccines, 65, 202–3
    polio vaccine, 62
    Recombivax (hepatitis B vaccine), 62
Vaccines and Autoimmunity (Shoenfeld and
    Agmon-Levin), 71
vaccine schedule
    American Academy of Pediatrics, 58, 237
    and autism, 82, 83f, 96
    and brain development, 151f
    Denmark, 59, 59f
    France, mandatory vaccination (2017),
        167
    proposed reduction, 236–37
    UK (chickenpox), 59–60
    US, 6, 56f–57f, 59f
    US (1962), 55, 85
    US (1983), 55, 85
    US (2017), 56, 86, 236
    and vulnerable children screening, 239
VAERS, 54, 63, 65, 120
    events reported (2016), 64
    inaccuracy, 73, 123
    incomplete data, 79, 79f, 114, 123, 175, 230
    Lazarus on, 64
    most common events (2012), 64
    multiple vaccines data, 65
    Plotkin on, 114
    and Vaccine Injury Circle of Denial, 79f
varicella vaccine, 52f, 56, 57f, 59, 86, 87f, 88,
    136, 181, 206, 236
Vaxxed (movie), 210
Vaxxed Bus, 209–10
Verstraeten study, 89–90, 230
Verstraeten, Thomas
    and CDC, 90
    and GlaxoSmithKline, 90
    on study limitations, 90, 230
Vioxx, 55, 128–29
vitamin B12, 244
vitamin D, 247–48
Voices for Vaccines, 109
    and Task Force for Global Health, 110

W

Wakefield, Andrew, 105, 222
    and General Medical Council (UK) trial,
        134

and getting Wakefielded, 127–28, 136–37,
    168, 230
and MMR vaccine (*Lancet* study), 132–36
and *Vaxxed* (2006), 230–31
Walker-Smith, John
    and General Medical Council (UK) trial,
        134
    and UK's High Court trial, 134–35
Waxman, Henry, on Omnibus Health Bill (S.
    1744), 54–55
Weil, Andrew, 50
Weldon, Dave, on CDC conflict of interest,
    239–40
"well baby" visit vaccines, 1, 57–58, 86
Wiesel, Elie, 221
wisdom of crowds and autism, 96–97
World Health Organization, 69
Wright, Bob, 214
    and Autism Speaks, 215
Wright, Katie, 214–216
    on vaccine–autism connection, 216
Wright, Christian, 215
Wright, Suzanne, 215
    and Autism Speaks, 215
    on vaccine–autism connection, 215

Z

Zimmerman, Andrew, 169
    on Cedillo case, 203
    as expert witness (Hazlehurst case),
        171–72, 191–92, 193, 232
    as expert witness (vaccine court), 170, 182
    Hazlehurst, Rolf, on 207–208
    on Hazlehurst, vaccines, and autism,
        193–94
    on immune activation and autism, 195–97
    on mitochondrial dysfunction and autism,
        193, 232
    and Omnibus Autism Proceeding, 170,
        172, 190
    on Omnibus Autism Proceeding, 203
    and Poling, Hannah, 171, 178, 181–82,
        250
    on Poling, Hannah, 178, 195
    and vaccine–autism connection, 171
    on vaccine–autism connection,178, 179,
        193–94, 201, 250

About the Author

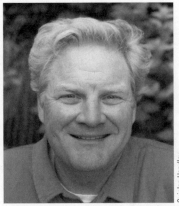

Quinlan Handley

J.B. Handley is the cofounder and chairman of Generation Rescue, a nonprofit organization focused on helping children recover from autism that was inspired by the journey of his son, Jamison, who was diagnosed with autism in 2004. He is also the coproducer of the documentary film *Autism Yesterday* and the cofounder of the *Age of Autism* blog. Handley cofounded Swander Pace Capital, a middle-market private equity firm with more than $1.5 billion under management, where he served as managing director for two decades. He is an honors graduate of Stanford University and lives in Portland, Oregon, with his wife, Lisa, and their three children.

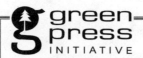

green
press
INITIATIVE

Chelsea Green Publishing is committed to preserving ancient forests and natural resources. We elected to print this title on 100-percent postconsumer recycled paper, processed chlorine-free. As a result, for this printing, we have saved:

316 Trees (40' tall and 6-8" diameter)
133 Million BTUs of Total Energy
137,000 Pounds of Greenhouse Gases
25,000 Gallons of Wastewater
1,000 Pounds of Solid Waste

Chelsea Green Publishing made this paper choice because we and our printer, Thomson-Shore, Inc., are members of the Green Press Initiative, a nonprofit program dedicated to supporting authors, publishers, and suppliers in their efforts to reduce their use of fiber obtained from endangered forests. For more information, visit: www.greenpressinitiative.org.

Environmental impact estimates were made using the Environmental Defense Paper Calculator. For more information visit: www.papercalculator.org.

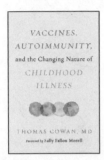
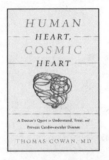
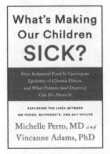
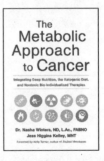
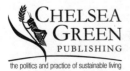

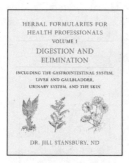
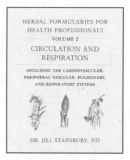
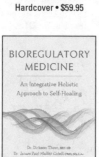
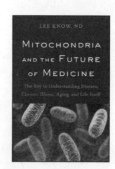
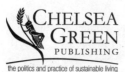